THE EPIDEMIOLOGICAL IMAGINATION
A READER

THE EPIDEMIOLOGICAL IMAGINATION
A READER

Edited by
John Ashton

Open University Press
Buckingham · Philadelphia

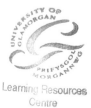

Open University Press
Celtic Court
22 Ballmoor
Buckingham
MK18 1XW

and

1900 Frost Road, Suite 101
Bristol, PA 19007, USA

First Published 1994

A catalogue record of this book is available from the British Library

ISBN 0 335 19100 2 (pbk)   0 335 19101 0 (hbk)

Library of Congress Cataloging-in-Publication Data
The Epidemiological imagination: a reader/edited by John R. Ashton.
          p.   cm.
    Includes bibliographical references and index.
    ISBN 0–335–19101–0   ISBN 0–335–19100–2 (pb.)
    1. Epidemiology.   I. Ashton, John, 1947–
  RA651.E62   1994
  614.4 – dc20   94–858
                                                                    CIP

Typeset by Type Study, Scarborough
Printed in Great Britain by
St Edmundsbury Press, Bury St Edmunds, Suffolk

This reader is dedicated to Martin Gardner, a friend and colleague of many of the contributors, an inspired researcher and well-loved teacher who epitomized the epidemiological imagination. Martin was a partner in the gestation of this book but did not live to see its appearance. His choice of papers is here and the introduction to them has been written by two of Martin's colleagues from Southampton.

Contents

CONTENTS

Preface

According to the History Man, in Malcolm Bradbury's novel of the same name, to understand the world you need a bit of Marx, a bit of Freud and a bit of social history. Those of us who have made the step from individual to population medicine and to public health might add – and a bit of epidemiology.

However, there is more than a bit of epidemiology in this reader. The need for such a book has seemed apparent to the editor for some time, based on the experience of organizing and teaching on Masters in Public Health courses in London and Liverpool. There are numerous formal textbooks of epidemiology, but perhaps less general discussion and interpretation. There is also a wealth of experience in our collective public health past, and as we shape the new public health there is a danger of ignoring lessons from the old. In 1989 the Pan American Health Organization produced a reader entitled *The Challenge of Epidemiology*, which brought together a large collection of important epidemiological papers in one place. That volume runs to almost 1000 pages and might seem to some rather intimidating. The current contribution is intended for use at the postgraduate Masters level as a way of introducing people to epidemiological thinking, to some of the masters and some of the classics.

The approach that has been adopted is to ask leading contemporary epidemiologists to select one paper in which they have been involved themselves and one classic paper, possibly historical, that seemed to them to convey the potential and excitement of the epidemiological approach. They have then been asked to write a short introduction explaining their choice. I hope that the resulting menu is as interesting to students and teachers as it has been to the editor.

The title is unashamedly borrowed from a social science classic of a similar name by C. Wright-Mills.[1] If this is plagiary then so be it – after all, all culture is plagiary, and it is my view that social science and the epidemiological method are part and parcel of the same culture of enquiry and understanding aimed at improving the human condition. I hope that students of all disciplines will find something here to stimulate them.

For the sake of ease of access and continuity a certain amount of abridging of these papers has taken place. Readers wishing to quote for the purposes of scientific publication are advised to check first with the original papers.

Royalties from the sales of this book will be used to support students of public health.

Reference

1 Wright-Mills, C. (1970) *The Sociological Imagination*. Harmondsworth: Pelican.

Acknowledgements

The editor would like to acknowledge the dedication of Carol Houghton in endeavouring to pull together a complicated set of contributions and to acknowledge assistance from Fran Bailey, Julie Hotchkiss and Alison Rylands. I would also like to thank Hazel Inskip and David Coggan for their contribution in undertaking to write the introduction to Professor Martin Gardner's choice of papers.

1 *Professor John Ashton*

Chave, S.P.W., (1958) John Snow, the Broad Street pump and after. Reprinted from *The Medical Officer*, 13 June, 99, 347–9.

Pickles, W.N. (1939) *The Commoner Diseases: Epidemiology in Country Practice* . Republished 1972, 1984. London: Royal College of General Practitioners.

INTRODUCTION

Not claiming to be an epidemiologist of any greatness myself, I have claimed the editor's privilege of choosing two papers to set the scene for the menu which follows.

The first is from the late Sidney Chave and is the classic description of Snow's work retold by the master story teller from the London School of Hygiene and Tropical Medicine, who introduced successive generations of students to the joy of synthesizing biography and socio-economic history with biological science and epidemiology. Nobody could have been more appropriate than Sidney to reinterpret Snow's work for the new era, for Sidney was a man who could really make the history of public health come alive and inspire people at the outset of their careers.[1,2]. I can clearly remember Sidney's introductory lectures to our Master's class at London and the feeling that I had come home to the social history that I had had to abandon when I chose the science path in the anachronistic British sixth form system.

It was in reconciling the dichotomy between the two cultures of humanities and science that Sidney was such a master. He began his working life as a laboratory boy in the Department of Chemistry at the London School of Hygiene, later becoming Chief Technician before taking an honours degree in psychology and carrying out research into the mental health of people living in Harlow New Town for his doctorate. His interests and expertise eventually spanned an amazing range, from water supplies, the disposal of sewage and his love for public health history to lifestyles, behaviour and health education, ornithology, numismatology and heraldry. There is much

talk today of the need for a new social epidemiology. I would argue that it is already there. Anyone who has studied at London has been introduced to an eclectic approach to epidemiology. The challenge to all of us is to ensure that this approach pervades research, teaching and the impact of epidemiology on policy and strategy. Snow's work contains many lessons for the new public health.

The second paper I have chosen is one of the chapters from Pickles's classic pre-war book, *Epidemiology in Country Practice*. The book describes how Pickles became infected with epidemiological curiosity and how his relationship with the London School of Hygiene and Tropical Medicine, Major Greenwood and others enabled him to carry out pioneering work on epidemiology in general practice as a working clinician. At a time when health systems all over the world are seeking to strengthen primary medical care and to push it towards real primary health care it is clear that an understanding of populations and of epidemiology is critical. When so many academic departments of general practice have failed to live up to their promise, it is salutary to consider that it is possible to do good research and teaching on the basis of sound day-to-day clinical practice in a service setting. It is hoped that the next few years will see a significant development of primary care epidemiology and, in this, Pickles's work should point the way.

References

1 Chave, S. (1987) *Recalling the Medical Officer of Health. Writings by Sidney Chave*. Edited by Michael Warner and

Huw Francis. London: King Edwards Hospital Fund for London.

2 Ashton J. (1989) Recalling the Medical Officer of Health. *Health Promotion*, 3(4), 413–19.

JOHN SNOW, THE BROAD STREET PUMP AND AFTER

On 19 June 1858, the following notice appeared among the announcements of deaths in *The Times*: 'On the 16th inst., at his residence 18 Sackville Street, Piccadilly, John Snow, MD, of apoplexy, aged 45.' For some weeks prior to his last illness Snow had been working on his book *On Chloroform and Other Anaesthetics*. According to his friend Benjamin Ward Richardson, he was drafting the concluding paragraph and was actually writing the word 'exit' when he was seized with a stroke from which he died ten days later.

It was nine years before his untimely death that Snow had first put forward his theory concerning the spread of cholera by polluted water. This he did in a small pamphlet of about 30 pages which was published at his own expense. But this first essay in the field of infectious diseases received only scant attention at the time. Five years later, in 1854, when cholera was sweeping across the country for the third time, he carried out his classic researches in South London. This investigation, which remains to this day a model of scientific inquiry, established beyond all reasonable doubt that cholera is a water-borne disease. Snow incorporated the substantial body of new evidence which he had gathered in the course of this inquiry into his 'much enlarged' volume of 162 pages: the so-called 'second edition' of his book *On the Mode of Transmission of Cholera*, which was published early in 1855. In the next three years only 56 copies of the book were sold, and in return for an outlay of £200 incurred in its preparation, the author was reimbursed with the princely sum of £3 12s. 0d.

Snow's theory ran counter to the prevailing view of his time, which attributed infectious diseases like cholera to the effluvia arising from filth and putrefaction. It is hardly to be wondered, therefore, that at first there were few who were disposed to accept this new explanation. In 1849, a reviewer commenting in the *Lancet* on Snow's first pamphlet on cholera wrote, 'The arguments adduced by the author against emanations causing the disease are not by any means conclusive.' Following the cholera epidemic of 1853–4, the Royal College of Physicians set up an investigation into its causes under Drs William Baly

and William Gull. They considered Snow's thesis and rejected it outright. 'The theory as a whole is untenable,' they reported and added, 'The matter which is the cause of cholera increases and finds the conditions for its action under the influence of foul or damp air.' So, too, the medical inspectors appointed by the General Board of Health in 1854 to inquire into the Soho outbreak, having examined Snow's views upon it, commented, 'we see no reason to adopt this belief.' The principal objections raised against Snow's theory were that it did not account either for the sudden onset or for the decline of the epidemics as satisfactorily as the current explanation in terms of miasmata.

In 1856, John Snow visited Paris with his uncle, Mr Empson of Bath. Empson, a dealer in curios, was known personally to the Emperor and Ward Richardson records that 'on this occasion special imperial favours were shown to him in which the nephew participated.' While in Paris, Snow entered his book at the Institut de France for a prize which was offered for the most outstanding contribution towards the prevention or treatment of cholera. Ward Richardson reports that no notice was taken of Snow's researches by the Institute. On the other hand Sir D'Arcy Power, the medical historian, writing of Snow in the *Dictionary of National Biography*, states that 'his essay upon the mode of communication of cholera which was first published in 1849 was awarded by the Institute of France a prize of £1,200.' In reply to a recent inquiry made by the writer, M. Pierre Gauja, the present Archivist of the Institute, confirmed that Snow did not in fact receive this award. It would appear that his theory was more acceptable abroad than at home, for about the same time Max Pettenkofer in Germany also rejected it.

In England two men of note, William Budd and William Farr, were almost alone in voicing their approval of Snow's thesis during his lifetime. In 1849, shortly after Snow had published his first paper on cholera, Budd brought out a pamphlet of his own on the same subject. He put forward a theory of causation and transmission of the disease similar to that of Snow, but in doing so he made a full acknowledgement of the priority of Snow's published work. In all his subsequent writings on cholera Budd stressed the water-borne nature of the disease and was at pains to give full credit to Snow for having first made this discovery.

William Farr at the General Register Office gave a more qualified support to Snow's theory. He himself had noted the high mortality from cholera which occurred in those districts of London whose water supplies were drawn directly from the sewage-laden reaches of the Thames. In the Report of the Registrar General for 1852 he discussed Snow's findings and reached the conclusion that the facts 'lend some countenance to Dr Snow's theory.' Four years later, in his letter to the Registrar General, Farr presented a long and detailed statistical account of the cholera epidemic of 1853–4. He concluded as follows: 'It is right to state that Dr Snow by his hypothesis and researches and by his personal inquiries; that the Registrar General by procuring information and by promoting inquiry; as well as the Board of Health by the Report, have all contributed in various ways to establish the fact that the cholera-matter, or cholerine, when it is most fatal, is largely diffused through water as well as through other channels.'

The report to which Farr referred was that made to the President of the General Board of Health by John Simon, in which he expressed the cautious view that 'fecalised drinking water and fecalised air equally may breed and convey the poison.' Simon remained for long an adherent of the old theory of the miasmata, and his acceptance of Snow's thesis came only gradually and after many years. In the month of Snow's death in 1858 he referred to his 'peculiar doctrine as to the contagiousness of cholera' and commented somewhat patronisingly that 'whatever may be the worth of the theory, it has been of use in contributing to draw attention to the vast hygienic importance of a pure water supply.' Sixteen years later he had moved his position, and in a report to the Local Government Board he remarked, 'Indeed, with regard to the manner of spread of the enterozymotic diseases generally, it deserves notice that the whole pathological argument which I am explaining grew amongst us in this country out of the very cogent facts which our cholera epidemics supplied, and to which the late Dr Snow 25 years ago had the merit of forcing medical attention, an attention at first quite incredulous, but which at least for the last 15 years as facts have accumulated has gradually been changing into conviction.' Later still in 1890, in his *English Sanitary Institutions*, Simon, looking back over the years to Snow's discovery, could write that it 'may probably still be counted the most important truth yet acquired by medical science for the prevention of epidemics of cholera.' This appreciation of Snow's work was handsome if somewhat belated.

In 1884 Koch announced his discovery of the cholera vibrio to the Berlin Conference and ten years later an English translation of his papers on cholera was published in this country. Koch made no mention of Snow although he fully accepted the water-borne nature of the disease. William Gairdner, Professor of Medicine at Glasgow, contributed an Introduction to the English edition in which he paid a fitting tribute to John Snow:

Since Dr Snow's researches were published and adopted by the Registrar General in England there has never been much doubt among us as to the water-communication of the choleraic infection, the evidence of which seemed to go on accumulating as the incidence of the disease, in respect of particular places, was more and more studied, and the severity of local epidemics was found to be strictly in accordance with the presence of dangerous impurities in the water supply.

The discoveries of the bacteriologists finally dethroned the doctrine of emanations, and served both to underline the soundness of John Snow's observations and to confirm the truth of his deductions.

The Broad Street pump

The name of John Snow is invariably associated with the Broad Street pump and with the outbreak of cholera which centred upon it. The story of this old pump forms an interesting chapter in the history of public health.

Just when it was set up in Broad Street is not known. The houses in this part of Soho were built between 1700 and 1740 and it is likely that the well was sunk about the same time. The district was a suitable one for shallow wells, for water could be obtained at a depth of about 20 feet almost everywhere. As a result wells were plentiful. There were at least 12 pumps within a radius of a quarter of a mile of Broad Street.

By 1850 two private companies – the New River and the Grand Junction – were supplying piped water to all the houses in the area. At that time these supplies were intermittent, the water being turned on for about two hours daily except on Sundays. Each household had to install a butt or cistern which was filled whenever the main supply became available. These storage butts were notoriously bad. They were usually uncovered, rarely if ever cleaned, and as a result the water drawn from them was generally dirty and often unsavoury.

By contrast the water from the well in Broad Street was clear, bright and sparkling, albeit through the presence of carbonic acid and nitrates, the end-products of organic contamination. Throughout the district around Golden Square its waters, always available and invariably cool and palatable, were most highly regarded. Not only did householders close at hand make extensive use of it, but many people living at a distance preferred to draw their water from Broad Street in preference to their local wells. It was commonly the duty of the children to fetch the water from the pump, and old people living alone bemoaned the fact that they had no one to fetch water for them. The pump-handle had a ladle attached to it from which the children were accustomed to drink, although we know that some parents disapproved of this practice. Many of the small workshops in the locality kept butts filled with the well water to be used for drinking purposes, especially in summer. The water was also used for mixing with spirits in all the taverns round about and it was supplied to customers in the coffee-shops and dining-rooms in the area. Some of the little shops used to bottle the water, add a little effervescent powder and sell it as 'sherbet' drink.

Perhaps the most striking testimony to the attractions of this water comes from Snow's account of the widow of Hampstead. This lady, whose husband had formerly owned the percussion-cap factory in Broad Street, had a bottle of the well water brought to her by a cart which travelled each day to St James. This was to prove her un-doing, for in the cholera epidemic she alone of the inhabitants of Hampstead contracted the disease and died.

The month of August 1854 was hot and dry and when cholera broke out in Broad Street it spread through the little neighbourhood like fire in a rickyard. Within ten days the population was literally decimated. It was without doubt, as John Snow himself described it, 'the most terrible outbreak of cholera which ever occurred in this kingdom'. At the time Snow was living in Sackville Street, about half a mile from the affected area, and although he was already fully engaged in his investigation in South London he hastened to the scene of this new outbreak. His suspicions quickly fell on the well in Broad Street and these were strengthened when he discovered that 'nearly all the deaths had taken place within a short distance of the pump'. He was able to establish that almost all the people who had died had consumed water from the pump. After pursuing his inquiries further, Snow recorded, 'I had an interview with the Board of Guardians of St James's parish on the evening of Thursday, 7 September, and represented the above circumstances to them. In consequence of what I said the handle of the pump was removed on the following day.'

It is interesting to note that the Minutes of the Board of Guardians and of the Vestry contain no reference to Snow's intervention. It is probable that he made his representation to the sanitary committee which had been set up by the Guardians to act during the epidemic, and that it was this body which ordered the pump to be taken out of use. By the morning of 8 September the epidemic had already declined sharply and the closure of the well did little to affect its course, although it may well have prevented a fresh outbreak. The removal of the handle was not by any means the end of the Broad Street pump, for within a short time it was brought back into service again.

Two further associates of John Snow enter the story at this stage – one a doctor and the other a clergyman. The doctor was Edwin Lankester, who in the following year became the first medical officer of health of St James; the clergyman was Henry Whitehead, the young curate at St Luke's church in Berwick Street. Lankester was a member of the Vestry and at his instigation a local inquiry into the epidemic was ordered to be carried out at the expense of the parish. Both John Snow and Henry Whitehead were co-opted on to the committee which was set up for this purpose. It was in the course of this investigation that Whitehead made the discovery which had till then eluded Snow and which brought a triumphant confirmation of his hypothesis. This was the elucidation of the way in which the well had become polluted.

Whitehead discovered that a baby living at 40 Broad Street, the nearest house to the pump, had died from what was described as 'exhaustion following diarrhoea' and that the child's illness immediately preceded the onset of the cholera epidemic. From his inquiries at the house he learnt that the baby's discharges had been disposed of into a cesspool which was less than three feet from the well. An immediate inspection revealed conspicuous evidence of the percolation of faecal matter from the ill-constructed cesspool through the decaying brickwork which lined the well. The chain of evidence incriminating the pump was now complete. Yet even this disclosure did not secure its final removal. Instead, the well was closed for six weeks while the brickwork was renewed, it was then pumped out completely three times, after which it was opened for use by the public once more.

In the following year, 1856, Edwin Lankester was appointed Medical Officer of Health of St James's parish under the Metropolis Management Act. One of the first matters to which he gave his attention was the water supply of the district. It was his aim to get rid of the numerous shallow wells in the area, and in his first annual report to the Vestry he complained that 'the most impure water in the parish is that of the Broad Street pump, and it is altogether the most popular.' This comment is all the more striking when it is recalled that it was made within two years of the great epidemic. Lankester went on to report that a chemical analysis had revealed that this water contained more inorganic salts (chlorides and nitrates) derived from organic pollution than the common sewer.

The Vestry appear to have been unmoved by these revelations, so in the following year Lankester wrote to every one of his fellow medical officers of health in the Metropolitan area asking their opinions about surface wells. Their replies, which he published in full, showed that the general consensus of opinion was in favour of closure. This seems to have led to a minor victory, for at the beginning of 1858 all the shallow wells in the Parish were closed by order of the Vestry. Lankester's success was short-lived, however, for in his report for that year he grumbled 'You did not think it advisable to continue the closing of the pumps.' And so, after an interval of four months all the wells were in use again.

Four years later Lankester took up the cudgels once more. In his customary forthright manner he informed the Vestry that all the wells in the parish were unsafe, with the single exception of the artesian near the church in Piccadilly. He reminded them that St James was now lagging behind most other districts for 'with the exception of our own parish these surface well-pumps have nearly all been closed throughout London.' He spoke of 'offering the public the filtered sewage of these pumps'. This seems to have prompted the Vestry to take some action, for in 1864 Lankester was able to report that 'the wells in the parish are gradually being abandoned – seven only remain.' But the Broad Street pump was among them. He remarked that drinking fountains had largely replaced wells in popular esteem but that St James had fewer of them than any other London parish.

It was in the next year that the threat of cholera returned to this country once again. Lankester thereupon urged the Vestry to lock the remaining pumps as a safety precaution, reminding them of the part that impure water, especially from surface wells, had played in the spread of cholera in the past. His warning went unheeded. The threatened outbreak materialized in the summer of 1866 when cholera broke out in the teeming slums of East London. Lankester promptly submitted to the Vestry a special report on the state of the wells which still remained in service in the area. This revealed abundant chemical evidence of organic contamination and once again he drew special attention to the Broad Street pump. Further support now came from another and perhaps unexpected source, for on 31 July a letter headed 'The Broad Street Pump' appeared in *The Times*. Signed by Dr W. Allen Miller, of King's College Hospital, and Professor E. Frankland, of the Royal College of Chemistry, it deplored the fact that the old pump was still in use and commented on the unfitness of its waters. The writers concluded with a solemn warning that the whole area could be infected 'by a single case of cholera occurring within the drainage area of the pump'.

Three days later a case of cholera was reported in No. 30 Broad Street. Lankester now sounded a note of alarm. He warned the Vestry yet again of the dangers of spreading the disease through the pollution of water: 'this can occur in no other way than by our pumps.' He pronounced the wells to be dangerous. 'I dare not take the responsibility of remaining quiet while these pumps are open, and, at the risk of offending you by my pertinacity, I implore you to order the pumps to be shut.'

This appeal seems to have been successful in bringing about, at long last, the final closure of the Broad Street pump. There are no further references to its use from that time.

Edwin Lankester died in 1874 and was succeeded as medical officer of health by James Edmunds. In his annual report for 1884, eight wells were mentioned by name, including the one in Broad Street which was said 'to have been covered but not filled in'. The rest is silence. Broad Street remained but its pump had passed into history.

Today, 100 years after the death of John Snow, the student of public health can still visit many of the places associated with his career. Bateman's Buildings, the little back street in Soho, where in 1836 Snow rented a room following his long walk to London to study medicine; Great Windmill Street, where a plaque on the wall of the Lyric Theatre marks the site of the Hunterian School of Medicine in which Snow was a student from 1836 to 1838; Frith Street, Soho, where in 1838 he 'nailed up his colours' and started his first practice; 18 Sackville Street, which was his home from 1852 until his death; and Brompton Cemetery, where stands a replica of the original monument erected to his memory by his friends. But perhaps it is fitting that the pilgrimage should end in Broad Street – now Broadwick Street, W1 – and at the old tavern which three years ago was renamed in honour of John Snow. For, below the inn-sign which bears his portrait, a tablet on the wall draws the attention of the passer-by to a red granite stone at the kerbside. This stone marks the site of the Broad Street pump.

Bibliography

The following are the principal sources which were used in the preparation of this article:

Richardson, B. W. 'John Snow, M.D.' *The Asclepiad*, 4, London 1887.

Snow, John. 'On the Mode of Communication of Cholera' Second edition. London, 1855.

Budd, W. 'Malignant Cholera.' London, 1849.

Reports on Epidemic Cholera, Royal College of Physicians, London, 1854.

Report of the Medical Council in relation to Epidemic–Cholera of 1854, General Board of Health, London, 1855.

Annual Reports, Registrar General. London, 1848 to 1856.

Report on the London Cholera Epidemics of 1848–9 and 1853–4, by the Medical Officer to the Board. General Board of Health. London, 1856.

Report on the Cholera Outbreak in St James, Westminster, 1854, by the Cholera Inquiry Committee, St James Vestry. London 1855.

Annual Reports of the Medical Officer of Health. St. James, Westminster, 1856 to 1884.

Koch, R. 'On the Bacteriological Diagnosis of Cholera and other papers.' Translated G. Duncan. Edinburgh, 1894.

Chave, S.P.W. 'John Snow and Cholera in London.' London School of Hygiene Library, 1955.

Chave, S.P.W. 'Henry Whitehead and Cholera in Broad Street.' *Medical History* (1958), 2(2), 92–110.

Acknowledgement

Chave, S.P.W. (1958) John Snow, the Broad Street pump and after. Reprinted from *The Medical Officer*, 13 June, 99, 347–9

THE COMMONER DISEASES

Having developed a technique for recording epidemic diseases, I now possess charts which contain all the instances of infectious diseases that have occurred in my practice during the last seven years, although from the epidemiological point of view these years have been comparatively dull. Speaking as a humanitarian and a medical officer of health this is, of course, most satisfactory, but as an epidemiologist it is rather unfortunate that I should have chosen seven years in which there has been only one large influenza epidemic, no extensive measles epidemic, no German measles, very little scarlet fever, and until recently, when we had six victims, only a single sufferer from diphtheria. I always remember Sir George Newman's quotation from Pasteur by way of solace, 'In the fields of observation chance only favours the mind which is prepared', and realize that when the inevitable epidemic of any particular disease does appear, the method of investigation will not have to be evolved to meet the occasion. If other country doctors feel disposed to keep similar charts, there will be many months in which the labour may seem to be in vain, but they will not only have their minds prepared, but will have a technique ready to hand to grapple with the epidemics as they come along. I do not forget that on the very first page of my chart book the connection between herpes and chicken-pox was plain for anyone to see.

Influenza

This chapter on the common infectious diseases naturally commences with the commonest and most important,

which is influenza. From the country doctor's point of view nothing alters the character of his work, with the possible exception of a measles epidemic, in the same way as this disease, for an influenza epidemic may transform a busy but orderly existence into a nightmare. As a tribute to his memory, and because it is possible that this book will be read by Wensleydale people, I cannot forbear to recall the heroic struggle for many weeks of my late partner, Dean Dunbar, in the pandemic of 1918, a struggle which greatly endeared him to his patients and which gave him a name that will be remembered for long in this dale. Such instances of self-sacrificing devotion were no doubt common in that period, when so many of us were required for the services. Since that dread time, in 1924, 1927, 1929 and 1931, we have had very extensive epidemics of this complaint, but with this difference, that there was hardly a patient in any of these epidemics who gave us a moment's anxiety, and the death-rate was providentially negligible. There was a return of our old enemy in 1937, when the epidemic spread more rapidly than in previous visitations, due probably to the improved methods of transport. This outbreak, however, was also not of a serious nature, although its very rapidity of spread made it one of the most difficult with which we have been confronted. To enter fifty or more houses and see probably three times the number of patients is no light task in a district with a scattered population. In addition some of these patients have to be visited a second time. Then, again, a large number of messages are received from those who *think* they have influenza, and also from our *malades imaginaires*, who feel that without a warning they are bound to be neglected in such a strenuous spell. There are also those who want a 'bottle' as a prophylactic 'rather to scale it away', as they say – 'scale', like so many of our North Riding words, being, I believe, good old Norse.

We read much at the present time in the press of the medicine-drinking habits of the population of this country, with special reference to those who come under the State Insurance Act, and therefore it is not surprising to find that in this district 'the bottle' is still very dear to the patient's heart. In all these epidemics our dispenser packed in our cars a large basket of appropriate remedies, which were doled out to our grateful patients, who had no possible means of sending for them.

I read not long ago that the appalling death-rate in the well-known epidemic of measles in Fiji was due not so much to its being a new disease for which there was not inherited resistance, as on account of the lack of nursing facilities, and that, owing to whole families going down simultaneously, the very necessaries of life could not be provided. The 'controls' in this epidemic were the members of the police force, whose conditions of living were entirely different, and who therefore showed a death-rate not above the normal. In some of our isolated farms during an influenza epidemic a state of affairs similar to that exhibited in Fiji was faithfully reproduced. The house was as cold as a vault, as not a single member of the family was in a fit state to crawl downstairs to light the kitchen fire. Food had been for days a difficult problem, and hot drinks an utter impossibility. Neighbours are very good, and at our request this was soon remedied, but with the inevitable result that the disease spread to the homes of the good Samaritans themselves.

There have been two small epidemics between 1931 and 1937. One of these, originating in a schoolmistress, raises a notable point. The area which suffered in this epidemic of 78 cases practically escaped in 1937, a circumstance which may indicate some degree of partial immunity in the inhabitants of the area.

There was something to be learned from the latest epidemic. As I have said it spread with a much greater rapidity than its predecessors, and its duration was barely three weeks, but in this time 10 per cent of our people were victims. Our previous epidemics lasted two months, and spread slowly from village to village, so that we were rarely busy in more than two or three villages at one time.

The few accurate observations I was able to make on the incubation period lead me to suppose that it was never less than two and never more than three days.

A curious little outbreak of this disorder occurred in June 1935 in one of our villages, when we thought we had escaped the pest for that year. The disease ran a normal course, and certainly appeared to be the typical form of influenza, and the form which would be likely to reproduce the disease in ferrets, but it left its victims, mostly children, with a spasmodic cough, which was definitely not whooping-cough, but to which it bore a striking resemblance. I was interested to notice that other epidemics with this sequela were reported in the medical press shortly afterwards.

In 1938 we again seemed to have escaped influenza altogether, but rumours of sufferers in surrounding districts reached us, and at last a few instances appeared in March, with a large incidence of lobar pneumonia.

Measles

The longer the incubation period in virus diseases, the longer the time before an epidemic comes to an end. A measles epidemic in this district usually lasts six months. When we come to discuss mumps we shall find that an epidemic of this disease lasted a year. Our measles epidemics seem to have a periodicity of about nine years, so that it is unlikely that we shall escape a similar outbreak in 1938 as our last one was in 1929. I wrote this sentence in 1936, and I have allowed it to stand, as in the present year (1938) the dawn of another epidemic is appearing. Two children, a brother and a sister, attended one of our schools feeling out of sorts on the first three days of the week commencing 28 February. The rash of measles commenced in each on 3 March. There were no other sufferers from measles in the whole district, but these children had been to a pantomime in Leeds, where measles was rife, on 15 February and no doubt were infected with the disease during this excursion. The prodromal symptoms in the little girl were negligible, and it is hard to state a date of commencement for her, but the boy's symptoms definitely began on 27 February, giving an incubation period of twelve days. The whole of the susceptible population of the school with two possible exceptions then contracted the disease.

The third wave is now in progress, and by attempting to make this the last, by a rigid policy of isolation of susceptible contacts, in which I am being loyally aided by my patients and the schoolmistress, I am hoping against hope that the epidemic will come to a dead end. This policy is, of course, interfering with nature, and it is practically certain that even if the rest of the dale is not infected from the patients in this village, it will have to suffer during the present or succeeding year, as the children are for the most part susceptible. (Figure 1).[1]

Sporadic cases have occurred in the interval, but they have been very few in number and there has been no spread, as all who were in contact, with very few exceptions known to me personally, had the disease in 1929–30, and the proportion of children born since the last epidemic is only now becoming of importance. I cannot say why we do not have the biennial epidemics which admittedly recur in the large towns, but I simply record, with an uneasy feeling that I am raising more points than I am able to solve, that the epidemics do recur about every nine years.

One large village and a small one, served by a single school, escaped in our last epidemic and remained free until a small boy, who had returned from a visit to his grandmother in another area, went to a school treat on 2 January 1932, in the early stages of the disease. Thereafter a large crop of cases occurred, and from these most of the remaining children in the immediate neighbourhood and some adults were infected.

During this epidemic I had an opportunity of arriving at an estimation of incubation period by one instance of infection when the only possible exposure was definite and of short duration. A man in a village remote from the

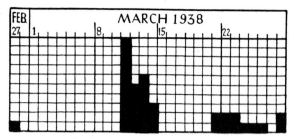

At School 28th February, 1st and 2nd March

Fig. 1 Measles.

prevailing epidemic exhibited the disease. Twelve days previously another man had called at my surgery, and, finding no one at home, repaired to the inn, conveniently situated on the other side of the road, and sat cheek by jowl with the first man over their pints. Returning to the surgery he was found to be suffering from measles. During the short visit to the inn he appeared to me, without a reasonable doubt, to have infected his companion. The incubation period was most accurately 12 days.

In an earlier epidemic, the following incident also suggested a twelve days' incubation period:

A boy in a farm 'place' arrived at the surgery on his bicycle, and announced that he had 'gitten mazzeles' (contracted measles). This was certainly the case, and he was told to go to his mother's home, and shout to her the same tidings outside the door in order that she might have the living-room cleared of his small brothers and sisters. He then repaired to his bedroom, where he remained a fortnight. On the twelfth day after his arrival, his aunt, and only his aunt, became a victim of the disease, although she had never seen the boy, and left the house the morning after his arrival. It was found that the boy's bedroom and the living-room directly below, by an unusual and capricious arrangement of the builder, were lighted by one long window, giving direct aerial access from one room to the other. The meal table was below this gap, and the aunt, who sat directly underneath at meals, was apparently thus infected.

The epidemic of 1929–30 in which the last incident occurred was remarkable for the number of adults which it attacked. There was a large number of young adults among the victims, many in their forties, and one veteran of 68, who to his dying day refused to believe he had suffered from measles, as ''twere but a childish complaint'.

Very few of our patients gave us any anxiety, and it is

worth nothing that there was not one instance of even the mildest ear trouble.

As regards incubation period, I believe instances such as those above are the only reliable ones on which to base incubation period in measles or any other disease, and are decidedly rare. Family outbreaks do not give accurate information, as it is not certain at what stage the original sufferers transferred the infection. Three years ago there was an outbreak of measles limited to one family, but that a family of ten children probably our largest at the present date. One child contracted the disease on a visit to relatives and commenced on 25 March. Five of the others began on 5 April, giving an incubation period of eleven days, three on 6 April, and one on 7 April. I have, however, seen crops in families, part of the family infected from the first patient and the rest from the second crop. This leads me to believe that measles is only infectious for a very short period, and I commend this as a subject for investigation to other doctors, as it certainly will be to me in any further epidemic. I can make no dogmatic statement on the small evidence at my disposal, but I believe that careful investigation will probably establish the very short infectivity in measles. I am confirmed in this belief by the fact that the statisticians have come to a similar conclusion from their examination of the records of epidemics. Acting on this assumption, I have never enforced isolation after a week from the beginning of the illness.

The incidence of a second attack in the same individual is said to be 1 in 200. I have no statistics to offer on this point, but I have never as yet attended to the same patient in two attacks in my 25 years in this practice.

In every epidemic a few babies under a year old have contracted this disease. In almost every instance the baby's mother was simultaneously a victim, both infected from the school child in the family, showing that the mother herself had no immunity to bestow on her offspring.

The disease is probably infectious, as is often stated, towards the end of the incubation period. As I have said, when I have been able to trace infection in a patient to a single exposure of short duration, the incubation period appears to be 12 days, but I find in families that this is frequently shortened to 10 or 11, which suggests that the infection is present one or two days previous to the advent of symptoms. In the present epidemic *Roland* and *Edith* first had symptoms on 11 March, their mother on 21 March, the baby brother and a little sister on 22 March. There has been little variation in the incubation period as I have observed it, and I believe that it is in the neighbourhood of what I have always seen when I could trace the infection to a single exposure, and that has been 12 days.

Life on the tidal beaches was governed by the phases of the moon, and a rhythm was implanted in living things which still holds good today. There is a little variation in the incubation period of a hen's egg, in the time of gestation in mammals, and even in the menstrual cycle of healthy women, and, although the parallel cannot be stressed too far, I believe that the great variation in the incubation periods of disease which has been taught is due to lack of opportunity in observation.

Scarlet Fever

Of this I have little personal experience, as there are very few entries in my charts, and in the whole of my time in this district we have had comparative freedom from this complaint. But 'what is scarlet fever for the clinician?' as F. G. Hobson asks in a valuable paper published in *The Lancet* in 1937, which all should read. There is the typical 'scarlet' with the throat and the strawberry tongue and the rash which looks hot and feels hot and only admits of one diagnosis, which at the present time gives us not the slightest anxiety. This, as Hobson points out, is the only form which we are under a legal obligation to notify, but there are other manifestations of infection by the same or very similar organisms which are just as infectious and give infinitely more trouble. It is said today that patients who are infected by the haemolytic streptococcus and do not develop a rash are those alone who are likely to cause anxiety from complications. My small experience is in complete accord with this expression of opinion.

Four years ago I attended a young married woman with a throat affection which appeared to be typical of scarlet fever, and which was followed by a septic pharyngitis and laryngitis with alarming symptoms, suggesting oedema of the glottis. Her elderly mother who nursed her also developed a sore throat, and then the worst attack of erysipelas I have ever seen, from which she only just managed to recover. The young woman who nursed this patient contracted a septic finger and an axillary abscess with cellulitis spreading to the breast, and was laid up for some weeks. These are much more serious conditions than the scarlet fever we see today, but all are due to a similar organism. I personally have never seen an acute nephritis following notifiable scarlet fever, but many of the instances of this disease which have come under my care have been connected with epidemics of sore throat of which the patient was a victim. Nine years ago I am convinced that practically the whole of the child population in one village suffered from scarlet fever in a mild form. The sole patient we attended was a poor little fellow with running ears, who, as he was the child of milk-sellers, was sent to hospital, where he nearly died of measles contracted after his admission.

This raises the point of hospitalization of sufferers from this disease in country districts, and my policy now is to keep all at home. I find that this can be done without detriment to the public health and I get no return cases. The problem for the medical superintendent of the fever hospital is a very different one from my own. He endeavours, quite rightly, to discharge his mild 'scarlets' at the earliest possible moment, fearing a superimposed infection by a more virulent strain. I find, therefore, that on their return these sufferers must continue to be watched and isolated. If isolation can be carried out after the patient's discharge from hospital, it can be carried out quite as effectively from the beginning of the illness. I have also thought it probable that the early stages of this disease are comparatively non-infective, and I can certainly produce evidence in support of this. Why, therefore, send the patients to hospital, subject them to the risks of infection by a more virulent strain of the same disease, not to mention the possibilities of measles or even diphtheria, until the cubicle system is adopted universally, for the very stage of scarlet fever which is least infective? In my early days in this practice, when we kept all our patients at home and relentlessly isolated them for long periods, the experience with few exceptions was one patient only in each house, and here are instances which, I believe, point to the comparative absence of infectivity of the disease in its early stages:-

1 A boy of ten commenced with scarlet fever on 23 November. I saw him on 26 November and promptly dispatched him to hospital. He had three small sisters, and although there had not been the slightest attempt at isolation, all escaped for the time being. The boy returned on the evening of 20 December and was suffering from paronychia and a very slight nasal discharge which escaped notice in hospital. On the morning of 24 December his three little sisters fell sick, and when I saw them on Christmas day were in full rash. Incidentally the whole family developed measles from infection at hospital.

2 Several years ago I saw another victim of this disease, a young man who had apparently commenced two days before. On the day of onset, though suffering from a sore throat and feeling rather ill, he kept a 'date' at a dance with his young woman, with whom he was presumably in a fairly close contact. He also danced with several other girls, but did not succeed in infecting any of them with scarlet fever. This, I suppose, proves nothing unless we have the certain knowledge, as we have in the incident quoted above, that the contacts were Dick-positive. I do not think, however, that this need trouble us, as most of our country people are susceptible to the disease, and given the opportunity of infection, which I believe is provided mainly by patients in a later stage of the disease, it is a common occurrence for quite elderly people to develop scarlet fever – witness a woman of 58 early in 1936, and two middle-aged people later in the same year.

3 A girl of ten, having commenced to be ill the previous day, with considerable fortitude attended a tea-party given to celebrate a public occasion and was found to have a rash on reaching home. There was a large number of children at this party as well as adults and not a single other case appeared, although her mother who nursed her developed the disease nine days after, and three days after the child had developed a nasal discharge.

I have had a few instances of a definite exposure of short duration. In no case was it less than three days or more than four, three days being the most usual.

Now that diseases of the typhoid group seem to have disappeared from this and most other rural areas, scarlet fever is the most difficult of all these maladies which we have to face as sanitarians. It is a platitude to repeat that epidemics are kept alive by the patients who escape notice either because of the extreme mildness of the attack or the absence of rash, and still more, despite our vigilance, by the discharging ears or nose of those long since convalescent. Some years ago I allowed one small girl, whom I had actually isolated for three months, and whose nose I thought had ceased discharging, to return to school. Curiously enough, she left all her schoolmates unscathed, but quite obviously infected an adult with whom she had taken tea during the first week of her release.

The necessary interference with the livelihood of the farmers makes this disease a very unpopular one in country districts, and, if all patients are sent to hospital, a very costly addition to the expenditure of the Rural District.

As is well known, scarlet fever has passed through many fluctuations in severity. I happen to possess John Pechey's edition of *The Whole Works of that Excellent Physician, Dr Thomas Sydenham*, printed in 1701, and it is interesting to see scarlet fever referred to as 'this name of a disease, for it is scarce anything more', and many of us in this period would hold the same opinion of the disease as we have seen it. It is good to have had a father in this profession, as I had, whose account of scarlet fever in his young days was very different, and whose opinion of the disease explains the very real fear which is still felt in our area, where memories are long and the tragedies of the

past are never forgotten. Scarlet fever in those days was 'fever', i.e. *the* fever, and required no qualifying adjective any more than, as Greenwood writes, the plague requires one. The disease must also have passed through a mild phase at the beginning of the last century, but the physicians of that period congratulated themselves complacently on the improved methods of treatment to explain the reduction in the death-rate. We ourselves have no such pleasing illusions, and can hope only that the reappearance of the malignant form will be long delayed.

Whooping-Cough

There are numbers of entries of whooping-cough in the charts, but nothing of much interest to record. The two large epidemics have been fortunately of a mild nature and few patients have received medical attention, the names and dates of the sufferers being obtained from inquiry at the schools or from the parents.

In this disease the onset is so often insidious that it is very difficult to fix an incubation period. However, I have no instance in my charts to support as short an incubation period as three days, such as has been suggested by R. E. Smith and others. I had one good instance of the short and only possible exposure in the last epidemic. Two children in different villages began with whooping-cough on 16 and 17 July respectively. They were the first patients in these villages, and I found that they had both been to Redcar on 1 July for the annual school treat, and that there were definitely sufferers from this disease in the train among the children from a village further down the dale. Even allowing for an insidious commencement, the incubation period in these two cases must have been more than a fortnight. From previous observations in families, I had fixed the period as from 10 to 12 days, but just as in measles, it is possible infectivity may be present prior to the exhibition of symptoms.

Of the duration of infectivity I have nothing to say, as I have no incidents fixing its length, and I have not as yet made use of cough-plates. I have always isolated the patients for six weeks after the beginning of whooping, and this appears to be satisfactory, although probably erring on the safe side.

Epidemics of whooping-cough do not show a tendency to spread from village to village like those of measles and influenza, possibly because the average age of the children is less and generally before the school age. Whooping-cough does not appear to be a serious disease in Wensleydale, probably because the children with few exceptions are of superior physique, well fed and well cared for, and there is a complete absence of rickets. I have entries of 146 sufferers during the last seven years, and among this number there has been no instance of pneumonia and no death. In the 1924 influenza epidemic, a baby died in a few days, and its death is the only one I have to record from whooping-cough.

Mumps

Mumps leaves us alone for long periods, and in my 25 years I have seen but one epidemic. This began in August 1935, consisted of exactly 100 cases, and lasted a whole year, due to its long incubation period. My own experience, however, does not support an incubation period as long as 21 days, and I have a few instances of the short and only possible exposure.

The first was an infection at a wedding outside the district. *Betty* was a bridesmaid at this wedding on 11 June. She was a rather sick little bridesmaid, and later was found to have this disease. On the evening of 26 June her mother first had symptoms, and a few days later showed me a letter from her sister, the bride of 11 June, stating that she also began on the selfsame evening. The incubation period in the case of the bride was definitely 15 days, and as the little bridesmaid was quite well the day before the wedding the duration in the mother's case was possibly the same.

The second incident was a family visiting the neighbourhood. *Anne*, infected at her boarding-school, commenced on 8 August, but was not isolated until 10 August. Her sister developed mumps on 23 August and her aunt, who was of the party, on 25 August. The possible days of exposure were 8 and 9 August, so the incubation period in the one case was 15 to 16 days, and in the second 17 or 18. In the aunt's case it was conclusive, as she did not join the party until 8 August.

The third incident was this: a boy of thirteen attended school on 5 and 6 March in the early stages of the disease. The next two sufferers in the school commenced respectively on 20 and 22 March, suggesting an incubation period of 14 or 15 and 16 or 17 days. These are the only instances I could find of dated infection in the whole of this extensive epidemic.

The period of infectivity appeared to be less than a fortnight. Grammar-school boys and girls were infected by their younger brothers and sisters at home, and by fixing a fortnight as the period of infectivity the school was kept clear until the girl mentioned before, who knew better than her mother, started the ball rolling.

As a precautionary measure, all home contacts, although allowed to continue at school for the fortnight following the appearance of the disease at home, were kept away for the next fortnight, during which time most of them succumbed themselves. The disease was of a mild type, and the only complications were orchitis in two adult males and swelling of the lachrymal glands in one little girl.

Note

1 Figure 1 represents the whole of the epidemic, as it did not spread to other villages.

Acknowledgement

Pickles, W.N. (1939). The commoner diseases. In *Epidemiology in Country Practice*. Republished 1972, 1984. London: Royal College of General Practitioners.

2 *Sir Donald Acheson*

Doll, R. (1955) Mortality from lung cancer in asbestos workers. *British Journal of Industrial Medicine*, 12, 81–6.

Acheson, E.D. (1976) Nasal cancer in the furniture and boot and shoe manufacturing industries. *Preventive Medicine*, 5, 295–315.

INTRODUCTION

I have chosen two widely different papers within the field of occupational cancer. Although Sir Richard Doll's paper on lung cancer in asbestos workers is much less well known than his work on smoking, it is a classic in its own right, which would have gained him a place in the history of epidemiology had it been his only publication. The first point of importance is that it provides the earliest conclusive evidence that asbestos fibres are carcinogenic. We now know that asbestos related lung cancer is not limited to severely exposed workers with asbestosis, but also occurs in people who have experienced lower exposures. If the other asbestos related tumours such as mesothelioma are taken into account, asbestos, and in particular its amphibole varieties – crocidolite (blue) and amosite (brown) – has proved to be among the most important occupational and environmental carcinogens of the twentieth century.

Almost as an aside Sir Richard's paper also gives one of the first and unquestionably one of the·simplest descriptions of the man-years method of calculating expected numbers. Subsequently this technique rapidly became established as a standard way to measure risk in cohort studies. Previously risk was usually estimated by a 'snapshot' of the situation at the beginning of the period of exposure, thus wasting much of the available information.

My own paper is not in the same class of importance. It is a cameo with a generous share of serendipity in its origins. It deals with the occurrence of nasal cancer in two industries: the furniture industry and the boot and shoe

industry. With the exception of one unfortunate woman who lived over her husband's cabinet making business, no non-occupational cases of cancers due to these dusts have been described.

The seminal observation that there is a link between work in the furniture industry and adenocarcinoma of the ethmoid sinus (the tumour probably originates in the mucosa of the middle turbinate) was made by Miss Esmé Hadfield, who was an otorhinolaryngologist in the furniture town of High Wycombe[1]. Epidemiological analysis showed that the tumours do not occur in the relatively dust-free parts of the furniture factories where paints, polishes and varnishes are used (as was originally thought) but on the contrary are concentrated among the areas where machinists, turners, cabinet-makers and sanders using high speed grinding machines work[2]. The common environmental factor is exposure to hardwood dust. Later it was shown that similar tumours occur in the furniture industries of many other countries. Workers outside the furniture industry, such as coopers, wheelwrights and parquet floor layers, who are also exposed to hardwood dust likewise experience a high incidence of adenocarcinoma of the ethmoid.

The discovery that in addition to the problem in the furniture industry there is an increased risk of nasal cancer in the boot and shoe industry was entirely due to the coincidence that the region within the Oxford Cancer Register where the studies mentioned above were conducted is also the site of a substantial part of the British boot and shoe industry. A concentration of cases of nasal adenocarcinoma stood out clearly in those parts of Northamptonshire where the boot and shoe industry is centred, and where there is no furniture industry. Further analysis showed that unlike the findings in furniture workers, boot and shoe operatives also have an excess of other histological types of cancers of the paranasal sinuses. Virtually all the cases occurred in the three small departments in the boot and shoe factories (the press and preparation rooms and the finishing room) where the workers encounter large quantities of the dust of leather used for heels and soles of shoes. These areas in the Northamptonshire factories contain only 20 per cent of the male and 5 per cent of the female operatives. A high incidence of nasal cancer has subsequently been found in other countries where shoes are made from leather by a similar process. These include Belgium and Italy. Shoe menders who use high-speed grinding machines to repair leather shoes also have an excess incidence of nasal cancer. Once again preconceived ideas about the nature of the carcinogen had to be abandoned. As chromates, which are used in the tanning of the soft upper parts of leather shoes, had long been known to be carcinogenic, these were at first suspected to be responsible[3]. But it turned out that the dust with which the tumours are associated comes exclusively from the soles and heels, which are tanned by a different process.

It is intriguing to note that there may be a stronger link than coincidence between the occurrences of nasal adenocarcinoma within the two industries. Unlike the soft leather of the upper parts of shoes, the hardened leather for soles and heels is tanned by the historic method of immersion in vegetable infusions from the bark, fruit, galls and leaves of trees including hardwoods. These not only contain natural insecticides but may also be the locus of metabolites of moulds or fungi. The tantalizing possibility remains that nasal adenocarcinoma within the two industries is caused by the same group of carcinogens.

References

1 Hadfield, E.H. Referred to in Macbeth, R. (1965) Malignant disease of the paranasal sinuses. *Journal of Laryngology*, 79, 592–612.

2 Acheson, E.D., Cowdell, R.H., Hadfield, E.H. and Macbeth, R.G. (1968) Nasal cancer in wood workers in the furniture industry. *British Medical Journal*, ii, 587–96.

3 Bidstrup, P.L. and Case, R.A.M. (1956) Carcinoma of the lung in workmen in the biochromates producing industry in Great Britain. *British Journal of Industrial Medicine*. 13, 260–4.

MORTALITY FROM LUNG CANCER IN ASBESTOS WORKERS

Sixty-one cases of lung cancer have been recorded in persons with asbestosis (Boemke, 1953; Hueper, 1952) since Lynch and Smith (1935) reported the first case. In view of the infrequency of asbestosis, the large number of cases suggests – but does not prove – that lung cancer is an occupational hazard of asbestos workers. The strongest evidence that it may be a hazard has been produced by Merewether and by Gloyne. Merewether (1949) found that lung cancer was reported at necropsy in 13.2 per cent of cases of asbestosis (31 out of 235) but in only 1.3 per cent of cases of silicosis (91 out of 6884) and Gloyne (1951), on personal examination, found lung cancer in 14.1 per cent of necropsies on subjects associated with asbestosis (17 out of 121) against 6.9 per cent in silicotics (55 out of 796). Neither author gave full details of the sex composition of the groups examined, but since women form a higher proportion of asbestos workers than of persons employed in occupations liable to give rise to silicosis (coal-miners, stonemasons, pottery workers, foundrymen, metal grinders) and since lung cancer is less common among women, the differences in the proportions of cancer cases cannot be accounted for by differences in sex distribution. In fact the proportions which are more properly comparable with the findings in silicotic subjects are the proportions of lung cancer found among men with asbestosis, 17.2 per cent in Merewether's series and 19.6 per cent in Gloyne's.

Animal experiments are inconclusive. A positive result was reported by Nordmann and Sorge (1941) who found that of 10 mice which had been exposed to asbestos dust and survived for 240 days, two developed lung carcinoma. Smith (1952), however considers that one of the 'carcinomas' was, in fact, an example of squamous metaplasia and that the other, an adenocarcinoma, may have developed spontaneously from the common mouse adenoma. A negative result has been reported by Vorwald and Karr (1938). The majority of workers (cited by Hueper, 1952) consider that a causal relationship between asbestosis and lung cancer is either proved or is highly probable and the reality of the relationship was agreed at the recent International Symposium on the Epidemiology of Lung Cancer (Council of the International Organizations of Medical Sciences, 1953). A minority, however, remains sceptical (Cartier, 1952; Warren, 1948), including, according to Hueper (1952), Lanza and Vorwald, so that it was thought desirable to undertake a fresh investigation.

Necropsy data

Since 1935, records have been collected of all the coroners' necropsies on persons known to have been employed at a large asbestos works.[1] Pathological diagnoses in 105 consecutive cases are summarized in Table 1. Details of the cases in which lung cancer was found are shown in Table 2. During the first half of the period eight deaths occurred in which lung cancer was found in association with asbestosis, while in the second half of the period there were seven such cases and a further three in which lung cancer was found without asbestosis. The number of asbestos workers employed at the works increased steadily from 1914, and a great increase in the number of lung cancer deaths was also recorded among the whole population of England and Wales over the same period.

It might, therefore, have been anticipated that a larger number of cases in which the two conditions were associated would have been found in the last 10 years. National regulations for the control of asbestos dust were, however, introduced in 1931 (Asbestos Industry Regulations, 1931) and the precautions taken to prevent dust dissemination in the works had become effective by the end of the following year. All the subjects in whom the two diseases were found together had been employed for at least nine years under the old conditions, and although 11 of the 15 men and women died within 30 years of their first exposure, the association of the two conditions has not yet been found in any person taken into employment during the last 31 years (1923–53). It is, therefore, possible that the reason more cases were not found in the second half of the period is that reduced exposure to dust has already begun to lessen the incidence and severity of asbestosis.

Method of estimation of risk

Although the necropsy data shown in Tables 1 and 2 suggest (1) that some groups of asbestos workers have suffered an increased risk of lung cancer, and (2) that the risk may now have decreased, it is not possible to be certain of either of these propositions without a more detailed knowledge of the whole mortality experience of the workers. The first proposition has, therefore, been tested by comparing the mortality experienced by that section of the male employees of the works referred to above, who had worked for at least 20 years in 'scheduled areas',[2] with the mortality recorded for all men in England and Wales; and the second proposition by comparing the incidence of lung cancer among men

Table 1 Causes of death diagnosed at necropsy among persons employed at an asbestos works (1933–52)

Cause of death	Asbestosis present	Asbestosis absent	All cases
'Heart failure'	34	11	45
Pulmonary tuberculosis	12	9	21
Lung cancer	15	3	18
Other diseases of the respiratory system	10	4	14
Other diseases	4	3	7
All causes	75	30	105

employed for different periods under the pre–1933 conditions. The investigation was limited to the small group of men who had been employed for at least 20 years, since the labour involved in searching out the individual records of men employed for shorter periods would be disproportionately great and, so far as was known from Table 2, would be comparatively unrewarding.

The date of birth, date of completing 20 years' work in the 'scheduled areas', and, where applicable, date of ceasing employment and date and cause of death were obtained, for each man, from the records of the firm's Personnel Officer. Full details were, in most instances, already available for the men who had ceased employment as well as for the greater number who continued to be employed, since some of those who had left were registered as having asbestosis and the attention of the firm had been drawn to the death of others, in view of the possibility of the cause of death being industrial in origin. All the remaining men were successfully traced and the relevant details obtained. This was not difficult since, by limiting the study to men who had been employed in one place for 20 years, few were found to have changed their job or to have moved out of the region.

From the data the numbers of men alive in each five-year age group were counted separately for each of the years from 1922 (the first in which a man was recorded as having had 20 years' service) to 1953. A man who had completed the 20 years before the beginning of a year and who was alive at the end of it was counted, for that year, as one unit; a man who completed the period before the beginning of a year but who died during it, and a man who completed the period during a year and who survived to the end of it, were each counted, for that year, as half a unit; the one man who died the same year as he completed his 20-year period was counted as a quarter of a unit.

Table 2 Occupational history and necropsy data of asbestos workers with primary lung cancer

Year of death	Sex and age	Occupation	Period of exposure	Years of exposure	Years of exposure before 1 January 1933	Years from first exposure to death	Years from last exposure to death	Pathological report	
								Asbestosis	Histological type of primary lung cancer
1935	M.62	Weaver	1919–32	13	13	16	3	Present	'Carcinoma'
1935	M.54	Weaver	1909–32	23	23	26	3	Present	Epithelial carcinoma
1936	M.65	Fiberizer	1913–36	23	19	23	Less than 1	Present	Endothelioma of pleura
1938	M.47	Weaver	1910–12 1920–37	19	14	28	1	Present	'Carcinoma'
1939	M.49	Disintegrater	1910–14 1919–39	24	17	29	Less than 1	Present	'Carcinoma'
1940	M.52	Disintegrater	1911–15 1919–21 1923–39	22	15	29	Less than 1	Present	'Carcinoma'
1941	M.52	Weaver	1913–19 1924–38	20	14	28	3	Present	Oat-celled carcinoma
1942	M.59	Bag carrier	1913–41	28	19	29	1	Present	Oat-celled carcinoma
1948	M.59	Weaver	1912–14 1918–48	32	16	36	Less than 1	Present	Anaplastic carcinoma
1948	M.53	Weaver	1922–35	13	10	26	13	Present	'Carcinoma'
1948	M.48	Spinner	1922–48	26	10	26	Less than 1	Present	'Carcinoma'
1948	M.65	Maintenance man	1919–48	29	13	29	Less than 1	Present[a]	Oat-celled carcinoma
1950	F.51	Spinner	1915–42	27	17	35	8	Present	'Carcinoma'
1951	M.74	Fiberizer	1917–43	26	15	34	8	Present	Adenocarcinoma
1951	M.60	Weaver	1919–25 1929–50	27	9	32	1	Present	'Carcinoma'
1944	M.36	Weaver	1942–44	2	0	2	Less than 1	Absent	Oat-celled carcinoma
1951	M.43	Fiberizer	1939–48	9	0	12	3	Absent	Anaplastic carcinoma
1952	M.51	Weaver	1941 (3/12) 1945–52	7	0	11	Less than 1	Absent	'Carcinoma'

[a] Also pulmonary tuberculosis.

The causes of death were recorded as they were given on the death certificate or, when available, as they were finally determined by necropsy. The causes were classified in five categories (see Table 4), and the numbers in each category were then compared with those which might have been expected to occur by multiplying the numbers of men alive in each five-year age group by the corresponding mortality rates for men in England and Wales over the same period. Because of the small numbers, however, the populations were not considered separately for each year, but were added together to form five groups living in the periods 1922–33, 1934–8, 1939–43, 1944–8, and 1949–53, and the mortality rates used for each group were those for the years 1931, 1936, 1941, 1946 and 1951. The rates for 1931 were used for the period 1922–33, rather than those for the mid-years, since disproportionately few men were under observation during the early part of the period. As an example of the method, the mortality rate for all neoplasms other than lung cancer among men in England and Wales aged 55 to 59 in 1951 was 2.778 per 1000. The numbers of years lived in this age group in the five years 1949–53 were 15, 15, 17.5, 19 and 19 years. The number of deaths expected in the period was, therefore, estimated to be $(15 + 15 + 17.5 + 19 + 19) \times 2.778/1000 = 0.238$. The total number of deaths expected from each category of diseases was obtained by adding the numbers thus calculated for each group for each of the five periods.

Table 3 Number of man-years lived by men with 20 or more years of work in a 'scheduled area'

Age (years)	Period					All periods
	1922–33	1934–38	1939–43	1944–48	1949–53	
30–34	0	0.5	1.5	0	0	2
35–39	4.5	2	11	17.5	9	44
40–44	9.5	16	33.5	48	55	162
45–49	9.5	19.5	50	78.5	84	241.5
50–54	6.5	25.5	39.5	85	96.5	253
55–59	12	6	30	52	85.5	185.5
60–64	15	3	5.25	25.5	36	84.75
65–69	1	13.5	3	10	21.5	49
70–74	0	2	9	3	3.5	17.5
75–79	0	0	1	1.5	0.5	3
All ages	58	88	183.75	321	391.5	1042.25

The great majority of the men lived and, when they died, died in the town in which the works was situated, so that it would have been preferable to have based the calculation of the expected deaths on the death rates observed in that town rather than on the rates for all England and Wales. These, however, were not known in sufficient detail. Little error in the expected number of deaths from lung cancer is likely to have been introduced on this account since, according to Stocks (1952), the age-adjusted death rate for lung cancer among men in the town concerned was 96 per cent of the rate for England and Wales. Stock's figure was calculated only for the period 1946–9, but the proportion is unlikely to have varied greatly over the longer period of the investigation. The expected number of deaths from all causes is, however, likely to be somewhat underestimated since the age-adjusted death rate from all causes for the town is about 25 per cent higher than the England and Wales rate (i.e. the excess was 22 per cent in 1950, 28 per cent in 1951, and 22 per cent in 1952).

Results

The number of men studied was 113; the numbers of man-years lived in each of the five periods in each age group are shown in Table 3. The total number of deaths from all causes and the number of deaths observed in each of the five disease categories, together with the expected number of deaths, are shown in Table 4. From Table 4 it appears that the men who had been exposed to asbestos dust suffered an increased mortality from lung cancer, other respiratory diseases and cardiovascular

diseases, in association with asbestosis, but that their mortality from other diseases was close to that expected.

Four explanations of the findings are possible:

1 That all the men who had died of lung cancer were recorded because of interest in the condition, but that some of the records of other men dying of other diseases or still alive were omitted, with consequent underestimation of the expected number of deaths.
2 That lung cancer was incorrectly and excessively diagnosed among the asbestos workers.
3 That lung cancer was insufficiently diagnosed among the general population of England and Wales.
4 That the asbestos workers studied suffered an excess mortality from lung cancer.

It certainly cannot be claimed that the records of the Personnel Office were necessarily complete, but they were believed to be complete and no deficiency on this score would account for the total excess of deaths unless it were so gross that more than half the defined population had been omitted. Moreover, the number of deaths due to conditions unrelated to asbestosis was close to the estimated number and this is unlikely to have happened unless the population had been estimated approximately correctly and the deaths from all causes fully reported.

All the 11 deaths attributed to lung cancer were confirmed by necropsy and histological examination so that the excess number cannot be attributed to incorrect diagnosis among the group of asbestos workers. Some of the excess may well be due to an underestimation of the expected deaths since part of the increase in mortality attributed to lung cancer over the past 30 years is certainly due to improvements in diagnosis and in therapy (Doll,

Table 4   Causes of death among male asbestos workers compared with mortality experience of all men in England and Wales

Cause of death	No. of deaths		Test of significance of difference between observed and expected (value of P)
	No. observed	Expected on England and Wales rates	
Lung cancer[a]			
with mention of asbestosis	11	–	} <0.000001
without mention of asbestosis	0	0.8	
Other respiratory diseases (including pulmonary tuberculosis) and cardiovascular diseases			
with mention of asbestosis	14	–	} <0.001
without mention of asbestosis	6	7.6	
Neoplasms other than lung cancer	4	2.3	} >0.1
All other diseases[b]	4	4.7	
All causes	39	15.4	<0.000001

[a] Including one case with pulmonary tuberculosis.
[b] Including two cases (benign stricture of oesophagus and septicaemia) in which asbestosis was present but was not thought to have been a contributory cause of death.

1953). Even, however, if it were postulated that the whole of the recorded increase between 1931 and 1951 was spurious and that the real mortality from the disease throughout was that ascribed to it in 1951, the expected number of deaths is increased to only 1.1 and the observed excess is still grossly significant. For the actual number of lung cancer cases to be so little in excess of the expected as to be reasonably attributable to chance, it would be necessary for the expected cases to be 6.2, that is 5.6 times the number of estimated on 1951 rates. In other words, it would be necessary to postulate that in 1951 (and throughout the previous 20 years) there was 5.6 times as much cancer of the lung as was recognized in 1931, which would mean that the condition would have to have been present and capable of detection in over 20 per cent of all men at death. Moreover, even if this were so, it would still not account for the fact that all the cases of lung cancer were found in association with asbestosis.

It is, therefore, concluded that the fourth explanation is the most reasonable one and that the asbestos workers who had worked for 20 or more years in the 'scheduled areas' suffered a notably higher risk from lung cancer than the rest of the population.

To test if the risk has altered since the 1931 regulations were introduced, it is not only necessary to make allowance for duration of employment before the end of 1932, but also to allow for the men's ages and for the total durations of their employment in the 'scheduled areas', since the men employed in the earlier periods can also

have been employed longer and lived to be older. On the other hand, there is no need to consider the changing incidence of lung cancer in the total population of England and Wales since the non-industrial risk has been shown to be small in comparison with the industrial one. The data required for comparing the risks among men employed for under 10 years, for 10 to 14 years, and for 15 years and over in the pre–1933 conditions are shown in Table 5. The ages shown are the ages at death of the men who have died and the ages in mid–1953 for the men who are still alive. The expected numbers of men in each pre–1933 employment group found to have asbestosis or asbestosis and lung cancer are estimated by multiplying the numbers in each age, total employment and pre-1933 employment subgroup by the proportions of men with asbestosis or with asbestosis and lung cancer in the same age and total employment group for all lengths of pre–1933 employment combined. For example, three out of the nine men aged 50 to 54 years who had been employed for 20 to 24 years in the areas in which they might be exposed to asbestos dust were found to have asbestosis and lung cancer. Since three men had worked for under 10 years in the pre–1933 conditions, three had worked for 10 to 14 years, and three had worked for 15 or more years, the expected number of cases in each of the pre–1933 employment groups would have been the same, **i.e.** $3 \times 3/9$ or 1. In fact, the numbers of cases found were 0, 1 and 2. The total numbers expected in each pre–1933 employment group are

Table 5 Numbers of men employed for different periods before 1933 and numbers known to have asbestosis and lung cancer in association with asbestosis divided by total duration of employment in a scheduled area and by age

Total length of employment in 'scheduled area' (years)	Age at 30 June 1953, or at death (years)	Length of employment before 1 January 1933									All lengths of employment before 1 January 1933		
		0–9 years			10–14 years			15+ years					
		No. of men	No. of men with asbestosis	No. of men with cancer of lung	No. of men	No. of men with asbestosis	No. of men with cancer of lung	No. of men	No. of men with asbestosis	No. of men with cancer of lung	No. of men	No. of men with asbestosis	No. of men with cancer of lung
20–24	35–39	1	–	–	1	1	–	0	–	–	2	1	–
	40–44	4	–	–	1	1	–	0	–	–	5	1	–
	45–49	7	1	–	0	0	–	1	1	1	8	2	1
	50–54	3	2	–	3	3	1	3	3	2	9	8	3
	55–59	5	3	–	2	1	–	0	0	0	7	4	0
	60–64	3	1	–	1	1	–	1	1	0	5	3	0
	65–69	2	0	–	0	–	–	1	1	1	3	1	1
	70–74	0	0	–	0	–	–	1	1	–	1	1	–
	75–79	1	1	–	0	–	–	0	–	–	1	1	–
25–29	40–44	3	–	–	0	–	–	0	–	–	3	0	–
	45–49	10	2	–	2	1	1	0	–	–	12	3	1
	50–54	6	2	1	0	0	0	0	–	–	6	2	1
	55–59	6	1	–	8	4	0	1	1	–	15	6	0
	60–64	3	–	–	1	1	0	3	3	1	7	4	1
	65–69	1	–	–	1	1	1	0	0	0	2	1	1
	70–74	0	–	–	0	–	–	1	0	0	1	0	0
	75–79	0	–	–	0	–	–	1	1	1	1	1	1
	80–84	0	–	–	0	–	–	1	0	–	1	0	–
30–34	45–49	2	–	–	0	–	–	0	–	–	2	0	–
	50–54	2	–	–	5	–	–	2	–	–	9	0	–
	55–59	1	–	–	1	–	–	3	2	1	5	2	1
	60–64	1	–	–	0	–	–	2	1	–	3	1	–
	65–69	0	–	–	0	–	–	0	0	–	0	0	–
	70–74	0	–	–	0	–	–	1	1	–	1	1	–
35+	55–59	0	–	–	0	–	–	1	–	–	1	0	–
	60–64	0	–	–	0	–	–	1	–	–	1	0	–
	65–69	0	–	–	0	–	–	2	–	–	2	0	–
All (20 years +)	35–39	1	–	–	1	1	–	0	–	–	2	1	–
	40–44	7	–	–	1	1	–	0	–	–	8	1	–
	45–49	19	3	–	2	1	1	1	1	1	22	5	2
	50–54	11	4	1	8	3	1	5	3	2	24	10	4
	55–59	12	4	–	11	5	0	5	3	1	28	12	1
	60–64	7	1	–	2	2	0	7	5	1	16	8	1
	65–69	3	0	–	1	1	1	3	1	1	7	2	2
	70–74	0	0	–	0	–	–	3	2	0	3	2	0
	75–79	1	1	–	0	–	–	1	1	1	2	2	1
	80–84	0	–	–	0	–	–	1	0	–	1	0	–
	All ages	61	13	1	26	14	3	26	16	7	113	43	11

obtained by adding the numbers calculated for each of the age and total employment groups within it. The results are shown in Table 6.

The differences between the numbers of men observed and the numbers expected in each employment group, had the incidence of the conditions remained steady throughout, are statistically significant (total asbestosis X^2 = 7.52, $n = 2$, $P = 0.025$; asbestosis and lung cancer X^2 = 8.74, $n = 2$, $P = 0.01$).[3] They are highly so if the trend,

that is the biologically important reduction in the proportion between observed and expected numbers as the length of pre–1933 employment is reduced, is also taken into consideration. It is clear, therefore, that the incidences both of asbestosis and of lung cancer associated with asbestosis have become progressively less as the number of years during which men were exposed to the pre–1933 conditions has decreased.

The extent of the risk of lung cancer over the whole

Table 6 Observed and expected asbestosis and lung cancer rates

		Length of employment before 1 January 1933		
		Under 10 years	10–14 years	15 years and over
Total number of men with asbestosis	observed	13	14	16
	expected	21.9	10.3	10.8
Number of men with asbestosis and lung cancer	observed	1	3	7
	expected	5.5	2.4	3.1

period among the men studied appears to have been of the order of ten times that experienced by other men. This agrees well with the data reported by Merewether (1949), but it is somewhat greater than that suggested by Gloyne's data (1951). The great reduction in the amount of dust produced in asbestos works during the period has been accompanied by a reduction in the incidence of lung cancer among the workmen so that the risk before 1933 is likely to have been considerably greater – perhaps 20 times the general risk. Whether the specific industrial risk of lung cancer has yet been completely eliminated cannot be determined with certainty; the number of men at risk, who have been exposed to the new conditions only and who have been employed for a sufficient length of time, is at present too small for confidence to be placed in their experience. It is clear, however, that the risk has for some time been greatly reduced. The extent of the reduction is particularly striking when it is recalled that between 1933 and 1953 the incidence of the disease among men in the country at large has increased sixfold.

Summary

The cause of death, as determined at necropsy, is reported for 105 persons who had been employed at one asbestos works. Lung cancer was found in 18 instances, 15 times in association with asbestosis. All the subjects in whom both conditions were found had started employment in the industry before 1923 and had worked in the industry at least nine years before the regulations for the control of dust had become effective.

One hundred and thirteen men who had worked for at least 20 years in places where they were liable to be exposed to asbestos dust were followed up and the mortality among them was compared with that which would have been expected on the basis of the mortality experience of the whole male population. Thirty-nine deaths occurred in the group whereas 15.4 were expected. The excess was entirely due to excess deaths from lung cancer (11 against 0.8 expected) and from other respiratory and cardiovascular diseases (22 against 7.6 expected). All the cases of lung cancer were confirmed histologically and all were associated with the presence of asbestosis.

From the data it can be concluded that lung cancer was a specific industrial hazard of certain asbestos workers and that the average risk among men employed for 20 or more years has been of the order of ten times that experienced by the general population. The risk has become progressively less as the duration of employment under the old dusty conditions has decreased.

Notes

1 Necropsies on asbestos workers are ordered by the coroner when in his opinion, there may be a question of asbestosis being a contributory cause of death.
2 By 'scheduled areas' is meant those areas where processes were carried on which were scheduled under the Asbestos Industry Regulations of 1931 as being dusty.
3 The expected numbers of lung cancer are small and the probability that the differences could arise by chance has consequently been somewhat, but not seriously, underestimated. If all men with more than ten years pre–1933 employment are grouped together and Yates' correction made for small numbers, $X^2 = 5.82$, $n = 1$, $P = 0.02$.

References

Asbestos Industry Regulations (1931) Statutory Rules and Orders 1931, No. 1140. HMSO, London.
Boemke, F. (1953) *Med. Mschr.*, 7, 77.
Cartier, P. (1952) *Arch. industr. Hyg.*, 5, 262 (contribution to discussion).
Council of the International Organizations of Medical Sciences. (1953) *Acta Un. Int. Cancr.*, 9, 443.
Doll, R. (1953) *Brit. Med. J.*, 2, 521.
Gloyne, S.R. (1951) *Lancet*, 1, 810.
Hueper, W.C. (1952) *Proceedings of the Seventh Saranac Symposium*.
Lynch, K.M. and Smith, W.A. (1935) *Amer. J. Cancer*, 24, 56.
Merewether, E.R.A. (1949) *Annual Report of the Chief Inspector of Factories for the Year 1947*. HMSO, London.
Nordmann, M. and Sorge, A. (1941) *Z Krebsforsch.*, 51, 168.
Smith, W.E. (1952) *Brit. J. Cancer*, 6, 99.
Vorwald, A.J. and Karr, J.W. (1938) *Amer. J. Path.*, 14, 49.
Warren, S. (1948) *Occup. Med.*, 5, 249.

Acknowledgement

Doll, R. (1955) Mortality from lung cancer in asbestos workers. *British Journal of Industrial Medicine*, 12, 81–6.

NASAL CANCER IN THE FURNITURE AND BOOT AND SHOE MANUFACTURING INDUSTRIES

Malignant disease of the nasal cavity and paranasal sinuses is rare in the general population. Recent estimates of the annual incidence of nasal cancer of various histological types are shown in Table 1 (3). If the commonest malignant tumours in England are used as a standard for comparison, the incidence in males of all histological types of nasal cancer taken together is approximately one-hundredth that of carcinoma of the bronchus, and in females one-hundredth that of carcinoma to the breast.

Squamous cell epithelioma is by far the commonest histological variety of intranasal malignant tumour. In a study of all 468 cases registered in southern England during the years 1961–5, 328 patients (70.1 per cent) were found to have squamous tumours, 39 (8.3 per cent) had adenocarcinomas and 19 (4.1 per cent) had transitional cell tumours (3). All other tumours together, including those in which histological material had not been examined, accounted for the remaining 82 (17.5 per cent) cases.

The purpose of this paper is to review the work published in the last 10 years which has shown that nasal cancer is a substantial risk in woodworkers in the furniture industry and certain workers in the boot and shoe manufacturing industry.

The mucociliary mechanism of the nose

Apart from the nasal vestibule in which the epithelium is of the stratified squamous variety, the nasal mucus membrane is similar to the rest of the respiratory tract and is lined with pseudostratified columnar ciliated epithelium interspersed with mucus secreting glands and islands of squamous epithelium (14). It has been known for many years that particles of dust and of dyes deposited in the nose are transported by ciliary action in a stream of nasal mucus into the nasopharynx. From here the mucus is despatched to the stomach through the wiping action of the soft palate during swallowing. Additional supplies of

mucus are passed into the nose through the apertures of the paranasal sinuses.

Until recently, progress in our knowledge of the various factors which influence the effectiveness of mucociliary transport within the nose, and the consequent rate of clearance of dust, has been extremely slow. The situation has now been transformed by the introduction of a technique by which the course of radioactive labelled resin beads may be followed accurately through the nasal passages (20). The use of this technique has shown that there is a wide range of variation in the rate of mucociliary transport in normal subjects but that the average appears to be about 5 mm/min (19). In the next few years we can expect rapid progress in our knowledge of mucociliary transport under various industrial conditions.

Nasal cancer in the furniture industry

Historical note

The clinical observation that there was probably an association between cancer of the nasal cavity and work in the furniture industry was made in 1964 by the British otorhinolaryngologist, Esmé Hadfield, who works in High Wycombe, Buckinghamshire. Her observation was reported by her colleague, R. G. Macbeth, in a general account of malignant disease of the paranasal sinuses published in the following year (17). He wrote:

> One striking small series must, however, be mentioned and I am indebted to Miss Esmé Hadfield of High Wycombe for drawing my attention to these patients. Out of a total of 20 patients from High Wycombe no less than 15 were associated with the making of wooden chairs.

At this point the significance of the observation was considered to be uncertain. In 1966, in a letter to the author of this review asking for epidemiological assistance, Macbeth noted that the tumours were all adenocarcinomas. The subsequent epidemiological work has confirmed Hadfield and Macbeth's clinical observation, clarified and extended our knowledge of the relationship, and shown that the risk is not limited to chairmakers in High Wycombe but occurs widely in the furniture industry in many countries.

In view of the fact that it has been the subject of the closest study so far, much of the material in this review will relate to the furniture industry which is located in High Wycombe and the surrounding area of Buckinghamshire, published in the report of an epidemiological survey of the southern half of the Oxford Hospital Region

Table 1 Incidence per million per annum of all types of carcinoma of the nasal cavity and sinuses in southern register areas of England (1961–1965)

| Age group | Average incidence per 10^6 per annum | | | | | |
| | Adenocarcinomas | | Squamous carcinomas | | All types | |
	Males	Females	Males	Females	Males	Females
15–64	0.5	0.2	4.3	1.9	5.8	3.1
65+	3.0	1.6	26.3	10.6	34.9	16.6
15+	0.8	0.4	7.0	3.5	9.4	5.6

(1, 2). Subsequently, a national survey of nasal adeno-carcinoma in England has been carried out and important additional clinical and pathological information relating to the pathogenesis of the tumour has been published (15).

The topography of the Oxford survey area

The survey was designed to test Hadfield and Macbeth's hypotheses that there was an association between nasal adenocarcinoma and the furniture industry. The area chosen for study was the southern part of the Oxford Hospital Region, which consists of Oxfordshire, including the city of Oxford, Reading and part of Berkshire, and High Wycombe and part of Buckinghamshire (Figure 1). Using the facilities of the Oxford Regional Cancer Register, with careful checks from all other possible sources of data, an attempt was made to ascertain all cases of nasal cancer diagnosed in residents since the register was established in 1951. The decade 1956–65 was used for the computation of annual incidence rates.

Figure 1 shows the geography of the area and the location of the furniture industry within it. The concentration of the furniture industry in High Wycombe and the surrounding villages owes its existence to the presence of an extensive beech forest on the slopes of the Chiltern Hills close to the growing population centre of eighteenth-century London. Since the second half of the eighteenth century and possibly from earlier times, chairs have been made from the Chiltern beeches, at first as a cottage industry, but in the last 100 years with an increasing degree of organisation and mechanisation. Manufacture of other types of furniture began towards the end of the nineteenth century and since that time there has been increasing utilisation of a wide variety of domestic and imported hardwoods. In the period before the Second World War the industry still consisted of a large number of small firms, most of which had fewer than

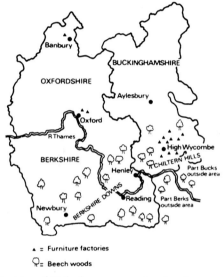

Fig. 1 Map of Oxford survey area showing diagrammatically the sites of furniture factories.

50 employees. Working conditions in these small firms were relatively poor by contemporary standards and the use of exhaust ventilation was unusual. At the time of the survey, High Wycombe and the surrounding area accounted for 12 per cent of the British furniture industry, and 80 per cent of the wooden chairs manufactured in the United Kingdom were made there.

Fortunately, from the point of view of the conclusions it was possible to draw from the data, a furniture industry making a different range of products has existed in Oxford and Banbury for at least 50 years, although on a very much smaller scale. This has been concerned with general office and ecclesiastical furniture, not chair making, the principal materials being oak and mahogany. Little beech is used in these factories.

21

Table 2 Distribution of male woodworkers in Oxfordshire and in the parts of Buckinghamshire and Berkshire in the Oxford Cancer Register area

Occupation	High Wycombe	Bucks. (incl. H.W.)	Berks.	Oxon.	Whole area	
					N	%
Carpenters and joiners	230	1760	2270	1810	5840	53.5
Cabinet and chair-makers	520	980	180	250	1410	12.9
Sawyers and woodworking machinists	650	1370	400	410	2180	20.0
Patternmakers	30	70	40	90	200	1.8
Woodworkers not elsewhere classified	250	580	430	270	1280	11.7
All	1680	4760	3320	2830	10910	99.9

[a] Source: Census of England and Wales, 1971; 10 per cent sample.

The population of the Oxford survey area

The population of the area at the time of the survey consisted of just over one million people. These were distributed in the cities of Oxford and Reading which each had a population of about 100000, the smaller towns of Aylesbury, Banbury and High Wycombe, and the rural countryside. Apart from a plant for the manufacture of motor vehicles in Oxford, there is little heavy industry in the area.

As the boundary of the survey had to follow the catchment area of the Oxford Cancer Register, and this unfortunately cut across the local county boundaries, it was not possible at the time of our original publication to obtain accurate estimates of the numbers of woodworkers for the whole survey area, although accurate estimates were available for the town of High Wycombe itself. Table 2 takes advantage of the fact that accurate occupational figures for the precise area of the survey became available following the 1971 census. The important point which emerges from this table is that slightly more than half of the population of male wood workers in this area are carpenters and joiners. These men are employed principally in the building trade, do not work in factories and, in general, work with softwoods. The 1410 cabinet- and chair-makers work in the furniture industry, three-quarters of them in Buckinghamshire. It is safe to assume that the majority of the sawyers and wood machinists and the unclassified workers in Buckinghamshire has been employed in the furniture industry. In the remainder of the area many of these men are concerned with preparing timber for the building and joinery trades. It is important to note that the Buckinghamshire furniture industry employs a substantial number of men and some women who are not woodworkers. In

Table 3 The histological type of the tumours in the Oxford survey by sex

Type of tumour	Males	Females	Total	Sex ratio
Squamous	36	24	60	1.5
Adenocarcinoma	33	3	36	11.0
Transitional cell	4	5	9	0.8
Anaplastic	10	10	20	1.0
Unclassified	15	8	23	1.9
Total	98	50	148	2.0

addition to clerks and labourers these include upholsterers and French polishers. In the town of High Wycombe in 1961 the furniture industry is thought to have comprised some 3000 men in all, but exact figures are lacking.

The incidence of nasal adenocarcinoma in the Oxford area

The survey yielded a total of 148 cases of nasal cancer of which 83 had been diagnosed during the decade defined for the calculation of incidence rates (1956–65). The relationship between histological type of tumour and sex is shown in Table 3. Adenocarcinoma in this area is seen to be almost an exclusively male disease. An analysis of the material by place of residence showed the expected concentration of the adenocarcinomas in the High Wycombe area. An analysis by age showed that it was distinctly unusual for adenocarcinoma to appear after the age of 65, while almost exactly half of the other classified tumours occurred after that age. The strength of the

Table 4 Relationship of work in the furniture industry (at any time) to histological type of tumour in men in Oxford survey area

	Woodworkers in f.i.[a]	Others in f.i.	Other woodworkers	Other work	Nature of work unknown	Total
Adenocarcinoma	22	4	2	4	1	33
Squamous, etc.	3	1	2	48	11	65
All	25	5	4	52	12	98

[a] f.i. = furniture industry.

relationship between work in the furniture industry and adenocarcinoma is demonstrated for males in Table 4. As many of the patients with non-adenocarcinomatous tumours were very old at the time of diagnosis it was more difficult to obtain occupational data from them or from their relatives. However, even when allowance is made for possible bias introduced by this factor, the relationship between intranasal adenocarcinoma and the furniture industry is remarkable.

The computation of incidence rates was complicated by the difficulties in estimating the population at risk in the various specific occupations (2). Our best estimates are that the risk of adenocarcinoma in High Wycombe cabinet- and chair-makers, and in wood machinists, was similar, namely 0.7 ± 0.2 per 1000 per annum during the decade 1956–65, that is to say at least 500 times the risk in adult males in southern England. As five cases of this normally rare tumour were found in the diminutive Oxfordshire furniture industry, which employs less than 500 workers, a similar magnitude of risk can be assumed to exist there. A small but significant number of cases were also found amongst other workers in the furniture industry (see Table 7). The primary conclusion of the Oxford survey was thus to prove Hadfield and Macbeth's hypothesis of an association between nasal adenocarcinoma and work in the furniture industry, and to demonstrate that the risk was not limited to furniture workers concerned in the manufacture of chairs in the High Wycombe area but extended to groups of furniture workers making other types of product. The evidence, so far as it went, also suggested that there was no comparable risk in carpenters and joiners.

In the year following the publication of the report, nasal adenocarcinoma became a prescribed industrial disease[1] for workers in the furniture industry in the United Kingdom. As a result, sufferers and their widows became eligible for compensation.

The latent period and the period of exposure

If the material from the Oxford and national surveys is

combined, there is a total of 49 men with adenocarcinoma in whom it is possible either to be certain of the year of entry to the furniture industry or to make a reasonable assumption about that date. If this date is taken as the point in time at which exposure to the carcinogenic substance began, it is possible to calculate the latent period. The average was found to be 42.8 years (range 27 to 69 years). This may be compared with an average of 40 years in 17 cases reported from Lyons, France (13).

Eighteen furniture workers in the Oxford and national surveys had left the industry some years before the diagnosis of the adenocarcinoma. A study of these cases shows that it is possible to develop an adenocarcinoma after as little as 3, 5 and 7 years' exposure, respectively, within the furniture industry and as much as 38 years after leaving it. Hadfield refers to an additional patient, diagnosed after the publication of the Oxford survey, whose period of exposure to dust within the furniture industry was only 18 months (14). This is the shortest known period of exposure.

The distribution of the years of exposure and the intervals after leaving the industry are shown in Table 5. It is interesting that there is no significant difference between the mean latent period in men who left the industry prior to diagnosis of the tumour and those who remained within it ($t(47, 0) = 0.5$, $P > 0.05$).

The period during which the factor has been present in the industry

A study of the occupational histories makes it possible to set limits on the *minimum period* during which the carcinogenic factor has been present in the industry (Figure. 2). Four men who subsequently developed nasal adenocarcinoma each worked in the industry for less than 10 years, and had left by 1927. We can therefore deduce that the factor was present in the early 1920s. At the other end of the scale six men have developed adenocarcinoma who entered the industry in the 1930s (the latest entering in 1935). In summary, it may be deduced from the epidemiological evidence that the

Table 5 The distributions of the intervals between entry to the furniture industry and departure (A); departure from the industry and diagnosis of the tumour (B); and the sums of these intervals (C) in 18 men who left the industry. D shows the distribution of intervals between entry to industry and diagnosis in 31 men who remained in the industry[a]

Number of years	Number of patients leaving industry prior to diagnosis			Patients still in industry at diagnosis
	A	B	C	D
1–4	1	0	0	0
5–9	3	3	0	0
10–14	4	2	0	0
15–19	1	2	0	0
20–24	4	2	0	0
25–29	0	4	0	2
30–34	2	4	3	4
35–39	0	1	5	4
40–44	1	0	3	10
45–49	1	0	3	6
50–54	0	0	1	4
55–59	1	0	2	0
60+	0	0	1	1
Total	18	18	18	31
Average	21.3	22.3	43.6	42.3

[a] All published English cases in which sufficient information is available.

Table 6 Nasal adenocarcinoma in the Oxford survey area by year of diagnosis, including 18 previously unpublished cases

Year of diagnosis	Number of cases
Up to 1949	3[a]
1950–1954	3
1955–1959	8
1960–1964	12
1965–1969	15
1970–1974	6
Total	47

[a] Excluding two cases without precise histological classification.

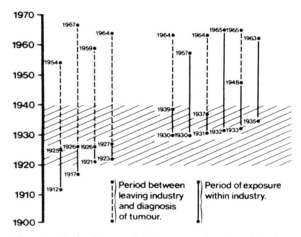

Fig. 2 Periods of occupational exposure in selected furniture workers from the Oxford survey.

factor was certainly present in the British furniture industry between about 1920 and 1940. It may or may not have been present previously or subsequently. In Britain no person who entered the industry after the Second World War (i.e. after 1945) is, so far, known to have developed a nasal adenocarcinoma. In France, however, one of the two patients with furniture makers' adenocarcinoma, reported by Fombeur, started work in 1941 (12). It is clear that materials introduced into the furniture industry since the Second World War cannot be responsible for the cases reported in this paper.

Another approach to this problem is to examine the distribution of the cases of adenocarcinoma in time.

Table 6 shows the total number of cases of adenocarcinoma in men who are known to have worked at any time in the furniture industry in the Oxford survey area up to the end of 1974. The table includes 18 cases which have occurred in the area since the original publication.

Table 6 suggests that nasal adenocarcinoma, as an occupational risk in the furniture industry, was rare before

Table 7 Published cases of nasal adenocarcinoma in workers in the English furniture industry according to occupation and putative exposure to wood dust, polishes, etc.

Occupation within furniture industry	Number of men	Nature of dust		Polishes, lacquers, sprays
		Wood dust	Adhesives	
Labourers, yardsmen, etc.	3	+	+	+
Turners	3	+ +	−	−
Wood machinists	17	+ +	−	−
Makers[a]	20	+ +	+	−
French polishers and stainers	3	+	+	+ +
Upholsterers	2	+	+	+
Furniture workers unsp.	3	?	?	?
Total	51			

[a] Cabinet- and chair-makers, benchmen, sanders and veneerers.

1950. The evidence and reasoning on which the conclusion was based that this appearance is not an artifact due to poor ascertainment prior to that date, have already been published. The decline in the number of cases diagnosed since 1970 is encouraging and may be a first indication of a decline in the epidemic. However, there is also evidence of a decline in the number of woodworkers in the Buckinghamshire furniture industry between the 1961 and 1971 censuses. If we assume that the latent period of the tumour is 40 years, the shape of the epidemic suggests that the factor appeared in the industry about 1910, reached a peak in the 1920s and, possibly, began to decline in the 1930s.

Woods, glues or polishes?

The working area of a furniture factory is generally divided into three parts: the machine shop where timber is sawn and turned into pieces of appropriate shape; the making shop where it is assembled into chairs, tables, etc.; and the finishing area where polish, sprays and varnishes are applied. In the machine shop the material used (at least in the area of the Oxford survey) is almost exclusively hardwood and there is a great deal of dust. Dust is also present in the making up area due to the use of sanding machines, and in this area volatile adhesives are also used. The effective use of polishes requires a relatively dust-free atmosphere. This means that men who work in this area are less exposed to dust than the other workers. However, the manual 'French' method of applying polish, in use until it was replaced by the use of polyethylene sprays after the Second World War, required the use of sandpaper and created a dust containing wood and polish (14).

Table 7 shows that the environmental factor common to all cases is wood dust. Wood machinists and turners are not exposed to polishes or adhesives to any appreciable extent and yet the evidence suggests (*vide supra*) that the risk in wood machinists is similar to that in cabinet- and chair-makers.

The nature of the woods responsible

Two almost insuperable difficulties stand in the way of the identification of species of tree which might bear carcinogenic wood. The first is that most furniture makers are exposed during their working life to a wide variety of timbers. The second is that the woodworker may not know the exact nature and origin of the timber, and these are often referred to in botanically imprecise terms. Table 8 shows information collected from occupational histories published in the Oxford and national surveys. As the epidemiological evidence showed that the factor concerned was definitely present between 1920 and 1940, in taking these histories attention was focused on the industrial environment as it existed before the Second World War. Case No. 010 is of interest because the man worked in a small firm of chair-makers which used almost exclusively local Chiltern beech seasoned in their own yard. This man's history seems to incriminate beech. Case No. 005 and two other men who could not be questioned all worked in a factory making dining room suites and piano stools where beech was not used, and the woods in common use were oak, mahogany and sapele. Case No. 002 was rarely in contact with beech, and Nos. 407, 408, and 416 never were. Of the cases reported from the continent of Europe, information about the nature of the timbers to which the worker was exposed is available for

Table 8 Types of wood to which 16 workmen in the English furniture industry were exposed, who subsequently developed nasal adenocarcinoma and for whom detailed occupational histories were obtained

Case No.	Types of wood to which exposed					
	Oak	Beech	Mahogany	Sapele	Walnut	Other
002	+	(+)[a]				+
005	+		+	+		+
006	+	+	+		+	
007	+	+	+			
008	+	+	+			
010	(+)[a]	+				(+)[a]
011	+	+	+		+	
031	+	+	+		+	+
032		+	+			+
405	+	+	+			
407	+		+		+	+
408	+					+
409	+	+	+			
410	+	+	+		+	+
416	+		+		+	+
419	+	+	+		+	

[a] Parentheses indicate that a small quantity of this wood was used.

two French cabinet-makers and one Danish furniture worker. Of the French cases, one man had been exposed to oak and deal only, the other to a variety of hardwoods including oak. Neither had been exposed to beech. The Dane had been exposed principally to beech and birch-wood. It may be concluded from the available data that beech, almost certainly, and oak, probably, are associated with the disease. The evidence does not exclude the possibility that the factor is also present in other woods. Data from industries where one type of timber is used exclusively (e.g. the Swedish pine furniture industry) would be of great interest. The fact that nasal cancer is rare in the much larger group of woodworkers who operate outside the furniture industry, principally in the building trade, and who are exposed largely to soft-woods, does not necessarily mean that these woods are not potentially carcinogenic. It may be that the conditions of work in these trades do not produce a sufficiently high concentration of dust of the approximate particle size to be harmful.

Furniture makers' adenocarcinoma outside the Oxford survey area

A national survey of nasal adenocarcinoma in England (excluding the Oxford area) published in 1972 revealed 24 men and one woman with these tumours who had at some time worked in the furniture industry (5). As this survey was based on national cancer register material which is known to be incomplete, notably in terms of histological classification, it was not possible to make an accurate estimate of incidence from the material. However, the number of cases of adenocarcinoma observed was 95 times the number expected on the basis of the relative size of the furniture industry, and the ratio of observed to expected cases was much higher in the furniture industry than in any other industry. It was possible to conclude from the distribution of the cases that there is certainly a high risk of nasal adenocarcinoma in the London and East Anglian furniture industry and probably elsewhere in the industry also.

Writing from Lyons, France, Gignoux and Bernard have described 17 cases of cancer of the ethmoid in woodworkers, which occurred over a period of 15 years (13). Fifteen of these tumours were adenocarcinomas. Of the 17 men, 12 were cabinet-makers, three were joiners, one was a sawyer, and one a cooper. Subsequently Fombeur has added two further cases of adenocarcinoma from France, one in a joiner–cabinet-maker (*menuisier-ébéniste*) and one in a joiner–carpenter (*menuisier-charpentier*) (12). It is not clear whether these men worked in the furniture industry. Writing from Louvain in Belgium, Debois published information about 20 nasal adenocarcinomas of which 15 were in woodworkers (11). There is also evidence that furniture makers' adeno-carcinoma exists in Denmark (6, 18). Mosbech and

Acheson examined the death certificates of all persons certified as having died of nasal cancer in Denmark during the period 1956–66 (18). In seven cases (five men and two women), woodwork was mentioned on the death certificate. Further enquiries showed that all four of the men had died of adenocarcinoma, and all of these had worked in the furniture industry, three as cabinet-makers and one as a chair-maker. In a survey of the Aarhus area of Jutland, Andersen found 12 cases of nasal adenocarcinoma in men who had been heavily exposed to wood dust (6). Ten had been furniture makers, one a turner, and one a coach maker. Andersen's estimate of the annual incidence (0.5 per 1000) was similar to that reported from High Wycombe. Ball was unable to find any evidence of an excess risk of death from nasal cancer in the Canadian woodworking industry (7, 8). This may be due to the fact that only a very small proportion of the Canadian wood industry is concerned with the manufacture of furniture.

The dust particles and their behaviour within the nose

Hounam and Williams have studied the size and concentration of dust particles in five High Wycombe factories (16). In spite of the presence of exhaust ventilation in all of the factories studied, the average concentration was similar to the threshold limit value of 5 mg/m^3 provisionally recommended by the American Conference of Governmental Industrial Hygienists. In a recent study of the Danish furniture industry the concentration exceeded this limit in more than half the samples (23). It can be assumed with safety that in the period between the two world wars, when exhaust ventilation was not in general use, the conditions of work were even dustier. No conclusions were possible from Hounam and Williams' survey about the relative dustiness of the various processes. Approximately three-quarters of the airborne dust particles were found to have an equivalent diameter in excess of 5 μm. With particles of this size, most of the dust is trapped in the nose and relatively little passes into the lungs. Examination of the particle by the scanning electron microscope showed that most of the particles are either fibrous or flaky in character with a high surface to volume ratio. Little or nothing is known of the chemical constitution of wood dust in furniture factories, the extent to which combustion takes place during machining, and the degree to which particles from grinding or sanding machines themselves contribute to the dust.

By carrying out careful nasal examinations of more than 3000 furniture workers in the High Wycombe area, Hadfield and Macbeth have made a number of important discoveries about the pathogenesis of furniture makers' adenocarcinoma (14, 15). Firstly, they have found that in the vast majority of subjects the dust is deposited in two areas: low down on the anterior part of the nasal septum and on the anterior end of the middle turbinate in an area about 1 cm in diameter. Secondly, they have found that smears taken from the region of the middle turbinate in woodworkers show evidence of squamous metaplasia significantly more commonly than do smears from men of similar age who do not work in the furniture industry. Black, Evans and their colleagues working with Hadfield and Macbeth in the High Wycombe industry have shown that mucociliary clearance of technetium 99m-labelled particles introduced into the nose is grossly impaired in woodworkers as compared with other men of the same age (10). Solgaard and Andersen confirmed these findings in the Danish furniture industry and in addition showed that the prevalence of mucostasis in woodworkers was correlated with the concentration of inhaled dust (23).

Hadfield and Macbeth's hypothesis is that wood dust in the furniture industry, either by inducing squamous metaplasia or for some other reason, depresses muco-ciliary clearance sufficiently to permit prolonged contact of the mucosa of the anterior end of the middle turbinate with the dust (15). A carcinogen in the dust penetrates the mucus glands and initiates carcinogenesis in the nasal mucosa itself. In the majority of instances this becomes clinically manifest when it has penetrated the ethmoid sinus, but Hadfield adduces clinical evidence to suggest that the point of origin of the tumours is in the mucosa of the middle turbinate (14).

Nasal cancer in woodworkers outside the furniture industry

In the original epidemiological survey of the Oxford area, a striking finding was that only two cases of nasal adenocarcinoma were found in woodworkers who had not worked in the furniture industry (a timber merchant's representative and a joiner), in spite of the fact that the population of these workers outnumbers all the wood-working trades in the furniture industry combined (see Table 2); but two cases of squamous carcinoma were noted, respectively, in a brewer's cooper and a crate-maker. The national survey revealed a small but significant excess of cases both of adenocarcinoma and of other histological types of nasal tumour in woodworkers who had not made furniture. These included four joiners who worked in the building industry, a wheelwright, a sawyer who had worked in a timber yard, a packing case maker and a carpenter. The authors from the continent of Europe have also reported a few cases of nasal cancer in woodworkers outside the furniture industry (6, 11, 13, 18). The collected published material suggests that a different histological spectrum of nasal tumours may exist in woodworkers not exposed to the furniture industry, but more material will require to be collected before any certainty is possible on this point.

Smoking and snuff taking

Snuff taking is a traditional habit in the Buckinghamshire furniture industry, perhaps because the men are not allowed to smoke at work on account of the risk of fire (2). Some of the men interviewed said they found the use of snuff helpful in clearing their nose of dust. However, only three of 17 furniture workers with adenocarcinoma, in whom it was possible to obtain information, had ever taken snuff, and Andersen found no history of snuff taking in his Danish cases (6). The use of snuff is therefore clearly not a necessary factor in the causation of the disease. However, in view of the occurrence of snuff taking in a few of the Northamptonshire cases also, this habit should still be considered as a possible contributory factor. The majority of the men were or had been smokers but the appropriate information concerning the population at risk is not available at present.

Nasal cancer in the boot and shoe manufacturing industry

The discovery that there is a substantially increased risk of nasal cancer in the boot and shoe manufacturing industry is due to the coincidence that the region covered by the Oxford Cancer Register contains not only a large element of the furniture industry, but a substantial share of the boot and shoe manufacturing industry in Britain. Thus when the original epidemiological survey reported in the first section of this paper was undertaken, a concentration of cases of nasal cancer was noted in Northamptonshire. As a study of the census revealed that there was no furniture industry in this county it was decided to set aside the Northamptonshire material for study at a later date. The subsequent survey, which was published in 1970, revealed an association between nasal cancer and dust in the Northamptonshire boot and shoe industry (3).

The county of Northamptonshire and the boot and shoe industry

The population of Northamptonshire at the time of the 1961 census was almost exactly 400 000, of whom about

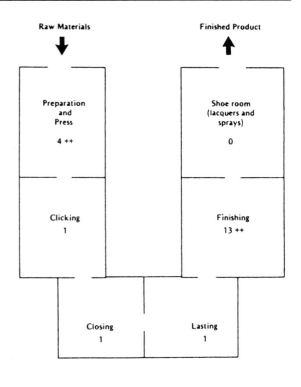

++ = dust

Fig. 3 Plan of a typical shoe factory indicating the principal dusty areas.

one-quarter lived in the city of Northampton. According to the census there were 16 030 male and 12 970 female leather workers actively employed in 1961. Most of these were workers in the boot and shoe industry, of which about one-third of the national manpower is situated in this county.

The boot and shoe manufacturing industry has been established in Northamptonshire for at least 150 years. It owes its origin there to the suitability of the land in this part of England for cattle raising and the consequent convenient supply of hides.

In most of the Northamptonshire boot and shoe factories the production process is divided into six departments (22). These are indicated in Figure 3. According to the Shoe and Allied Trades Association, the operations which have been particularly dusty in the past have been as follows:

(a) sorting leather in the rough stuff room;
(b) revolution press operating;
(c) insole surface scouring;

(d) heel building;

(e) heel and sole trimming and scouring.

The first two of the operations considered take place in the *preparation and press rooms*, the remainder in the *finishing room*, and it is principally the workers in these departments who are exposed to dust. On the whole, workers in the closing, making and lasting rooms and in the shoe room are not exposed to dust. About 20 per cent of the men and 5 per cent of the women employed in the Northamptonshire industry work in the two dusty departments. The fact that exposure to dust takes place in relatively few of the processes involved in the manufacture of shoes made it possible to demonstrate the association between nasal cancer and dust by studies within the factories as well as by comparison between the industry and other Northamptonshire workers.

The risk in boot and shoe operatives as compared with workers in other industries

The survey set out to identify every case of nasal cancer diagnosed in Northamptonshire residents since the setting up of the Oxford Cancer Register in 1951. Sixty-one patients with nasal cancer were ascertained, and are distributed by sex and histological type in Table 9. Twenty-four of the men and two of the women had worked at some time in the boot and shoe industry. Forty-six of the cases were diagnosed during the period 1953–67 when ascertainment is thought to have been complete. These cases were used in the computation of incidence.

Of the 29 men whose cases could be used in the calculation of incidence, 17 (59 per cent) had been employed in the boot and shoe trade either when the tumour was diagnosed or, if they had retired prior to the diagnosis of the tumour, in retirement. If these cases are

related to the estimated population in 1961 of 15 600 men, the average annual incidence of all histological types of tumour taken together is 0.07 ± 0.02 per 1000. As only 17 per cent of the male working population in Northamptonshire are active or retired boot and shoe operatives, it seemed possible that there might be a relationship between the occurrence of these tumours and work in this industry. The arrangement is taken a step further in Table 10. Here the number of cases observed in the boot and shoe workers is given and also the number which would have been expected if the average incidence rates for men in the south of England had prevailed. An excess is demonstrated for both adenocarcinomas and squamous carcinomas, but the numbers are small. When formal tests of significance were made using Fisher's exact test of the differences in incidence rates between (a) Northamptonshire boot and shoe workers (population 1) and other Northamptonshire men (population 2), and (b) Northamptonshire boot and shoe workers (population 1) and men in the south of England (population 3), the probabilities were all significantly low. This was in spite of the fact that two of the men with tumours classified amongst the 'other Northamptonshire men' (population 2), on the basis of their current occupation, had worked in the boot and shoe trade in earlier life. In addition to the 17 men, two women whose tumours were diagnosed in the 15 year period are known to have worked in the industry prior to marriage, but it is not possible to obtain an estimate of an appropriate expected number for comparison.

The conclusion of the comparisons described above is that there is probably an excess risk of nasal cancer in male boot and shoe operatives as compared with other men in the population, and that this excess risk includes both adenocarcinoma and squamous cell carcinoma.

Comparisons within the industry

The distribution of the 26 published cases of nasal cancer occurring in workers in the Northamptonshire boot and shoe industry (including two women), by occupation and histological type, is shown in Table 11. It can be seen that no fewer than 17 of 20 patients in whom classification is possible worked either in the preparation and press rooms or the finishing room. Using information which became available subsequently from the British Footwear Manufacturers Federation about the size of the population at risk in the dusty sectors of the industry, it was possible to make estimates of incidence based upon 20 men working in the industry at the time of diagnosis or on retirement between 1950 and 1969 (4). It was shown (Table 12) that in the dusty areas the average annual

Table 9 Nasal cancer in Northamptonshire by sex and histological type of tumour

Type of tumour	Males	Females	Total	Male/ female ratio
Adenocarcinoma	13	4	17	3.3
Squamous	20	9	29	2.2
Transitional	6	4	10	1.5
Other and unclassified	0	5	5	—
All	39	22	61	1.8

Table 10 Number of cases observed in male boot and shoe operatives (1953–1967) and the number expected according to the incidence rates experienced in southern England

Age groups	Adenocarcinoma			Squamous carcinoma			All types		
	Obs	Exp	O/E	Obs	Exp	O/E	Obs	Exp	O/E
15–64	2	0.1	20	4	0.9	4	9	1.2	8
65+	5	0.1	50	3	0.7	4	8	1.0	8
Total	7	0.2	35	7	1.6	4	17	2.2	8

Table 11 Classification of occupations in 26 workers in the Northamptonshire boot and shoe industry with nasal cancer

	Type of tumour			
	Adeno-carcinoma	Squamous carcinoma	Other	All
Preparation, sorting, bottom works, revolution press	2	2		4
Clicking			1	1
Closing			1[a]	1
Lasting/making		1		1
Finishing (including heel scouring and trimming)	7[a]	5	1	13
Shoe room				
Other, maintenance, etc.	1			1
Boot and shoe operatives unsp.	2	1	2	5
All	12	9	5	26

[a] One female worker in each group.

incidence was 0.14 per 1000 (equally distributed between adenocarcinomas and all other types) while for the remainder of the workers the incidence (0.01 per 1000) was approximately as expected in the male population in general. Of the six men in Table 11 for whom a precise attribution to one of the six departments is not possible, three had been exposed to dust. These were a general maintenance worker, a man who had worked in all departments and a worker engaged in assembling and finishing surgical boots, who had been exposed to a great deal of leather and cork dust. Since publication of the survey in 1970, 11 further cases of nasal cancer have been reported in boot and shoe operatives in Northamptonshire. Of eight in which sufficient information is available to classify the occupation, five are known to have been exposed to dust, four in the preparation or finishing rooms.

The analysis of the location of the cases within the industry very much strengthens the evidence in favour of a causal relationship between the inhalation of dust associated with the manufacture of boots and shoes and nasal cancer.

Latent period, period of exposure and secular trend

Assuming that exposure began on entry to the industry, it can be calculated that the average period from commencement of exposure to diagnosis differed significantly between men with adenocarcinomas (mean 54.6 years) and men with squamous, transitional and anaplastic tumours (mean 41.7 years). The latent period for men with nasal adenocarcinoma in the boot and shoe industry is also substantially longer than for men with the same histological type of tumour in the furniture industry. The meaning of these differences is obscure.

Ten patients had left the industry prior to the development of the tumour. Of these, three are worthy of special mention. One, a woman, worked as a heel sander for a period of three years (1896–8), left the industry, and developed her adenocarcinoma 59 years later in 1957. The second, a man, worked as a heel sander from 1932 to 1938 and developed a squamous carcinoma in 1968, 30 years after leaving the industry. By studying these and other cases it is possible to conclude that the factor or

Table 12 Estimates of the comparative incidence of nasal cancer in dusty and other departments of the Northamptonshire boot and shoe industry (1950–1969)[a]

| | Population at risk | Cases of nasal cancer | | | | | |
| | | Adenocarcinoma | | Others | | All | |
		(N)	%	N	%	(N)	%
Preparation and finishing departments	5000	7	0.07	7	0.07	14	0.14
Other departments	10 500	–	–	2	0.01	2	0.01
Unclassified	–	2	–	2	–	4	–
All	15 500	9	0.03	11	0.04	20	0.06

[a] Source of data concerning population was the British Footwear Manufacturing Federation.

Table 13 Cases of nasal cancer in workers in the Northamptonshire boot and shoe manufacturing industry by year of diagnosis and histological type of tumour, including 11 cases occurring since the original survey

	Adenocarcinoma	Squamous carcinoma	Other	All
1950–4	3	2	1	6
1955–9	3	3	0	6
1960–4	2	3	3	8
1965–9	4	3	1	8
1970–4	3	4	2	9
All	15	15	7	37

factors were present in the industry at least as early as the beginning of the century and as late as the 1930s. A third man worked for only six months in the shoe industry in the First World War, subsequently serving in the Army and as an engineer in a lift company. He developed an intranasal adenocarcinoma in 1953. The three cases demonstrate that, as in furniture makers' adenocarcinoma, it is possible to develop a tumour after a relatively short period of exposure and many years after leaving the industry.

Table 13 shows all the cases known to have occurred in the Northamptonshire industry, including 11 cases occurring since the original survey was published in 1970, by year of diagnosis. Although the degree of ascertainment prior to the establishment of the cancer register in 1951 is suspect, a systematic search of the death register in the city of Northampton revealed no death from nasal cancer in the boot and shoe industry prior to 1950, and supports the conclusion that occupational cases of nasal cancer were rare before that date. Unlike the situation in the furniture trade there is so far no indication of any decline in the epidemic.

Nasal cancer in the boot and shoe industry outside Northamptonshire

The national survey of cases of nasal adenocarcinoma diagnosed in the years 1961–6 in England, excluding the Oxford region, revealed seven additional adenocarcinomas in shoe workers (5). The number of cases of adenocarcinoma was 14 times larger than would have been expected if the cases of the tumour had been distributed randomly in men throughout England. Five of the cases of adenocarcinoma were in men working in the footwear repairing industry. As there were approximately 10 000 boot and shoe repairers in England and Wales in 1966, the figures suggest an average annual incidence rate of this tumour in this group of 0.08 per 1000, about 100 times the average rate of this tumour in adult males. The material therefore suggests that the excess risk of nasal cancer extends to these men, who often work in small shops under dusty conditions without adequate ventilation. The appearance, on the survey undertaken with different objectives, of a cluster of cases of nasal adenocarcinoma in shoe repairers gives a further line of

Table 14   Approximate crude incidence rates per 1000 per annum of intranasal cancer in various groups of men

Occupational group	Adenocarcinoma	Other types	All types
Woodworkers in f.i.[a]	0.7		0.7
Cabinet and chair-makers	0.6		0.6
Wood machinists	0.7		0.7
Boot and shoe operatives	0.03	0.04	0.07
Prep. and finishing	0.07	0.07	0.14
Other	–	0.01	0.01
Men in southern England	0.0008	0.0086	0.0094

[a] f.i. = furniture industry.

support for the hypothesis of a relationship with dust. The survey did not attempt to ascertain all the cases of nasal squamous carcinoma, but four cases of this histological type of tumour were found in boot and shoe operatives.

Two of the patients with adenocarcinoma reported from Louvain by Debois were shoe workers (11). These are the only reported cases of nasal cancer in shoe makers outside England.

Snuff taking and smoking

In view of the finding that some of the furniture workers had taken snuff, we enquired about this habit in as many of the Northamptonshire cases as possible. Of the 26 patients in whom it was possible to obtain data, eight had been snuff takers. Five of these were boot and shoe operatives and three were not. The occurrence of the habit in patients from a wide range of occupations with nasal cancer is suggestive that it may be a contributory factor and deserves further study.

Nature of the dust in boot and shoe factories

So far as is known no formal studies of the composition of the dust in boot and shoe factories have been undertaken. The principal materials used until the last 20 years were leather, rubber, shoe fibreboard (made of a mixture of wood and leather fibres, the former derived from waste paper) and, to a lesser extent, cork. In recent years plastic materials have been introduced but these were not in use prior to 1960 and cannot therefore account for this epidemic. The presence of wood fibres in fibreboard used in building up soles and heels provides a possible link between shoemakers' and furniture makers' nasal cancer. Another possible link lies in the vegetable infusions from wood bark, fruit, leaves, galls, etc. used in tanning leather for soles and heels, or in the dyes used in the preparation of fibreboard. The only type of dust mentioned by all the patients in the detailed occupational

histories was that of leather, but it is possible that they were not able clearly to distinguish the dust of leather and fibreboard. Rubber and cork dust was mentioned, in addition, by a few and the presence of particles of dye in the dust was mentioned by one worker.

Chromate salts have been used in the tanning of leather mainly for the upper parts of boots and shoes since the latter part of the nineteenth century. Calcium chromate is a potent carcinogen for the subcutaneous tissues of the rat, and bronchial carcinoma is known to occur in some workers in the chromates-producing industry (9). However, in general the operations involving leather for the upper parts of shoes are much less dusty than those involving heels and soles, and are unlikely to be a factor.

The association of dusts from organic materials with nasal cancer, particularly nasal adenocarcinoma, raises the possibility that carcinogenic metabolites of moulds or fungi might be relevant in this connection as they have been shown to be in hepatic and other cancers in man (21).

Conclusion

The work reported in this review has established the existence of substantial risks of nasal cancer in furniture workers, and in the minority of workers (in Northamptonshire these workers are principally men) who are concerned with the dusty operations used in the manufacture and repair of leather footwear. A summary of the prevailing incidence rates in the areas subjected to the most intensive survey is shown in Table 14. In the case of furniture workers, the incidence until recently has approximated that of carcinoma of the bronchus; in the boot and shoe operatives exposed to dust, the incidence is similar to that of carcinoma of the rectum. In both these groups, therefore, these are important causes of illness and death. In furniture makers' cancer, the increase in incidence is virtually limited to one histological type of tumour – the adenocarcinoma – but in boot and shoe operatives, the incidence of all histological types of tumour is increased.

In both industries there is overwhelming evidence that the causative factor is in or associated with particles of dust. In the former case the dust comes from hardwoods, certainly from beech and probably from oak and other varieties. In the latter case the dust comes from leather, fibreboard, rubber and cork. The fact that fibreboard contains wood fibres is a possible link between the two industrial tumours.

It is important to point out that the environmental conditions which gave rise to the cases of nasal cancer reported in this paper existed in the industry many years ago, and we have no direct evidence to determine whether or not such conditions still exist. Over the past 30 years substantial improvements have taken place in exhaust ventilation in the larger factories in both industries and have led to a reduction in the quantity of dust inhaled by the workers. Improvement in hygiene in the smaller factories and in repair shops has probably been less effective. There have also been changes in the composition of the dust in both industries following the introduction of new materials. Nevertheless, further studies of the composition of the dusts should be made and steps be taken to minimise the exposure of the workers. As is now the practice in the United Kingdom, compensation should be offered affected workers in the furniture industry and the right of compensation should be extended to the boot and shoe manufacturing and repairing industries.

Note

1 The National Insurance Regulations of the United Kingdom list the diseases including pneumoconiosis, for which workers are entitled to compensation (so-called prescribed diseases). In 1969 'adenocarcinoma of the nasal cavity or associated air sinuses in persons whose attendance for work is in or about a building where wooden furniture is manufactured' was added to the list by regulation 2 of Statutory Instrument 619/1969.

References

1 Acheson E.D., Hadfield E.H. and Macbeth R.G. Carcinoma of the nasal cavity and accessory sinuses in woodworkers *Lancet* 1967: 1; 311–12.
2 Acheson E.D., Cowdell R.H., Hadfield E.H., and Macbeth R.G. Nasal cancer in woodworkers in the furniture industry *Brit. Med. J.* 1968: 2; 587–96.
3 Acheson E.D., Cowdell R.H., and Jolles B. Nasal cancer in the Northamptonshire boot and shoe industry *Brit. Med. J.* 1970: 1; 385–93

4 Acheson E.D., Cowdell R.H. and Jolles B. Nasal cancer in the shoe industry. *Brit. Med. J.* 1970: 2; 791.
5 Acheson E.D., Cowdell R.H. and Rang E. Adenocarcinoma of the nasal cavity and sinuses in England and Wales. *Brit. J. Ind. Med.* 1972: 29; 21–30.
6 Andersen H.C., Eksogene ar sager til cancer cavi nasi. *Ugeskr. Laeg.* 1974: 137; 2567–70.
7 Ball M.J. Nasal cancer and occupation in Canada. *Lancet* 1967: 2; 1089–90.
8 Ball M.J. Nasal cancer in woodworkers. *Brit. Med. J.* 1968: 2; 253.
9 Bidstrup, P.L. and Case R.A.M. Carcinoma of the lung in workmen in the biochromates producing industry in Great Britain. *Brit. J. Ind. Med.* 1956: 13; 260–4.
10 Black A., Evans J.C., Hadfield E.H., Macbeth R.G., Morgan A. and Walsh M. Impairment of nasal mucociliary clearance in woodworkers in the furniture industry. *Brit. J. Ind. Med.* 1974: 31; 10–17.
11 Debois J.M. Tumoren van de neusholte bij houtbewerkers. *Tijdschr v Geneeskunde* 1969: 2; 92–3.
12 Fombeur J.P. A propos de cas recents de tumeurs ethmoido-maxillaires chez les travailleurs du bois. *Arch. Mal. Prof.* 1972: 33; 453–5.
13 Gignoux M. and Bernard P. Tumeurs malignes de l'ethmoide chez les travailleurs du bois. *J. Med. Lyon* 1969: 50; 731–6.
14 Hadfield E.H. A study of adenocarcinoma of the paranasal sinuses in woodworkers in the furniture industry. *Ann. Royal Coll. Surg. Engl.* 1970: 46; 301–19.
15 Hadfield E.H. and Macbeth R.G. Adenocarcinoma of ethmoids in furniture workers. *Ann. Otol. Rhinol. Laryngol.* 1971: 80; 699–703.
16 Hounam R.F. and Williams J. Levels of airborne dust in furniture making factories in the High Wycombe area. *Brit. J. Ind. Med.* 1974: 31; 1–9.
17 Macbeth R. Malignant disease of the paranasal sinuses. *J. Laryng.* 1964: 9; 592–612.
18 Mosbech J. and Acheson E.D. Nasal cancer in furniture makers in Denmark. *Dan. Med. Bull.* 1971: 18; 34–5.
19 Proctor D.F., Andersen I. and Lundqvist G. Clearance of inhaled particles from the nose. *Arch. Int. Med.* 1973: 31; 132–9.
20 Quinlan, M.F., Salman S.D., Swift D.I., Wagner H.N. and Proctor D.F. Measurement of mucociliary function in man. *Ann. Rev. Resp. Dis.* 1969: 99; 13–23.
21 Schoental R. Aflatoxins. *Ann. Rev. Pharm.* 1967: 7; 343–56.
22 Shoe and Allied Trades Association, Kettering, England. (Personal communication to the author).
23 Solgaard J. and Anderson I. Airway function and symptoms in woodworkers. *Ugeskr. Laeg.* 1975: 138; 2593–9.

Acknowledgement

Acheson, E.D. (1976) Nasal cancer in the furniture and boot and shoe manufacturing industries. *Preventive Medicine*, 5, 295–315. (Copyright © 1976 by Academic Press, Inc.)

3 Professor David Barker

Barker, D.J.P., Winter, P.D., Osmond, C., Margetts B. and Simmonds, S.J. (1989) Weight in infancy and death from ischaemic heart disease. *Lancet*, 2, 577–80.

Woolf, B. (1946) Studies on infant mortality. Part II. Social aetiology of stillbirths and infant deaths in county boroughs of England and Wales. *British Journal of Social Medicine*, 2, 73–125.

INTRODUCTION

It has become clear that differences in adult 'Western' lifestyle do not explain differences in people's risk of having coronary heart disease (CHD), and research into the causes of CHD requires a new direction. A number of studies have suggested that the environment in childhood and adolescence may be important, in terms of both 'excesses', such as physical inactivity and obesity, and deprivation. The accompanying paper, however, suggests that it is the environment *in utero* and during infancy that is important. This environment is essentially that afforded by the mother, rather than housing and other influences that affect children after birth.

The study described in the paper from our Southampton group was carried out following an ecological study which showed that, without exception, those areas of England and Wales that have high death rates from coronary heart disease had high neonatal death rates, deaths within the first month after birth, 70 and more years ago. At that time high neonatal death rates in a population were associated with a high incidence of babies born with low birthweight. An inference from these observations, therefore, is that poor growth *in utero* is in some way associated with the development of coronary heart disease in adult life.

In order to examine this hypothesis it was necessary to find groups of men and women whose birthweight and other measurements of early growth were recorded. In this way early growth could be related to the occurrence of coronary heart disease and its risk factors in adult life. Accordingly, the Medical Research Council carried out a systematic search of archives and record offices throughout Britain. A number of collections of records were found, the largest and most important of which contained details of all babies born in the county of Hertfordshire since 1911. The paper describes the first of a series of studies carried out on Hertfordshire people. Over 5000 men born in the east of the county during 1911–30 were traced. As predicted by the hypothesis, men with lowest weights at birth and at one year had the highest death rates from coronary heart disease.

Following publication of this paper the findings were confirmed in a larger study of men and women born in Hertfordshire, and in a study in Sheffield. Examination of samples of men and women living in those areas and in Preston, another place where birth records have been preserved, have shown that low growth rates *in utero* and during infancy lead to the appearance of cardiovascular risk factors in adult life, including raised blood pressure, impaired glucose tolerance, raised serum cholesterol concentrations and abnormal blood coagulation. Understanding the processes initiated *in utero* that lead to these abnormalities is now the focus of a large multidisciplinary research programme.

The second paper, on the social aetiology of stillbirths and infant deaths in county boroughs of England and Wales, was written by Dr Barnett Woolf in 1946. This interesting paper, written by an anthropologist, was one of the first to be published by the *British Journal of Social Medicine*. It describes Dr Woolf's meticulous analyses of infant mortality in the large towns of England and Wales during 1928–38 showing how poor social conditions lead to infant deaths. The paper is in many ways a model study of inequalities in health. Out of 30 social indices he selected seven that he found to predict infant mortality most closely. These indices related to overcrowding, poverty, industrial employment of mothers, family size, population density and latitude. He examined the associations between these indices and specific causes on infant death, for example bronchitis and diarrhoea, and deaths at different ages during the neonatal and post-neonatal periods. Having established associations he then considered how the social factors actually exert their effect on the life of the baby. It is the linking of specific social influences, such as low income, with specific processes such as fetal undernutrition and disorders such as prematurity that makes the paper so fascinating. Such data are needed for accurately targeted social policies.

Woolf anticipated modern epidemiology in a thoughtful discussion of the possible effects of diagnostic misclassification, the scope and limitations of the multiple regression method and the usefulness or otherwise of tests of statistical significance.

Woolf's analyses pointed up a series of important problems that are still being resolved. He concluded that the close relation between poverty, stillbirths and neonatal deaths derived from maternal malnutrition. He also suggested that maternal malnutrition before birth contributed to mortality from infection during infancy. He showed that infant deaths from infectious diseases were related to overcrowding, especially when the crowding was by other children rather than adults. He speculated on the risks to infants whose mothers worked and who had to be cared for by neighbours, often in the company of a number of other children. He cleverly deduced that the higher infant mortality in the north of the country was due to influences acting through the mother and bearing directly on the infant.

The practical conclusion of the study was that infant mortality was mostly preventable and that improving maternal nutrition was considerably more important than improving housing. Woolf realized that many of the hypotheses from his analyses would need to be tested by specific investigations. His conclusion that 'it is only by the close interweaving of statistical and field enquiries that a true science of social medicine can be built up' still applies today.

WEIGHT IN INFANCY AND DEATH FROM ISCHAEMIC HEART DISEASE

Introduction

The known causes of ischaemic heart disease explain only part of the differences in risk between populations and between individuals, and do not explain why in Britain the highest rates of the disease are in the poorest areas and lowest income groups.[1,2] The geographical differences in death rates from ischaemic heart disease in England and Wales are related to differences in infant mortality seventy years ago.[3] This relation is with both neonatal mortality (deaths before one month of age) and post-neonatal mortality (one month to one year).[4] Impaired growth and development in prenatal and early postnatal life may be an important risk factor for ischaemic heart disease. To investigate this hypothesis, we have studied death rates in men born in Hertfordshire during 1911–30, whose weights at birth and one year were recorded.

Subjects and methods

The registration districts of Royston, Bishops Stortford, Ware, Hertford, Hatfield and Barnet are grouped in east Hertfordshire. At the 1921 census most of the men were employed in agriculture or in trade and services.[5] There were no major industries. The combined population of the districts was 103 211. Infant mortality in the county was below the national average. In 1921–5 the rate was 49 deaths per 1000 births, 27 neonatal and 22 post-neonatal.[6] The corresponding figures for England and Wales were 76, 33 and 43.

From 1911 the attending midwife was required to notify every birth to the county medical officer of health within 36 hours. Almost all births occurred at home. The name and address of the mother, the date of birth and the birthweight were registered. The local health visitor recorded her observations on a form when she visited the home periodically throughout the first year. After a year the form was returned to the county health visitor and data were abstracted on to the register, including weight at one year and whether breast fed from birth, bottle fed or both.

More deaths were expected in men than in women and men were more readily traced because they did not change their surnames. A total of 17 464 boys were born alive in the six districts from 1911 to 1930. Of these, 1477 died during childhood. We excluded twins and triplets, leaving 15 664 singletons of whom 7991 had both birthweight and weight at one year recorded. Boys whose weights were recorded at ages other than one year, but not at one year, were excluded. Weights were measured in pounds (2.2 pounds = 1 kg) and were often rounded to the nearest half pound or pound. We therefore used the original units. Where forenames were missing or other data required for tracing were incomplete, we sought additional information from the national birth index,

Table 1 SMRs according to weight at one year of age and birthweight

Weight (pounds)	Cause of death						
	Ischaemic heart disease		Chronic obstructive lung disease		Lung cancer		All causes
One year old							
≤ 18 (n = 324)	111	(37)[a]	129	(6)	98	(11)	89 (85)
19–20 (n = 971)	81	(76)	86	(11)	99	(31)	89 (238)
21–22 (n = 1850)	98	(163)	41	(9)	87	(48)	85 (405)
23–24 (n = 1464)	71	(98)	61	(11)	57	(26)	68 (265)
25–26 (n = 769)	68	(49)	52	(5)	97	(23)	73 (150)
≥ 27 (n = 276)	42	(11)	29	(1)	70	(6)	58 (43)
Birthweight							
≤ 5.5 (n = 251)	104	(25)	93	(3)	113	(9)	101 (69)
6–6.5 (n = 752)	77	(51)	59	(5)	101	(22)	69 (131)
7–7.5 (n = 1598)	90	(129)	75	(14)	68	(32)	83 (340)
8–8.5 (n = 1757)	85	(141)	50	(11)	85	(47)	80 (380)
9–9.5 (n = 868)	62	(53)	69	(8)	67	(19)	70 (170)
≥ 10 (n = 428)	81	(35)	33	(2)	109	(16)	77 (96)
Total (n = 5654)	82	(434)	61	(43)	83	(145)	79 (1186)

[a] Number of deaths in parentheses. 2.2 pounds = 1 kg.

which lists all births in the country, and from local registers of baptisms. For 7613 men identification data were sufficient for submission to the National Health Service Central Register at Southport: 5654 (74 per cent) were traced, of whom 1186 died at age 20–74 years between 1 January 1951 and 31 December 1987. The average birthweight of men who were not traced was 0.1 pounds less than those who were traced, and the weight at one year was 0.2 pounds less.

We analysed cause of death in relation to birthweight, weight at one year, and infant feeding. The numbers of deaths were compared with those expected from national rates for men of corresponding age and year of birth.[7] Death rates were expressed as standardised mortality ratios (SMRs) with the national average as 100. Ischaemic heart disease was defined by *International Classification of Diseases* (ninth revision) numbers 410–414, chronic obstructive lung disease by 491–493 and 496, and lung cancer by 162–164. The social class of all except 22 of the men who died was derived from the occupation recorded on the death certificate.

Results

Four hundred and thirty-four of the 1186 deaths were due to ischaemic heart disease; 328 occurred below the age of 65 years. The overall death rate from this condition (**SMR 82**) was below the national average.

The average weight of the men when they were one year old was 22.4 pounds (SD 2.6). **SMRs** for ischaemic

Table 2 SMRs for ischaemic heart disease according to weight at one year and method of feeding

Weight (pounds)	Breast fed		Bottle fed	
≤ 18	112	(33)	105	(4)
19–20	81	(71)	79	(5)
21–22	100	(154)	72	(9)
23–24	69	(85)	97	(13)
25–26	61	(40)	144	(9)
≥ 27	38	(9)	89	(2)
Total	81	(392)	94	(42)

heart disease fell steeply with increasing weight at age one (Table 1). This downward trend was significant ($P < 0.002$, X^2 for trend). Of the other leading causes of death only chronic obstructive lung disease showed a similar trend (Table 1). There were only 43 deaths from this cause and the trend was not significant. There was no trend in death rates from lung cancer in relation to weight at one year (Table 1). Death rates from all causes showed a significant downward trend with increasing weight ($P < 0.001$). Exclusion of deaths from ischaemic heart disease and chronic obstructive lung disease abolished this trend.

The men's average birthweight was 7.9 pounds (SD 1.3). Men who weighed 5.5 pounds or less had the highest **SMR** for ischaemic heart disease, at 104 (Table 1). The downward trend in **SMRs** with increasing birthweight was not significant. Men who weighed 5.5 pounds or less also had the highest **SMRs** for obstructive lung disease, and for all causes of death (trend not significant). There was no trend in **SMRs** for lung cancer.

Table 3 SMRs for ischaemic heart disease according to birthweight and weight at one year in men who were breast fed

Weight at one year (pounds)	Weight at birth (pounds)			
	Below average (≤ 7)	Average (7.5–8.5)	Above average (≥ 9)	Total
Below average (≤ 21)	100 (80)	100 (77)	58 (17)	93 (174)
Average (22–23)	86 (34)	87 (67)	80 (29)	85 (130)
Above average (≥ 24)	53 (14)	65 (42)	59 (32)	60 (88)
Total	88 (128)	85 (186)	65 (78)	81 (392)

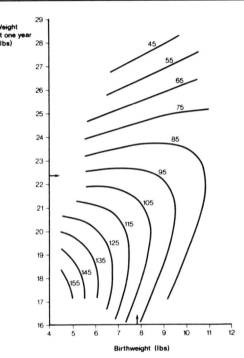

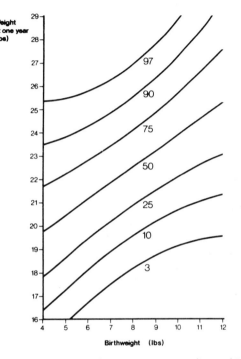

Fig. 1 Relative risks for ischaemic heart disease in men who were breast fed according to birthweight and weight at one year (lines join points with equal risk; arrows show mean weights).

Fig. 2 Percentiles of weight at one year according to birthweight in men who were breast fed.

Four hundred and twenty-nine (7.6 per cent) of the men were bottle fed. On average they gained 0.4 pounds more between birth and one year than did those who were breast fed (*P* < 0.001, two sample *t*-test). Among the bottle fed men death rates from ischaemic heart disease did not fall with increasing weight at one year (Table 2). This difference in trend between men who were breast and bottle fed was not significant. Because of the different weight gain of men who were bottle fed and the suggestion of a different association with ischaemic heart disease, we restricted analysis of the interrelation of birthweight and weight at one to the 5225 men who were breast fed. The lowest **SMRs** occurred in men who had above average birthweight or weight at one year (Table 3). The highest **SMR** (100) was in men for whom both weights were below average. Men for whom both weights were lowest, 5.5 pounds or less and 18 pounds or less, respectively, had an **SMR** of 220 (12 deaths, 95 per cent confidence interval 114–384).

The simultaneous effect of birthweight and weight at one [year] on **SMRs** is shown in Figure 1, derived with Cox's proportional hazards method.[8] The lines join points with equal risk of ischaemic heart disease and are truncated to define an area within which lie 95 per cent of the weights. The values are risks relative to the value of 100 for those with average birthweight and weight at one [year]. Figure 2 shows the percentiles of weight at one year according to birthweight.[9] Fewer men with lower birthweights attained the heaviest weights at one year and hence the lowest risks of ischaemic heart disease (Figure 1). For example, only 10 per cent of men whose birthweight was 5 pounds attained the median weight at one for those whose birthweight was 10 pounds.

Among the men who died mean birthweight was not related to social class at death (Table 4). There was no downward trend in mean weight at one year with lower social class, but men in social class V had a lower than average mean weight ($P < 0.05$). The standard deviations in each social class were similar.

Table 4 Mean birthweight and weight at one year according to social class at death

Social class	Mean weight at birth (pounds)	Mean weight at one year (pounds)
I ($n = 38$)	7.7	21.9
II ($n = 177$)	7.8	22.2
III non-manual ($n = 125$)	7.8	22.4
III manual ($n = 430$)	7.9	22.3
IV ($n = 264$)	7.8	21.9
V ($n = 130$)	7.8	21.6
Total ($n = 1164$)	7.9 (SD 1.3)	22.1 (SD 2.7)

Discussion

We have traced a population of men born in one part of Hertfordshire during 1911–30 whose weights in infancy were recorded. Hertfordshire is a prosperous part of England, and rates of ischaemic heart disease in the population are 18 per cent below the national average. Weight at one year of age predicted death from ischaemic heart disease. Among those whose weights were 18 pounds or less death rates were almost three times greater than among those who attained 27 pounds or more. These large differences were reflected in differences in deaths from all causes and hence life expectancy. Of the men, 92.4 per cent were breast fed and so these results cannot be extrapolated to bottle fed populations.

Of the 15 664 singleton boys born in the area during the study period, 7991 were weighed both at birth and at one year. Those who were not weighed at these ages may have differed from those who were. However, our analysis was based on internal comparisons and bias would be introduced only if the relation between infant growth and death from ischaemic heart disease differed in the two groups; this is unlikely. We traced 71 per cent of the 7991 boys, despite the lapse of more than sixty years. Again bias from exclusion of those untraced is unlikely because the comparisons were internal. The variation within the data enabled us to make comparisons across a wide range of weights. Two hundred and fifty-one men had birthweights below 5.5 pounds. They had the highest death rates from ischaemic heart disease and chronic obstructive lung disease, and from all causes combined. Other evidence linking child growth with ischaemic heart disease comes from the inverse relation between adult height and cardiovascular mortality in England,[10] Norway[11] and Finland.[12] Also average height is inversely related to cardiovascular mortality in the countries of England and Wales and in social classes.[13]

From our findings it could be argued that an environment which produces poor fetal and infant growth is followed by an adult environment that determines high risk of ischaemic heart disease. The adult influence is a matter of speculation. It is unlikely to be cigarette smoking, since early growth is unrelated to death from lung cancer; nor is growth related to any other leading cause of death except obstructive airways disease. We have information on social class only for a selected group of men, namely those who died. Among these men birthweight was unrelated to social class at death. Although average weight at one year was lower in men in social class V, the difference was small and there was no downward trend through all the social classes. These results argue against persistence of an adverse environment from intrauterine life to death.

The relation between weight at one year and death from ischaemic heart disease is strong: it spans more than sixty years, and it is graded. Among other leading causes of death only chronic obstructive lung disease shows a similar relation. Both prenatal and postnatal growth were important in determining weight at one year, since few infants with below average birthweights reached the heaviest weights at one. The combination of poor prenatal and postnatal growth led to the highest death rates from ischaemic heart disease. We conclude that processes linked to growth and acting in prenatal or early postnatal life strongly influence risk of ischaemic heart disease. Birthweight is inversely related to adult blood pressure, and fetal growth can therefore be linked with hypertension, a known risk factor.[14] Experiments on animals have shown that infant feeding programmes lipid metabolism throughout life.[15]

Our results suggest that greater early growth will reduce deaths from ischaemic heart disease. In England and Wales past trends in infant mortality, an indicator of infant growth and health, correlate with subsequent trends in ischaemic heart disease in the same generations.[16] The large falls in cardiovascular mortality in the United States,

Canada, Australia and New Zealand during the past twenty years may also have resulted from improved child growth and health, reflected in the fall in infant mortality sixty and more years ago.[17]

The benefits associated with postnatal growth are greatest for babies with below average birthweight (Figure 1): heavier weight at one year is accompanied by large reductions in death rates. Promotion of infant growth in babies of below average birthweight may therefore be a priority. Among babies with above average birthweight the risk of ischaemic heart disease is below average, irrespective of infant growth. Measures that promote infant growth may have additional benefit. Birthweight is strongly influenced by maternal height,[18] which is itself largely determined by growth in early childhood.[19] Increased growth of infant girls may lead to improved prenatal growth in their babies and may further reduce deaths from ischaemic heart disease.

References

1 Gardner, M.J., Crawford M.D., Morris, J.N. Patterns of mortality in middle and early old age in the country boroughs of England and Wales. *Br. J. Prev. Soc. Med.* 1969: 23; 133–40.

2 Registrar General's decennial supplement, occupational mortality in England and Wales 1970–72. London: HM Stationery Office, 1978.

3 Barker, D.J.P., Osmond, C. Infant mortality, childhood nutrition, and ischaemic heart disease in England and Wales. *Lancet* 1986: i; 1077–81.

4 Barker, D.J.P., Osmond, C., Law, C. The intra-uterine and early postnatal origins of cardiovascular disease and chronic bronchitis. *J. Epidemiol. Community Health* 1989: 43(3); 237–240.

5 Registrar General for England and Wales. Census of England and Wales 1921: county report for Hertfordshire. London: HM Stationery Office, 1923.

6 Registrar General's statistical review of England and Wales: part 1 tables, medical. London: HM Stationery Office, 1921 and following years.

7 Berry, G. The analysis of mortality by the subject-years method. *Biometrics* 1983: 39; 173–84.

8 Cox, D.R. Regression models and life-tables. *J. R. Stat. Soc. Ser. B* 1972: 34; 187–220.

9 Cole, T.J. Fitting smoothed centile curves to reference data. *J. R. Stat. Soc. Ser. A* 1988: 151; 385–418.

10 Marmot, M.G., Shipley, M.J., Rose, G. Inequalities in death – specific explanations of a general pattern? *Lancet* 1984: i; 1003–6.

11 Waaler, H.T. Height, weight and mortality: the Norwegian experience. *Acta Med. Scand.* 1984: 679; (suppl.); 1–56.

12 Notkola, V. Living conditions in childhood and coronary heart disease in adulthood. Helsinki: Finnish Society of Science and Letters, 1985.

13 Barker, D.J.P., Osmond, C., Golding, J. Height and mortality in the countries of England and Wales. *Ann. Hum. Biol.* 1990: 17(1); 1–6.

14 Barker, D.J.P., Osmond, C., Golding, J., Kuh, D., Wadsworth, M.E.J. Growth in utero, blood pressure in childhood and adult life, and mortality from cardiovascular disease. *Br. Med. J.* 1989: 298; 564–67.

15 Mott, G.E. Deferred effects of breastfeeding versus formula feeding on serum lipoprotein concentrations and cholesterol metabolism in baboons. In: Filer L.J. Jr, Formon, S.J. (eds), *The breastfed infant: a model performance.* Report of the ninety-first Ross conference on paediatric research. Columbus, Ohio: Ross Laboratories, 1986: 144–9.

16 Osmond, C. Time trends in infant mortality, ischaemic heart disease and stroke in England and Wales. In: *Infant nutrition and cardiovascular disease.* Southampton: MRC Environmental Epidemiology Unit (Scientific report no. 8) 1987: 28–34.

17 Barker, D.J.P. The rise and fall of Western diseases. *Nature* 1989: 338; 371–2.

18 Butler, N., Alberman, E. *Perinatal problems: the second report of the 1958 British perinatal mortality survey.* Edinburgh: Livingstone, 1969.

19 Tanner, J., Healy, M., MacKenzie, J., Whitehouse, R. Aberdeen growth study I: the prediction of adult body measurements from measurements taken each year from birth to 5 years. *Arch. Dis. Child.* 1956: 31; 372.

Acknowledgement

Barker, D.J.P., Winter, P.D., Osmond, C., Margetts B. and Simmonds, S.J. (1989) Weight in infancy and death from ischaemic heart disease. *Lancet* 1989: 2; 577–80.

STUDIES ON INFANT MORTALITY
Abridged by Ms Julie Hotchkiss

Introduction

The object of this series of papers is to give as complete and detailed a quantitative account as the data allow of the way in which infant mortality and stillbirth rates are influenced by social conditions. In the first paper (Woolf and Waterhouse, 1945) multiple regression equations were given showing the relation between the infant mortality rate and five indices of social conditions in the county boroughs of England and Wales for the eleven years 1928 to 1938 inclusive. The indices used were:

H: Percentage of families living more than one person per room (Census, 1931).

U: Average monthly percentage unemployment among adult males (Ministry of Labour, 'Local Unemployment Index').

P: Percentage of occupied males in social Classes IV (semi-skilled workers) and V (unskilled workers) (Census, 1931).

F: Percentage of females aged fourteen and over employed in manufacture (Census, 1931).

L: Degrees of latitude north of 50° 30'.

From the various equations a detailed balance sheet of infant deaths was drawn up and a number of calculations were made, which may be broadly summarized as follows.

The infant mortality rate to be expected if overcrowding, low income and industrial employment of women could have been entirely eliminated was 23.1. The difference between this figure and the observed mean rate of 65.4 represents preventable deaths. Of these, about one-third were associated with overcrowding, one-quarter with low-paid occupations, one-fifth with unemployment and one-eighth with industrial employment of women.

The paper by Woolf and Waterhouse contained statistical tests showing the undoubted significance of the various parameters, and social and medical reasons for regarding the relation between infant mortality and the social variables as a real one, in the sense that improvements in social conditions might really be expected to reduce infant deaths. But the paper did not deal with questions of social aetiology, of how overcrowding, low earnings and so on actually exert their influence on the life of the baby. The total infant mortality is a complex phenomenon, made up of deaths at different periods of the first year of life attributable to different diagnostic categories. The previous paper expressly postponed discussion of aetiology until the total mortality had been dissected by age at death and by cause as stated on the death certificate. This further analysis has now been carried out, and the present paper gives regression equations for the separate diagnostic groups and age-periods (including stillbirth) during which death occurs. The number of social indices has been increased to seven by the addition of family size and the local density of population.

The degree to which total infant mortality can be subdivided for purposes of analysis obviously depends upon the availability of the relevant figures. For age at death in county boroughs the information is given in considerable detail. In every yearly issue of Part I of the Registrar-General's *Statistical Review* over the period 1928 to 1938 there is a table giving for each county borough the actual numbers of infants reported as dying at ages: under one day, one to seven days, one to four weeks, four weeks to three months, three to six months, six to nine months and nine to twelve months. For the analysis by cause of death, however, the published data are not quite so favourable. The only figures available for the individual county boroughs are contained in a table giving actual numbers of registered deaths at various ages throughout the whole span of life, divided into 32 cause categories until 1930, and thereafter into 36 groups. Most of these categories relate to deaths in higher age-groups, so the information about infants is not very detailed. It is particularly unfortunate that a number of different causes responsible for the majority of neonatal deaths are lumped together under the one heading of 'congenital causes, etc.' Nor is there any tabulation for individual county boroughs of deaths by cause at different periods of infancy. More detailed analyses are available for the country as a whole, and for various larger subdivisions by geographical region, type of municipal area, and occupation and social class of the father. Some of the valuable ancillary information in these tables will be presented in the next section, as an introduction to the regression equations for the county boroughs.

Infant mortality by cause and age at death

Causes of infant death, as stated on the death certificate, may conveniently be classified under the following five headings: (1) 'developmental and wasting diseases', which are sometimes referred to by the Registrar-General as 'congenital causes'; (2) 'infectious diseases'; (3) 'bronchitis and pneumonia'; (4) 'diarrhoea and enteritis'; (5) 'other causes'. The main individual diagnostic categories included under these headings, and their contributions to the infant mortality rate, are shown in Table 1.

As will be seen from the table, the Registrar-General's grouping of 'developmental and wasting diseases' comprises five separate causes. Sometimes the heading is 'congenital causes', which may include some or all of the following: injury at birth, diseases of the umbilicus, pemphigus neonatorum and other diseases of early infancy. As Table 1 shows, the addition of these items would put only an extra 3.01 on to the death-rate in this group, bringing the total from 28.53 to 31.54. Nevertheless, this variation in methods of grouping and tabulation is apt to cause difficulties and unfortunately it is not always possible from the published data to make them refer to the same list of causes of death.

Similar caution is necessary in interpreting figures for the infectious disease group. In his annual *Statistical*

Table 1 Infant mortality by cause: mean death-rates per 1000 live births, England and Wales, 1928–1938

'Developmental and wasting diseases'	
Congenital malformations	5.71
Congenital debility	2.92
Premature birth	17.57
Atelectasis	1.79
Icterus neonatorum	0.54
Total	28.53
'Congenital causes' in addition to above	
Injury at birth	2.27
Other diseases of early infancy	0.74
Total	3.01
'Common infectious diseases'	
Measles	0.94
Whooping cough	1.85
Diphtheria	0.15
Others	0.05
Total	2.99
'Other infectious diseases'	
Influenza	0.53
Meningitis	0.38
Cerebrospinal fever	0.29
Total	1.20
'Bronchitis and pneumonia'	
Bronchitis	2.67
Pneumonia	9.45
Total	12.12
'Diarrhoea and enteritis'	5.56
'Other causes'	
Convulsions	1.90
Tuberculous diseases	0.82
Hernia, intestinal obstruction	0.57
Suffocation	0.47
Cellulitis and other diseases of skin	0.46
Syphilis	0.42
Diseases of ear and mastoid	0.32
Inattention at birth	0.31
Inflammation of stomach	0.30
Other respiratory diseases	0.23
Miscellaneous	2.50
Total	8.30
Total infant mortality	61.71

Review the Registrar-General classifies under the title 'common infectious diseases' the following: measles, whooping-cough, diphtheria, scarlet fever, varicella and smallpox. Table 1 shows that in this group the most important are measles and whooping-cough, which together account for 2.79 out of the total mortality rate of 2.99. But in the 1931 Decennial Supplement, the heading 'infectious diseases' covers a much wider field. If one adds only three important diseases – influenza, meningitis and cerebrospinal fever – it will be seen from Table 1 that the death-rate in this group is increased by 1.20 from 2.99 to 4.19. Here again it is not safe to compare the death-rates from different tables or reports without a preliminary inquiry as to the actual diseases grouped under the general heading.

'Bronchitis and pneumonia' are usually included in the Registrar-General's 'miscellaneous' group of causes of death, but as they contribute nearly 20 per cent to the mortality rate we have singled them out for separate investigation. 'Other causes' is of course the most unstable of all the group headings, as its content depends on what is included in or left out of all the other groups. In the Registrar-General's annual *Statistical Review*, the content of the 'miscellaneous diseases' group differs widely from 'other causes' as given in Table 1. He does not include tuberculous diseases, which he tabulates separately. On the other hand, he does include injury at birth and other diseases of early infancy, all the infectious diseases such as influenza and meningitis, left out of his list of common infectious diseases, and also bronchitis and pneumonia.

In this paper the individual causes included in a general group will always be indicated, and the tabulated causes of death will be taken at their face value. The probable degree of reliability of the different diagnostic categories will be discussed in a later section.

In Table 1 are shown the average yearly death-rates attributed to the main individual causes and groups of causes, for the whole of England and Wales during the eleven years 1928 to 1938. Table 2 shows the percentage of the total death-rate for each group of causes. It will be seen that the most important group is 'congenital causes',

Table 2 Infant mortality by cause: percentages of total rate, England and Wales, 1928–1938

Congenital causes	
Registrar-General's 'Developmental and wasting diseases'	46.2
Other congenital diseases	4.9
Total	51.1
Infectious diseases	
Registrar-General's 'Common infectious diseases'	4.9
Other infectious diseases	1.9
Total	6.8
Bronchitis and pneumonia	19.6
Diarrhoea and enteritis	9.0
Other causes	13.5
Total	100.0

Table 3 Infant mortality by age at death: mean death-rates per 1000 live births, England and Wales, 1928–1938

Age at death	Mortality rate	Cumulative mortality rate	Percentage	Cumulative percentage
Under 1 day	10.51		17.0	
1–7 days	11.58	22.09	18.8	35.8
1–4 weeks	8.83	30.92	14.3	50.1
4 weeks to 3 months	9.83	40.75	16.0	66.1
3–6 months	8.54	49.29	13.8	79.9
6–9 months	6.66	55.95	10.8	90.7
9–12 months	5.76	61.71	9.3	100.0
Total	61.71		100.0	

responsible for over half the deaths. Within this group the largest individual item is premature birth, with a rate of 17.57, constituting 28.5 per cent of the total mortality. The next largest group is 'bronchitis and pneumonia', covering almost one-fifth of all deaths. 'diarrhoea and enteritis' accounts for about one-eleventh of the deaths, and 'infectious diseases' for about one-fifteenth. Whooping-cough is the most deadly disease in this group, followed in diminishing order by measles, influenza, meningitis, cerebrospinal fever and diphtheria. Among 'other causes' the largest single item is convulsions – an uncertain and unsatisfactory diagnostic category whose occurrence on death certificates is steadily diminishing. 'Tuberculous diseases', formerly a prominent cause of infant deaths, has now become a relatively minor class, with a rate of 0.82. A big improvement in the general standard of mothercraft is indicated by the rates for suffocation and inattention at birth, which together amount to 0.78 – a figure that is of course much too high, but nevertheless is a great advance on the state of affairs even a generation ago. The average number of births per annum for the period 1928 to 1938 was about 613 000, so that a death-rate of one corresponds to about 613 deaths a year.

Risk of death is greatest immediately after birth, and diminishes steadily thereafter. Table 3 gives the figures for England and Wales during the period 1928–38. Deaths on the first day were 17 per cent, or more than one-sixth, of those during the whole first year of life. Deaths in the first four weeks are often referred to as neonatal deaths. The neonatal rate was 30.9, just over half the total infant mortality. Almost two-thirds of the deaths occurred during the first three months of life, and four-fifths in the first six months.

In the Registrar-General's Decennial Supplement (DS, 1931) there are tables showing infantile mortality by cause and age with the social class of the father. All deaths

of legitimate infants during the three-year period 1930–2 were assigned to the appropriate social class according to the father's occupation as stated on the death certificate, and the average numbers of yearly deaths were related to live births within the social class registered in 1931. Mortality rates per 1000 live births by cause groups for each social class are shown in Figure 1. 'Congenital causes' comprises all the items shown under the first two headings in Table 1, and 'infectious diseases' covers a comprehensive list including all the diseases under headings 'common infectious diseases' and 'other infectious diseases' in Table 1, with the exception of meningitis. 'Other causes' in the figure differs slightly from the list in Table 1, since deaths from meningitis have to be added and a few deaths from the rarer infectious diseases have to be subtracted. All these adjustments, however, are quite small, and the cause groups in the figure are substantially the same as those shown in Tables 1 and 2. Another consideration affecting strict comparability is the fact that Tables 1 and 2 refer to all infants born during 1928–38, while Figure 1 relates only to legitimate infants during 1930–2, though the differences are very small and do not affect the general conclusions.

For infant mortality as a whole and for each group of causes there is a steady increase in the rate between class I and class V, but the relative disparities differ greatly for the various diagnostic headings. 'Congenital causes' shows by far the smallest relative class gradient, the ratio of the rates for class V and class I being approximately 1.5:1. The greatest contrast occurs in the bronchitis and pneumonia group, where the rate for class V is about 6.75 times that for class I. Next comes the infectious diseases group, with a ratio of about 5.4:1, and then diarrhoea, with a disparity of nearly 4:1. For 'other causes' the ratio is 2:1. The relative importance of the cause groups alters as one passes down the social scale. Congenital causes, for example, were responsible for over two-thirds of the

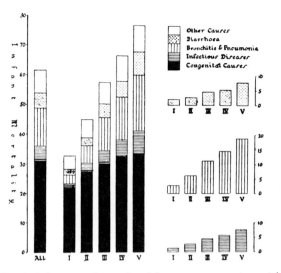

Fig. 1 Infant mortality analysed by cause groups in social classes of England and Wales, 1930–1932.

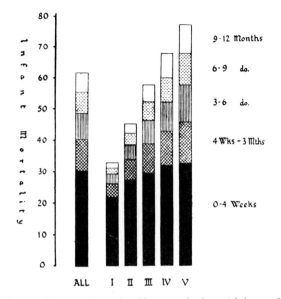

Fig. 2 Infant mortality analysed by age at death; social classes of England and Wales, 1930–1933.

deaths in class I and about three-sevenths in class V, as compared with the national average of just over half the deaths. Conversely, bronchitis and pneumonia, which have the steepest class gradient, were assigned as the causes of about one-quarter of the deaths in class V as compared with about one-twelfth in class I. There is a steady increase in mortality with increasing poverty for every individual cause listed by the Registrar-General, with two exceptions, both of which are included in the 'congenital causes' group. One is congenital malformations, which is substantially the same in classes II to V, though the rate in class I is a little lower. The other is injury at birth, which is slightly in excess in classes I and II as compared with classes IV and V.

Figure 2 depicts the social class mortalities divided according to age at death. The rates are given for five periods of infancy: the neonatal deaths; four weeks to three months; three to six months; six to nine months; and nine to twelve months. During each of these periods there is a class gradient, but it grows relatively steeper as the baby gets older. For the neonatal period the ratio of class V to class I is 1.5 : 1. For the remainder of the first quarter, it is about 3 : 1. During the second quarter, infants in class V have nearly four times the death-rate of infants in class I, and for the rest of the first year the disparity is about 5.4 : 1. Neonatal deaths are about half the total for all classes combined, two-thirds for class I, and three-sevenths for class V. The figures for neonatal deaths correspond very closely to those for deaths from congenital causes.

It is instructive also to compare the mortality experience of babies born in towns and in rural areas. For purposes of local government, the country is divided into county boroughs, municipal boroughs, urban districts and rural districts. The county boroughs are the larger towns, mostly with populations of over 50 000. At the time when the local government divisions were made, the municipal boroughs were the smaller towns, urban districts were areas of predominatingly urban character and rural districts were mainly country. Later extensions of industrial and residential building have in many cases altered the character of local government divisions. In particular, it frequently happens that urban districts are really the outer suburbs of a large town or conurbation of towns, while rural districts, especially in the mining areas, may quite often be densely populated and primarily industrial. London forms an exception to these municipal arrangements. The inner portion is the administrative county, divided into 29 semi-autonomous boroughs, and the outer built-up ring is carved into municipal boroughs and urban districts whose boundaries are based upon past conditions and have no relation to present social realities. It is nevertheless true that rural districts, taken as a whole, cover the agricultural population and its ancillaries with some admixture of mining, outer suburban and other urban elements; urban districts and municipal boroughs are less densely populated than county boroughs; and these in turn are on the whole relatively small towns compared to the continuous built-up area of Greater London, with its population of over 8 000 000.

The Registrar-General gives annual infant mortality rates, by cause and age, for the following four aggregates of municipal areas: (1) Greater London; (2) County Boroughs outside Greater London; (3) Other Urban Districts, comprising 'municipal boroughs' and 'urban districts' outside Greater London; (4) Rural Districts outside Greater London. This classification dates from 1931. Until 1930 the method of subdivision was slightly different, but not so as materially to affect comparability with the later series of figures. Figure 3 shows these data for the eleven-year period 1928–38 for England and Wales as a whole and for the four types of municipal area, by cause of death. A few minor items included in 'congenital causes' in Figure 1 are excluded in Figure 3, and 'infectious diseases' contains meningitis but does not contain some very rare infectious conditions. On the whole, however, the categories in Figures 1 and 3 are reasonably comparable. Figure 3 also shows stillbirth rates. To make them comparable with the infant mortality rates they are calculated per 1000 live births.

The phenomena displayed in Figure 3 may be summarized as follows.

For the total infant mortality, the order is county boroughs, urban districts, Greater London, rural districts. The rate for county boroughs, 70.8, is twelve units higher than that for urban districts. Urban districts and London had approximately the same mortality, and rural districts had a rate more than four units lower.

For congenital causes and also for other causes, London had by far the lowest rate. County boroughs had the worst figure, then urban districts, and then rural districts, but the rates for the three extra-metropolitan divisions differed little among themselves compared with the gap between them and London.

For infectious diseases and also for bronchitis and pneumonia, county boroughs were worst, followed by London, urban districts, rural districts.

For diarrhoea, London was markedly worse than county boroughs. There must be some radical difference in social aetiology between diarrhoea on the one hand and infectious diseases and bronchitis and pneumonia on the other, since diarrhoea is the only category where the death rate goes up with increasing degree of urbanization.

The relative distribution of stillbirths resembles that of congenital causes, except that urban districts are slightly higher than county boroughs. The superiority of London over the other areas is even greater for stillbirths than for congenital causes.

London is best for stillbirths, congenital causes, and

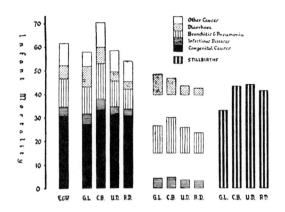

Fig. 3 Infant mortality analysed by cause groups, and stillbirths, in different types of local government areas, England and Wales, 1928–1938. EW, England and Wales; GL, Greater London; CB, county boroughs outside Greater London; UD, other urban districts outside Greater London; RD, rural districts.

other causes, and worst for diarrhoea. County boroughs are worst for everything except stillbirths and diarrhoea. Stillbirths are highest in urban districts, but county boroughs run them close. Rural districts are best for infectious diseases, bronchitis and pneumonia, and diarrhoea. The child born in the country thus has the least risk of death from zymotic diseases, while the London baby fares best in relation to the risks of birth and early infancy.

Some of these results, such as the lower rates for the three infectious groups in smaller towns and rural areas, will probably seem obvious and natural. Other features, such as the low stillbirth and congenital rates and the high diarrhoea rate in London, may appear anomalous and puzzling. It will be shown below that these anomalies can be satisfactorily explained by the aetiological considerations suggested by the regression equations for the county boroughs.

When mortality in the four classes of administrative area is analysed according to age at death the results are quite regular. During the neonatal period county boroughs show the highest rate, followed closely by urban districts and rural districts, with London well behind. The difference between county boroughs and rural districts is 2.1; between rural districts and London it is 6.3. For the remainder of the first quarter and for the rest of the year, the order is county boroughs, London, urban districts, rural districts.

The simultaneous analysis of infant mortality by cause and age at death is illustrated in Figures 4 and 5. The data used are the mean rates during 1928–38 in county boroughs, but the figures for other types of area of

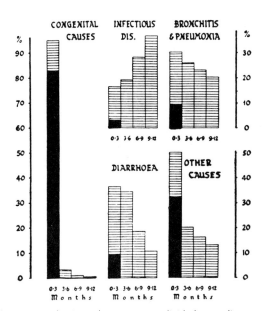

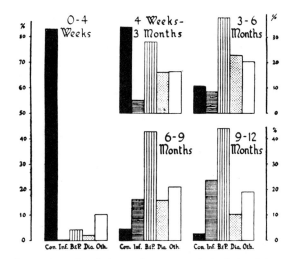

Fig. 5 Mortality during various age periods during infancy divided according to cause group, county boroughs, 1928–1938. Total mortality rate in each group is taken as 100.

Fig. 4 Mortality in each cause group divided according to age at death, county boroughs, 1928–1938. Total mortality rate in each group is taken as 100. Black area, neonatal rate (0–4 weeks).

England and Wales as a whole show the same essential features. In both figures the ordinates represent percentages of the relevant partial mortality rate. In Figure 4 the mortality in each cause group is divided according to age at death. The solid black rectangle represents the percentage of the deaths occurring during the neonatal period, and the shaded area above it those during the remainder of the first quarter. It will be seen that the great majority of deaths from congenital causes occur during the neonatal period, deaths from infectious diseases increase with age and deaths in the other cause groups go down. Figure 5 shows the percentage of the deaths in each of the periods attributable to the various cause groups. In the neonatal period deaths from congenital causes greatly predominate, and these also claim the largest single share during the rest of the first quarter, with bronchitis and pneumonia a close second. Thereafter 'bronchitis and pneumonia' is always in the lead, and as the baby gets older the relative importance of diarrhoea recedes and that of infectious diseases advances. It was seen from Figure 1 that infectious diseases and bronchitis and pneumonia are the cause groups with the steepest class gradient. These become more and more important as the baby grows older, accounting for the increasing disparity in relative class mortality with increasing age.

Regression equations for county boroughs

In order to estimate the influence of social conditions on stillbirths and infant mortality at different ages and from different causes, multiple regression equations were computed by the product-moment method between the appropriate mortality rates for the individual county boroughs and the seven selected indices of social conditions. If M is the mortality rate for a county borough (technically the 'dependent variable') and A, B, C . . . are the numerical values for that borough of the various social indices (the 'independent variables'), then the regression equation is of the general form:

$$M = K + Aa + Bb + Cc + \ldots \pm d,$$

where a, b, c . . . are constants (the 'regression coefficients') and d is the difference between the observed value of M and that calculated from the regression equation. The mathematical procedure ensures that the constant K and a, b, c . . . are so fixed that Σd^2 is a minimum. Woolf and Waterhouse (1945) give a full and critical discussion of the applicability of the method to the study of infant mortality, and of the effects of imperfections or errors in the raw figures on the trustworthiness of the equations obtained. Errors in the dependent variable, provided they are random and uncorrelated with the social indices, do not in general affect the equations, although they lower their degree of statistical significance. But imperfections in the independent variables will distort the equations, both by giving an

45

incorrect picture of the relative influence of the various social conditions, and by underestimating the total effect of all the social indices acting together. Before the equations can be calculated, therefore, it is necessary to make a preliminary examination of all the variables with respect to their accuracy and relevance. They must be subjected to a process of social and medical questioning: how accurately do they measure the social phenomenon to which they allegedly refer; are they likely to be relevant to the topic under investigation, and, if so, are they more closely applicable than any other available measure of the same phenomenon? This cross-examination of the data is aided and guided by objective mathematical tests. Out of various possible groups of indices of social conditions, that group is the most relevant which gives the highest multiple correlation with the dependent variable.

Stillbirth and infant mortality rates

All the mortality rates used for the regression equations were calculated from figures of numbers of live births, stillbirths and infant deaths in the individual county boroughs, as published in the annual *Statistical Review* of the Registrar-General. The death-rate from each cause group or during each period of infancy was calculated thus:

$$\frac{\text{Total relevant deaths during 1928–38 inclusive}}{\text{Total live births during 1928–38 inclusive}} \times 1000$$

In general, the pooled rates used in the regressions will be higher than the mean of the yearly rates, since mortality rates have tended to fall, and in the earlier years, when mortality was higher, there were also more births, giving these years a greater influence on the final figures.

As already stated, figures for death by age are given for seven subdivisions of the first year of life. These periods, with the symbols used in this paper, are as follows:

DAY	Under 1 day
WK	1–7 days
MON	1–4 weeks
1Q	4 weeks–3 months
2Q	3–6 months
3Q	6–9 months
4Q	9–12 months

For death by cause, only an abridged list of causes is available, and this was revised in 1931. The groupings used in this paper, together with their symbols, are as follows:

CON   The Registrar-General's category of 'congenital causes, etc.', comprising all the items under the first two headings in Table 1.

INF   Infectious diseases, comprising:
        Typhoid and paratyphoid fevers (called 'enteric fever' before 1931).
        Measles.
        Scarlet fever.
        Whooping-cough.
        Diphtheria.
        Influenza.
        Encephalitis lethargica.
        Cerebrospinal fever (called 'meningococcal meningitis before 1931).

B & P   Bronchitis and pneumonia.

DIA   Diarrhoea.

OTH   Other causes, being total deaths less all those in above groups.

Total infant mortality will be denoted by the symbol IM and stillbirths by the symbol STI.

The ultimate source of all these figures is the individual birth, stillbirth or death certificate, and it is necessary to inquire into the reliability of these certificates and of the rates calculated from them. It is of course possible that a few births are not registered at all, or that the date or other particulars are wrongly stated, but it seems likely that birth figures are on the whole highly accurate. One source of error is the difficulty of differentiating between a stillbirth and a death in the first few minutes of life; affecting the figures for stillbirths and deaths on the first day, and number of live births. A further difficult area is the demarcation between a stillbirth, a foetus at least 28 weeks since fertilization, and an abortion, a foetus of lesser maturity.

Figures for cause of death are also subject to a degree of uncertainty which is hard to assess. It must be very difficult in many cases for the doctor to assign the cause of infant death with any confidence, especially as necropsies are rarely performed. Some diagnostic categories, such as congenital debility or convulsions, are little more than a record of the presence of symptoms of unknown origin. The margin of uncertainty will probably not be so great when causes are grouped as in this paper. The congenital group as a whole may be expected to be fairly easily distinguishable from the group of infectious diseases, while diarrhoea is also likely to be more or less uniformly diagnosed by different doctors. There is, however, much more doubt about the discrimination

Table 4 Infant mortality and stillbirth rates per 1000 live births in county boroughs, 1928–1938

	Unweighted mean	Weighted mean	Highest C.B.	Lowest C.B.	Total deaths	% of IM	% of IM + STI
Infant mortality	66.6	70.4	97.6	41.9	164 414	100.0	61.7
Stillbirths	44.5	43.6	69.7	32.7	101 859	62.0	38.3
By cause							
Congenital causes	32.9	33.1	47.0	22.9	77 255	47.0	29.0
Infectious diseases	3.9	4.7	8.2	1.2	10 880	6.6	4.1
Bronchitis and pneumonia	14.2	15.4	26.6	6.0	36 084	21.9	13.6
Diarrhoea	5.5	7.0	13.2	1.1	16 424	10.0	6.2
Other causes	10.0	10.2	20.5	5.9	23 771	14.5	8.9
By age at death							
0–1 day	10.9	11.1	15.2	7.4	25 994	15.8	9.8
1–7 days	12.3	12.0	16.6	7.8	27 953	17.0	10.5
1–4 weeks	9.8	9.8	16.8	4.4	22 941	14.0	8.6
4 weeks to 3 months	10.7	11.5	16.7	4.8	26 953	16.4	10.1
3–6 months	9.3	10.5	15.9	4.1	24 541	14.9	9.2
6–9 months	7.3	8.2	14.1	2.9	19 211	11.7	7.2
9–12 months	6.4	7.2	11.8	2.9	16 821	10.2	6.3

between infectious diseases and bronchitis and pneumonia, especially when lung infection is secondary to a disease in the infectious group. The Registrar-General has rules for selecting one cause when the certificate indicates multiple causation, but it seems likely, nevertheless, that a death that would be certified by one doctor so that it counted as measles or whooping-cough might be so described by another doctor that it counted as pneumonia. The 'other causes' group, which includes some of the most dubious diagnostic headings, will also suffer from lack of precision.

In so far as differences in diagnostic practice are randomly distributed among boroughs and not correlated with poverty, overcrowding or the other social indices, they will merely add to the error variance without imparting any systematic bias to the regression coefficients. There seems to be no special reason to suppose that method of certification will vary markedly with social conditions. It is fortunate that in the two cause groups most subject to errors of demarcation – infectious diseases and bronchitis and pneumonia – the relative influence of the various social indices as computed from the regression equations is so similar that moderate differences in certification procedure between the various county boroughs can have no appreciable distorting effect on the general conclusions.

Some figures indicating the distribution of mortality to be accounted for by the regression equations are given in Table 4. The mean mortality rate is obtained by averaging the rates for the individual county boroughs. The second column gives the rate obtained by dividing the aggregate of deaths by the aggregate of births, which has the effect of weighting the contribution of each borough by its total of births. Where the weighted mean is larger than the unweighted, the more populous county boroughs tend to have a higher mortality rate than the smaller places, and vice versa. It will be observed that large population is positively associated with infant mortality, and negatively with stillbirths. Congenital and 'other' causes, and neonatal deaths, have unweighted and weighted means that are substantially identical; in the other cause groups and in deaths after the first month, high mortality is associated with large population. Table 4 next gives the range of mortality rates for each heading. The ratio of the highest to the lowest for total infant mortality, stillbirths and congenital causes is just over 2:1. For all the other cause groups the ratio is much bigger, being about 3.5 for other causes, 4.5 for bronchitis and pneumonia, 7 for infectious diseases and 12 for diarrhoea. Figure 6 shows the range of variation among county boroughs for each cause group, in comparison with the difference in 1930–2 between social classes I and V. It will be seen that in each case the range in county boroughs is greater, showing that the Registrar-General's analysis of infant deaths by social class by no means expresses the full extent of the contrasts. Table 4 also shows the total number of deaths within each category, and the percentage contribution of these deaths to (a) all deaths of live-born babies, and (b) all infant deaths plus stillbirths, the total wastage of lives associated with birth and infancy. It will be seen that

47

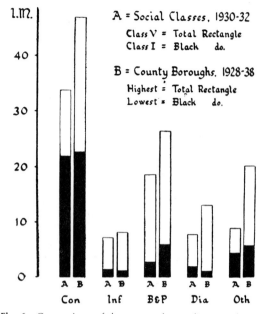

Fig. 6 Comparison of the range of mortality rates by cause groups in the Registrar-General's social classes and in county boroughs.

stillbirths constitute nearly two-fifths of this wastage, neonatal deaths nearly three-tenths and deaths during the postnatal period nearly one-third. Among these the biggest single cause group is bronchitis and pneumonia.

Indices of social conditions

The five social indices used by Woolf and Waterhouse (1945) are listed in the first paragraph of this paper. Woolf and Waterhouse gave a full description of the criteria and procedure by which this group of five was selected from about thirty indices tried. For reasons stated in their paper, they were unable to obtain a satisfactory measure for a number of other presumably relevant social conditions, including size of built-up area, density of population on the site and efficiency of infant welfare services.

Size of family

The measure used is G, the gross reproduction rate in 1931, as calculated by Charles (1938) from Census data. The gross reproduction rate is the computed average number of girl babies produced by a woman during the whole of her reproductive period. It is not a perfect measure of size of family, for several reasons. In the first place, the calculations are made by postulating equal numbers of women in each reproductive age group, so

that if the female populations in two places have different age-compositions the index will tend to misrepresent the relative mean family sizes. Secondly, the index takes no account of infant and child mortality, so that in places with a high death rate the family size will be exaggerated. Thirdly, the index refers only to current births, whereas the existing families were produced over a period during which the reproduction rate may have been different. Lastly, and probably most important, the index is highly sensitive to the proportion of women who are married. Two places might have exactly the same average family size, but if one has a higher ratio of married to single women, it will have a correspondingly bigger gross reproduction rate. This distorting effect is especially likely to be important in well-to-do places and holiday resorts, where there is a concentration of unmarried domestic servants, and in centres of mining and heavy industry, from which girls migrate to take up domestic work. The former will have an unduly low index, and the latter one that is too high. Since the well-to-do places have low infant and child mortalities, the last two effects will tend to cancel out. These criticisms, except possibly the last, do not apply to the gross reproduction rate when used for its primary purpose, as an indicator of population trends in the future, but only to its use as a measure of the mean size of actually existing families at the time of computation. Nevertheless, the gross reproduction rate is probably the best available index of relative family size, and, by the objective test of the amount of variance it is able to explain, it seems to be highly relevant in accounting for the observed distribution of infant mortality and stillbirth rates.

Density of population

Successive reports from the Registrar-General's office have been pointing to the positive relation between mortality and density of population ever since the time of William Farr. But the construction of an accurate index is a formidable task. The usual criterion – persons per acre – cannot be applied to big areas like county boroughs. Some cities – Leeds and Birmingham, for example – have extended their boundaries to include undeveloped land to be used for future housing schemes. The value of the index will depend on exactly where the borough boundary runs in relation to open spaces or factory areas on the outskirts. A person-per-acre index gives a distorted picture of comparative densities of population, and its correlation with infant mortality was negligible (Woolf and Waterhouse, 1945).

The ideal index would be constructed as follows. With the location of each individual as centre, draw a circle with an area of one acre, and count the number of people

Table 5 First order correlations among social indices

	U	P	F	L	G	D
H	0.6378	0.6870	−0.0218	0.5348	0.7256	0.4311
U	–	0.5353	−0.0985	0.4743	0.5496	0.2657
P	–	–	0.0768	0.5015	0.6987	0.2836
F	–	–	–	0.2681	−0.2404	−0.0628
L	–	–	–	–	0.3120	0.1447
G	–	–	–	–	–	0.4244

it encloses. Add all these figures and divide by the number in the population. This would give the average number of people within one acre's surround of any individual, and so be a true measure of crowding as it is likely to influence spread of infection or of other effects of closeness of packing on infant mortality. The calculation of such an index is obviously entirely impracticable, but it is possible to obtain an approximation to it, as follows. An imaginary municipality is divided into two wards, A and B, each of 100 acres, A with a population of 9000 and B with 3000 inhabitants. The usual method of calculating density would give a figure of sixty persons per acre (12 000/200 = 60). But in Ward A there are three people suffering crowded conditions for every person enjoying comparative spaciousness in Ward B, so the figure of 60 is an underestimate of the crowding when measured as centring on each individual. If, however, one is prepared to assume that within each ward the population is evenly distributed, so that each single acre in A contains 90 and each acre in B contains 30 people, one can easily calculate the corrected or weighted index. In Ward A, 9000 people are each surrounded by 30. The average density, measured round people, is found by multiplying for each ward the population by the density, and dividing the total of such products by the total population. The weighted index is always higher than the unweighted, and the more unevenly the population is distributed the greater the difference between the two indices.

For the successful application of this method to actual county boroughs, it would be necessary to have figures of area and population relating to subdivisions small enough to justify the assumption that density of settlement within each division was substantially constant. This condition is not very well satisfied by the available data. In the 1931 Census, figures of area and population are given for each county borough by wards and sometimes by other kinds of sub-areas. From these the weighted density in each borough was calculated by the method described. On average, the weighted density exceeds the unweighted by about 76 per cent. But for some places, such as East

Ham, the difference is much less. These are boroughs which are fully built up, and which are fairly homogeneous in density of occupation in the different wards. In other cases the weighting process increases the density several fold. Examples are Barrow, where the figure is raised from 6 to 26; Leeds, from 13 to 38; and Brighton, from 12 to 66. These are boroughs containing undeveloped land or localized areas of factories, docks or shipyards. The correlation between weighted and unweighted density is about 0.84. This weighted index, as shown later, gives appreciable correlation and regression coefficients with the various components of infant mortality. Although it is probably only a rough approximation to the true average density per person as defined above, it is nevertheless a relevant index in respect of infant death rates. The weighted index of persons per acre is denoted by the symbol D.

First order correlations among the social indices are set out in Table 5. One of the new indices, G, shows quite a high correlation with H. Size of family is strongly associated with overcrowding in the house. The correlations with P and U, though lower, are also considerable. Poverty and unemployment tend to be highest in boroughs where family sizes are above the average. The correlation with F is negative, and rather small. On the whole, industrial employment of women is associated with small numbers of children. The other new index, D, gives unexpectedly low correlations with H and G. Density on the site is not the same social phenomenon as overcrowding in the house or large family size. The small correlations between D and the other variables indicate that its inclusion in the regression equations may add appreciably to the amount of variance accounted for. Table 6 shows the first order correlations between the social indices and the various mortality rates.[1]

The regression constant, K, gives the computed value of the dependent variable when each of the independent variables is at some chosen origin. The value of K in each of the equations therefore gives the mortality rate to be

Table 6 First order correlations between mortality rates and social indices

	H	U	P	F	L	G	D
IM	0.7353	0.6651	0.6686	0.3428	0.6634	0.5655	0.3394
STI	0.2004	0.4734	0.2898	0.4221	0.4000	−0.0966	−0.1981
CON	0.4650	0.4691	0.4821	0.4875	0.6061	0.2436	−0.0134
INF	0.6438	0.4832	0.5901	0.1956	0.4493	0.5623	0.5265
B & P	0.7566	0.6659	0.6988	0.2299	0.5587	0.6701	0.3912
DIA	0.6101	0.3554	0.4303	0.1812	0.3841	0.5529	0.5748
OTH	0.5171	0.6738	0.4693	0.1248	0.5896	0.3273	0.1688
DAY	0.2323	0.1634	0.1508	0.4265	0.3453	−0.0167	−0.1174
WK	0.3369	0.4544	0.3632	0.4371	0.6521	0.0688	−0.1940
MON	0.6806	0.6298	0.6116	0.2846	0.6586	0.4750	0.1899
1Q	0.6477	0.5818	0.6167	0.2613	0.5404	0.5560	0.4325
2Q	0.7465	0.6624	0.6583	0.1621	0.5547	0.6885	0.5375
3Q	0.7447	0.6215	0.6329	0.2794	0.5431	0.6442	0.4812
4Q	0.7626	0.6171	0.7206	0.2081	0.5007	0.6947	0.4536

expected, if the equation is a true description of the facts, in an ideal population with:

- no families living more than one person per room;
- no men unemployed;
- no men in low-paid occupations;
- no women employed in industry;
- a latitude of 50° 30′, that of the extreme south of England;
- a gross reproduction rate of 0.6;
- a weighted density of twenty persons per acre.

The value of K in this paper may be expected not to correspond exactly with that given by Woolf and Waterhouse, for two reasons. First, the mortality rates used here are based on pooled births and deaths over the eleven years, and so give slightly more weight to the years of high mortality, when births were also higher. This will tend to increase the value of K calculated on the new basis. Secondly, the value of K will vary with the exact levels arbitrarily chosen as the origins for G and D. If, as is in fact the case, the rates of 0.6 for G and 20 persons per acre for D are higher than those actually obtaining among the best-off section of the population, the value of K will be increased on this score also. There is another point to be noted about the values of K in the various equations. For reasons stated by Woolf and Waterhouse, all the county boroughs were given equal weight in the computations, irrespective of their populations. The values of K calculated from these unweighted rates are those given in Table 7 and we return to this point in a later section.

The regression equations

Table 7 shows the regression equations for the various mortality rates for 82 out of the 83 county boroughs in England and Wales over the eleven years 1928 to 1938. Bootle had to be omitted because of lack of unemployment data. The table is arranged in four sections. The first gives the equations for total infant mortality (IM) and for stillbirths (STI), and the sum, constituting the equation for the total wastage of life during birth and infancy. Next comes infant mortality, divided into the five cause groups, with a check total. Then the seven periods of infancy are given, again with a check total. Finally the equation for the neonatal period – the first four weeks of life (NEO) – is obtained by summing the three equations for DAY, WK and MON, and compared with the expression for the postnatal period, the rest of the year of infancy (POST), which is the sum of the equations for 1Q, 2Q, 3Q and 4Q. The two check totals should correspond with the equation for infant mortality at the top of the table, and do so fairly well; the small discrepancies arise from rounding errors.

Each regression coefficient gives the change in the mortality rate to be expected for an increase of one unit in the social index in question. The coefficient is therefore inversely proportional to the unit of measurement, so the relative sizes of the coefficients for the different social indices are no guide to their relative importance in relation to infant mortality. If, for example, latitude had been measured in minutes instead of degrees, its regression coefficients would have been one-sixtieth of those shown in the table. G is another social variable with

Table 7 Regression equations

IM	$= 26.805 + 0.357\,H + 0.441\,U + 0.153\,P + 0.407\,F + 2.14\,L + 11.98\,G + 0.044\,D$
STI	$= 25.660 + 0.058\,H + 0.535\,U + 0.351\,P + 0.195\,F + 0.14\,L - 22.43\,G - 0.113\,D$
IM + STI	$= 52.465 + 0.415\,H + 0.976\,U + 0.504\,P + 0.602\,F + 2.28\,L - 10.45\,G - 0.069\,D$
CON	$= 19.807 + 0.102\,H + 0.153\,U + 0.090\,P + 0.183\,F + 0.98\,L - 0.36\,G - 0.065\,D$
INF	$= 0.211 + 0.029\,H + 0.015\,U + 0.030\,P + 0.029\,F + 0.08\,L + 1.33\,G + 0.028\,D$
B & P	$= 0.031 + 0.118\,H + 0.147\,U + 0.073\,P + 0.127\,F + 0.26\,L + 7.83\,G + 0.021\,D$
DIA	$= 2.002 + 0.083\,H - 0.018\,U - 0.072\,P + 0.064\,F + 0.23\,L + 5.55\,G + 0.060\,D$
OTH	$= 4.743 + 0.023\,H + 0.136\,U + 0.034\,P + 0.011\,F + 0.55\,L - 2.16\,G - 0.001\,D$
Total	$= 26.794 + 0.355\,H + 0.433\,U + 0.155\,P + 0.414\,F + 2.10\,L + 12.19\,G + 0.043\,D$
DAY	$= 9.068 + 0.066\,H + 0.015\,U - 0.023\,P + 0.054\,F + 0.19\,L - 1.13\,G - 0.023\,D$
WK	$= 7.452 + 0.030\,H + 0.089\,U + 0.032\,P + 0.055\,F + 0.75\,L - 2.46\,G - 0.046\,D$
MON	$= 3.376 + 0.076\,H + 0.071\,U + 0.031\,P + 0.048\,F + 0.45\,L + 0.52\,G - 0.012\,D$
1Q	$= 3.975 + 0.030\,H + 0.069\,U + 0.044\,P + 0.064\,F + 0.27\,L + 2.70\,G + 0.031\,D$
2Q	$= 2.091 + 0.043\,H + 0.084\,U + 0.013\,P + 0.059\,F + 0.31\,L + 4.92\,G + 0.045\,D$
3Q	$= 1.343 + 0.063\,H + 0.062\,U - 0.008\,P + 0.075\,F + 0.14\,L + 4.17\,G + 0.027\,D$
4Q	$= 0.266 + 0.057\,H + 0.046\,U + 0.056\,P + 0.054\,F - 0.01\,L + 3.42\,G + 0.018\,D$
Total	$= 27.039 + 0.365\,H + 0.436\,U + 0.145\,P + 0.409\,F + 2.10\,L + 12.14\,G + 0.040\,D$
NEO	$= 19.896 + 0.172\,H + 0.175\,U + 0.040\,P + 0.157\,F + 1.39\,L - 3.07\,G - 0.081\,D$
POST	$= 7.143 + 0.193\,H + 0.261\,U + 0.105\,P + 0.252\,F + 0.71\,L + 15.21\,G + 0.121\,D$

a very small numerical range of variation, the highest value being 1.43 and the lowest 0.55. Its regression coefficients are accordingly quite large figures. Before any aetiological conclusions can be drawn from the equations, the influences of the various social agencies must be exhibited on a comparable basis. This is done in the next section.

Tests of the statistical significance of the various equations, involving the conventional assumptions about random sampling from a normally distributed universe, are set out in Table 8. For each equation there is shown:

The coefficient of multiple correlation, denoted by R.

The *explanation*, or proportion of total variance accounted for by the equation (R^2), denoted by E.

The *non-explanation*, or residual variance, which equals $1 - E$.

The value of Snedecor's F calculated for the appropriate number of degrees of freedom, according to the formula

$$F = \frac{74E}{7(1 - E)}$$

It is clear from Table 8 that the level of explanation is high. With one exception, all values of R are above 0.75, and of E above 0.56. The exception is mortality during the first 24 hours, which would be expected to have a large error variance owing to uncertainty of timing of births and deaths. But even this equation has an F of 4.8 as compared with the 0.1 per cent point of 3.9 ($P < 0.001$). For the other equations the F values are much higher, rising to 43 for total infant mortality. The equations as a whole may therefore be regarded as highly significant.

The last column of Table 8 gives the standard error of estimate for each equation. If the mortality rates for the individual county boroughs are calculated from the equations, the differences between the computed and the actual figures will be less than the value shown in approximately two-thirds of the cases. The equations enable total infant mortality rate to be estimated for any county borough with a standard error of about six units, and stillbirth rate within ± 4.5. For the seven periods of infancy the standard error varies between 1.05 and 1.53. The various cause groups have standard errors of estimate ranging from 0.93 for infectious diseases, whose mean rate is the smallest at 3.85, to 3.14 for congenital causes, whose mean rate is the highest at 19.81.

An example of how the equations may be applied to analysing the mortality in an individual county borough is shown in Table 9, for the largest borough, Birmingham. The top part of the table shows the detailed calculation of the expected infant mortality and stillbirths, expressed both as rates and as numbers of deaths, from the values of the seven social indices. As might be expected from its large population and consequently low sampling variance, Birmingham gives closer agreement between calculated and observed deaths than the last column of Table 8 might lead one to expect. Infant mortality agrees

Table 8 Significances of equations

Equation	R	$E = R^2$	$1 - E$	F	SE of estimate
IM	0.8960	0.8027	0.1973	43.0	6.03
STI	0.8079	0.6527	0.3473	19.9	4.51
CON	0.7920	0.6272	0.3728	17.8	3.14
INF	0.7707	0.5940	0.4060	15.5	0.93
B & P	0.8781	0.7711	0.2289	35.6	2.35
DIA	0.7664	0.5874	0.4126	15.0	1.75
OTH	0.7526	0.5664	0.4336	13.8	1.56
DAY	0.5608	0.3145	0.6855	4.8	1.45
WK	0.8233	0.6778	0.3222	22.2	1.27
MON	0.8301	0.6891	0.3109	23.4	1.27
1Q	0.8002	0.6403	0.3597	18.8	1.53
2Q	0.8834	0.7804	0.2196	37.6	1.35
3Q	0.8809	0.7759	0.2241	36.6	1.13
4Q	0.8763	0.7679	0.2321	35.0	1.05

0.1 per cent point for $F = 3.9$.

to within 146 deaths, and stillbirths to within 22 deaths. Similar calculations were made for the deaths-by-cause groups and by periods of infancy, and the results are summarized at the bottom of Table 9. In three cases out of twelve the difference between observed and calculated rate exceeds the standard error of estimate.

Similar computations performed for other county boroughs indicate that on the whole the larger the place the closer the concordance between expected and observed mortality rates. It is fair to claim that the equations are of quite high efficiency as a means of accounting for infant deaths from a knowledge of the measures of social conditions.

Social aetiology of stillbirths and infant deaths

A set of calculations similar to those for Birmingham in Table 9 can be made for the country as a whole by substituting in the various equations the mean value of each social index among county boroughs. There is, of course, no question here of finding any difference between calculated and observed rates, since the value of K is fixed by equating these two rates when the independent variables are all at their means. The object of such computations for the aggregate of county boroughs would be to obtain estimates of the amount of mortality associated with each social index. This procedure is justified only in so far as the individual regression coefficients, as distinct from the equations as a whole, can be regarded as 'significant'. The discussion of this point is best deferred until after the presentation of the results. For the moment the regression coefficients will be provisionally regarded as reliable measures of the relative influence of the various social agencies on infant deaths.

The results of the computations are set out in Table 10. For each equation there is shown the mean mortality rate, the value of K (representing the expected rate among the 'better-off'), the difference in mortality associated with each social variable for the average county borough (as compared with the baseline population used for calculating K), and finally the total amount of mortality 'explained' by the equation, which is of course the mean minus K. Approximately three-fifths of the total infant mortality and two-fifths of the stillbirths are associated with the differences in social conditions between the average county borough population and the better-off section. For infant mortality and stillbirths together, just over half the deaths are attributable to the specified social agencies.

Among the cause groups, almost the whole of the mortality from infectious diseases and from bronchitis and pneumonia is socially conditioned. For diarrhoea more than a third, and for other causes nearly a half, of the average mortality rate are found at the better-off level. For congenital causes, K is about three-fifths of the mean, just as it is for stillbirths.

When mortality is dissected by age at death, the proportion explained steadily rises throughout the year of infancy. Indeed, in the fourth quarter the computed mortality for the arbitrarily chosen baseline population (-0.27) is not significantly different from zero. Neonatal deaths, like stillbirths and congenital causes, give a K about three-fifths of the mean, while in the postnatal

Table 9 Birmingham, 1928–1938: Stillbirths and infant deaths observed and calculated from regression equations

	Rates			Deaths		
	IM	STI	Total	IM	STI	Total
Unexplained	26.81	25.66	52.47	4894	4684	9578
H 25.1%	8.97	1.46	10.43	1638	267	1905
U 11.2%	4.93	5.99	10.92	900	1094	1994
P 32.3%	4.94	11.32	16.26	902	2067	2969
F 23.9%	9.73	4.65	14.38	1776	849	2625
L 52.2°	4.28	0.28	4.56	781	51	832
G 0.972	4.45	−8.34	−3.89	813	−1523	−710
D 41.1	0.92	−2.38	−1.46	168	−435	−267
Total calculated	65.03	38.64	103.67	11 872	7054	18 926
Observed	65.83	38.76	104.59	12 018	7076	19 094
Excess observed	0.80	0.12	0.92	146	22	168

	Rates		
	Observed	Calculated	Excess observed
CON	32.28	31.81	0.47
INF	5.00	4.03	0.97
B & P	12.03	13.93	−1.90
DIA	7.73	6.87	0.86
OTH	8.79	8.47	0.32
DAY	12.72	10.92	1.80
WK	10.51	11.16	−0.65
MON	7.61	9.04	−1.43
1Q	10.47	10.66	−0.19
2Q	9.98	9.34	0.64
3Q	8.01	7.58	0.43
4Q	6.53	6.42	0.11
NEO	30.84	31.12	−0.28
POST	34.99	34.00	0.99

period more than three-quarters of the deaths are associated with adverse social conditions.

Directing attention to the individual social indices, one notices the following. For stillbirths, neonatal deaths, and congenital causes and other causes, both G and D have negative effects. Other things being equal, the equations indicate that the bigger the family and the greater the density of people on the site, the lower are the mortality rates in these categories. In a later communication it will be shown that the same thing is true for maternal mortality. In all cases the negative contribution of D is coupled with a positive influence of H. Overcrowding in the home is still associated with increased rates in these, and indeed in all, the various divisions of infant mortality. The equations enable one to distinguish the separate effects of these two related aspects of town life. For postnatal deaths and for the three zymotic cause groups, crowding in the house and crowding on the site seem to act in the same direction. For stillbirths and deaths in early infancy, at a given degree of crowding in the home, the higher the density per acre the lower the death rate. This is one unexpected outcome of the equations that will require aetiological discussion.

Another unexpected result is the negative effect computed for the two indices of low income, U and P, in the equation for diarrhoea. If these figures truly represent the facts, it would seem that, for equal degrees of overcrowding, family size, latitude and employment of women, the better-off the people in the borough the higher the death-rate from diarrhoea.

Three other negative figures appear. Two are associated with P, and relate to deaths on the first day and in the

Table 10 Mortality rates associated with the various social indices

	Mean	K	H	U	P	F	L	G	D	Total expl.
IM	66.60	26.81	9.82	8.64	5.46	6.13	5.12	4.02	0.60	39.79
STI	44.48	25.66	1.60	10.49	12.52	2.93	0.34	−7.52	−1.54	18.82
IM + STI	111.08	52.47	11.42	19.13	17.98	9.06	5.46	−3.50	−0.94	58.61
CON	32.93	19.81	2.80	3.01	3.20	2.75	2.36	−0.12	−0.88	13.12
INF	3.85	0.21	0.81	0.30	1.08	0.43	0.19	0.45	0.38	3.64
B & P	14.24	0.03	3.24	2.89	2.62	1.91	0.63	2.63	0.29	14.21
DIA	5.54	2.00	2.29	−0.36	−2.58	0.96	0.55	1.86	0.82	3.54
OTH	9.99	4.74	0.62	2.66	1.23	0.16	1.31	−0.72	−0.01	5.25
Total	66.55	26.79	9.76	8.50	5.55	6.21	5.04	4.10	0.60	39.76
DAY	10.94	9.07	1.83	0.28	−0.81	0.81	0.46	−0.38	−0.32	1.87
WK	12.33	7.45	0.82	1.74	1.14	0.82	1.80	−0.82	−0.62	4.88
MON	9.75	3.38	2.08	1.38	1.11	0.72	1.07	0.18	−0.17	6.37
1Q	10.67	3.98	0.82	1.35	1.58	0.96	0.64	0.91	0.43	6.69
2Q	9.28	2.09	1.19	1.65	0.45	0.89	0.74	1.65	0.62	7.19
3Q	7.26	1.34	1.73	1.22	−0.27	1.13	0.34	1.40	0.37	5.92
4Q	6.39	−0.27	1.57	0.90	2.00	0.81	−0.02	1.15	0.25	6.66
Total	66.62	27.04	10.04	8.52	5.20	6.14	5.03	4.09	0.56	39.58
NEO	33.02	19.90	4.73	3.40	1.44	2.35	3.33	−1.02	−1.11	13.12
POST	33.60	7.14	5.31	5.12	3.76	3.79	1.70	5.11	1.67	26.46

third quarter. The other negative is for L in the fourth quarter, but the computed effect on the average mortality rate – namely, −0.02 – is so small that it can be taken as not significantly different from zero.

For the negative effect of G in stillbirths, congenital and other causes, and neonatal deaths, there is a reasonable explanation available. The risk of stillbirth and of neonatal death is known to be higher for first births than for immediately subsequent parities. Thanks to the additional details at registration required under the Population Statistics Act of 1938, we now have comprehensive information about parity and age of mother in relation to all births, including stillbirths, and various tabulations of the new data have been published for 1939 and 1940. This shows that, for each age-group of mothers, the stillbirth rate is much higher among the firstborn than for second births. Thereafter it rises with increasing birth rank, but only at very high parities does the stillbirth rate approach that for first babies. For any given parity, the stillbirth rate increases with age of mother. The lower the value of G the larger the proportion of first births to total births. Low G also involves a higher average age of the mother at maternity. For both these reasons, G would be expected to have the negative association with stillbirths that is shown by the regression equation.

There are no similar recent data, on a nationwide scale, to show how neonatal death rates vary with parity and age of mother. But there is abundant evidence that first births have a higher rate than those immediately next in parity. Burns (1942), in a study of infant and maternal mortality in Durham from 1930 to 1936, found that the neonatal death rate in different social groups varied with parity as follows:

Parity	Miners	Other manual workers	Non-manual workers
1	39.1	28.5	34.5
2–3	32.2	25.3	25.7
4–6	44.4	34.2	20.7
7+	51.2	47.3	21.2

She also reported that neonatal mortality was high among the youngest mothers, decreased until the age-group 25 to 30, and thereafter increased with age of mother. Woodbury (1925) also found a higher neonatal mortality in first-born babies than among the succeeding parities in eight American cities between 1911 and 1916. His figures for the first nine birth-ranks were: 54, 39, 42, 36, 40, 40, 40, 49, 47. For the tenth and the later parities the rate was 69. His figures for neonatal death by age of mother also seem to show a minimum in the age-group 25 to 30. Baird (1945) also found that first-born babies were the most and second babies the least liable to neonatal death. Since the difference in mortality between first and subsequent parities is less marked for neonatal deaths than for stillbirths, and since higher average age of mother (which

Table 11 Means and standard deviations of social indices

Social index	Unit of measurement	Unweighted mean	Standard deviation	Weighted mean	Weighted mean − unweighted mean
H	% families living more than 1 person per room	27.49	9.61	28.20	0.71
U	% men unemployed	19.62	9.28	19.23	−0.39
P	% males in classes IV and V	35.72	6.88	36.27	0.55
F	% women in industry	15.05	12.15	17.00	1.95
L	Degrees latitude N of 50° 30′	2.40	1.21	2.40	0
G	Gross reproduction rate	0.935	0.190	0.959	0.024
D	Weighted density in persons per acre	33.66	16.20	41.36	7.70

is associated with low G) has a much more marked influence on stillbirths than on neonatal deaths, it would be expected that the effect of a given increment in reproduction rate would be much greater for stillbirths than for neonatal mortality. Table 10 shows that the regression equations faithfully reproduce this aetiological differential.

Both Burns and Woodbury found that postnatal mortality was lowest in first babies and increased steadily with birth-rank. Woodbury gives mortality rate by parity for each month of infancy, and from his figures it is possible to calculate the ratio that mortality at all parities bears to mortality of first-born in the periods corresponding to 1Q (second and third months), 2Q, 3Q and 4Q in Table 10. The ratios are 1.26, 1.54, 1.32 and 1.22, showing a maximum in the second quarter. The figures for the effect of G in Table 10 are also at a maximum in the second quarter.

The equations display a negative effect for D in relation to stillbirths, neonatal deaths, congenital causes and other causes; precisely the categories in which mortality rates for London are lower than for other localities. London has a higher D value than anywhere else in the country, 90.4 – nearly three times the mean of the county boroughs, and considerably higher than the largest individual value among the boroughs. London is also the most extensive built-up area, and there is a marked association between high D and large size of conurbation. This is brought out in Table 11, which shows the unweighted and the weighted mean value of each social index in the county boroughs. As in Table 4, the difference between the two kinds of mean is a measure of the association between the index and population size. It will be seen that H (crowding in the house) tends to be only very slightly greater in large than in small boroughs. The difference between the two means − 0.71 − is a small

fraction of the unweighted mean, which is 27.49. Similarly, P, F and G are a little higher in the more populous boroughs, L is indifferent and U is on the whole slightly excessive in the smaller municipalities. But D shows an excess of 7.70 – nearly 23 per cent – of its weighted over its unweighted mean. It is therefore quite highly associated with population size. Woolf and Waterhouse (1945) have previously discussed the feasibility of an index expressing size of built-up area, but were unable to devise a suitable measure. Now it happens that the index D is a fairly good measure of size of built-up area. In interpreting the role of D in the various equations, one must bear in mind that it expresses two social phenomena: close packing of population and, less efficiently, size of conurbation.

Although the negative coefficients for D may have been unexpected, they are seen to be consistent with other data. After due allowance has been made for other variables, the larger and more closely packed a conurbation, the lower its rates for stillbirths, neonatal mortality, congenital causes and other causes. Therefore London, the largest and most closely packed area, has an exceptionally low rate for each of these categories of mortality. On the other hand, the D effect is positive for postnatal mortality, for infectious diseases and bronchitis and pneumonia, and especially for diarrhoea. In all these cases, London has a rate markedly above that for the rural areas.

It is now possible, and necessary, to attempt to group the social indices into aetiological categories, and this is done in Table 12. It is reasonable to suppose that the mortality from these diseases will depend on two processes: (1) exposure to infection, which will determine the case-incidence; (2) case-fatality rate, which will vary with the stamina and resistance of the infected infants. Probability of infection will be positively associated with

Table 12 Mortality rates associated with social indices grouped into aetiological categories

	'Better-off' rate K	Crowding H & D	Poverty U & P	Size of family G	Work by women F	Latitude L	Total expl.
IM	26.81	10.42	14.10	4.02	6.13	5.12	39.79
STI	25.66	0.06	23.01	−7.52	2.93	0.34	18.82
IM + STI	52.47	10.48	37.11	−3.50	9.06	5.46	58.61
CON	19.81	1.92	6.21	−0.12	2.75	2.36	13.12
INF	0.21	1.19	1.38	0.45	0.43	0.19	3.64
B & P	0.03	3.53	5.51	2.63	1.91	0.63	14.21
DIA	2.00	3.11	−2.94	1.86	0.96	0.55	3.54
OTH	4.74	0.61	3.89	−0.72	0.16	1.31	5.25
Total	26.79	10.36	14.05	4.10	6.21	5.04	39.76
DAY	9.07	1.51	−0.53	−0.38	0.81	0.46	1.87
WK	7.45	0.20	2.88	−0.82	0.82	1.8	4.88
MON	3.38	1.91	2.49	0.18	0.72	1.07	6.37
1Q	3.98	1.25	2.93	0.91	0.96	0.64	6.69
2Q	2.09	1.81	2.10	1.65	0.89	0.74	7.19
3Q	1.34	2.10	0.95	1.40	1.13	0.34	5.92
4Q	−0.27	1.82	2.90	1.15	0.81	−0.02	6.66
Total	27.04	10.60	13.72	4.09	6.14	5.03	39.58
NEO	19.90	3.62	4.84	−1.02	2.35	3.33	13.12
POST	7.14	6.98	8.88	5.11	3.79	1.70	26.46

H (the crowding of the house), D (the size and density of the herd) and G, which measures the extra risk when the crowding is by other children rather than adults. There is some independent evidence on each of these points. Halliday (1928) found that pre-school children from Glasgow tenements were four times more likely to be infected with measles than those in good-class residential areas. Wright and Wright (1942), studying the incidence of diphtheria, measles and whooping-cough in London boroughs, found that a low mean age of infection was highly correlated with substandard housing, while the association with poverty was much lower. Cheeseman, Martin and Russell (1939) gave reasons for attributing the rise in the age-incidence of diphtheria during the present century to the steady diminution of mean family size, with a consequent lessened exposure of infants to infection by other children; and the same arguments would doubtless apply to the other infectious diseases. It seems likely that female employment (index F) is also partly a measure of increased exposure to infection, as babies whose mothers go to work are left in the care of neighbours or family. Such infants would be exposed during the day to an artificial loading of the H effect – crowding in the home – and the G effect – crowding by other children – with a consequent increased liability to infection.

Once infected, the baby's chance of survival would depend upon a number of circumstances, including: (a) its state of nutrition; (b) the quality of the care and nursing it received; and (c) its prenatal and postnatal history, and especially whether it was born prematurely.

All such effects would be quite efficiently measured by the poverty indices, U and P. While there is a paucity of direct studies on the relation between nutrition in infants and their case-mortality from infectious diseases, there is abundant indirect evidence, and a consensus of opinion among medical authorities (Cruickshank, 1945; Spence, 1933; Young, 1945), that the nutritional aspect is of very great importance.

It seems probable that premature babies will be less able than full-term infants to recover from infectious diseases; but here again direct evidence is scarce. There are several studies, including those quoted by Crosse (1945), showing that premature babies have a very high mortality during the neonatal period. Woodbury (1925) found that premature infants also had a 50 per cent higher death-rate from respiratory diseases and a 120 per cent higher rate from infectious diseases than babies born at full term. It will be shown below that prematurity is probably largely influenced by the poverty indices, U and P, and relatively little by the crowding indices. It is also appreciably influenced by F, so that part of the effect of F in the equations for INF and B & P may be ascribed to the

Table 13 Percentages of 'explained' deaths from infectious diseases and bronchitis and pneumonia associated with the social indices

	INF (per cent)		B & P (per cent)	
Exposure to Infection				
H	22		23	
D	11		2	
H + D		33		25
G	12		19	
H + D + G		45		44
Resistance				
U	8		20	
P	30		19	
U + P		38		39
F	12		13	
L	5		4	
Total	100		100	

deleterious effect of female labour, acting on the child through the mother.

In default of the full scientific inquiry, the regression equations allow of an estimate of the relative importance of the various social agencies in relation to mortality from infectious diseases and bronchitis and pneumonia. From Tables 10 and 12 it will be seen that in both cause groups the contribution of the poverty indices (U and P) is rather greater than that of the crowding indices (H and D), though if G is included as an element in the crowding complex the order is reversed. The relative influence is more clearly brought out in Table 13, where the contribution to the mean mortality of each index, as given in Table 10, is expressed as a percentage of the total explained mortality in the two cause groups. It will be seen that the indices expressing exposure to infection account for 44 and 45 per cent of the respective mortalities, and those associated with resistance for 38 and 39 per cent. The conjecture of Spence, that the two aspects are of about equal importance, is supported by the equations. Within the exposure complex there is a difference between the two cause groups. In the infectious diseases, the size of density of the herd, expressed by D, is of more weight than in the respiratory diseases which, however, are more strongly influenced by G, infection by other children in the home. In the resistance complex, also, bronchitis and pneumonia appear to be the more strongly influenced by extreme poverty, as measured by U. All these differences are consistent with the known aetiology of these diseases, and with their relative mortalities in social classes and in the different types of locality, as shown in Figures 1, 2 and 3. The F

effect is about the same in each group, and the small L effect will be discussed later.

The aetiological picture for stillbirths to be deduced from Tables 10 and 12 is easily summarized; the big effects are large positive contributions by the poverty indices, U and P, and a large negative effect associated with G, small families being more subject to the biological risks attaching to first births and older mothers. There is also a substantial extra mortality when the mother works in industry. The positive influence of poverty outweighs the negative effect of G, so on the whole stillbirths are higher among the poor. But the disparity between rich and poor is much less than for infectious diseases, where poverty and large families act in the same direction with respect to mortality.

All these relationships are in accord with independent evidence or currently held specialist opinion. The modern view on the relation between maternal nutrition and child health is summed up by Young (1945) as follows:

> It has long been known that the pregnant state results in a marked increase in food requirements and the greatest demand for food occurs during the last months when the growth curves of the foetus and of the maternal organs are at the steepest. It was for long believed that the foetus was protected against the influence of undernourishment in an undernourished mother by drawing almost indefinitely on the mother's tissues. Animal-breeders, on the contrary, have long recognized that the health and vigour of the offspring are critically dependent on the antenatal nutrition of the mother animal. The Toronto (1941), Oslo (1939), and People's League of Health (1942) investigations in London suggest that the same holds true in the human field. Thus there is now a considerable body of evidence to suggest that the standard of the antenatal nutrition of the mother influences the incidence of prematurity and stillbirth and that in the poorer sections of the community prematurity and stillbirth of the antenatal origin are commoner than in the higher economic grades (Baird, 1945; Report on Infant Mortality in Scotland, 1943; Ebbs, Tisdall, and Scott, 1941).

To the references quoted by Young one may add a paper by Theobald (1946), who puts forward the reasons for regarding toxaemias of pregnancy, which so often result in stillbirth or premature birth of the infant, as largely determined by deficiencies in the maternal diet extending over the whole period of parturition.

The F effect in neonatal deaths is consistent with the figures for infant mortality by occupation of father in

1930–2, given by the Registrar-General (DS, 1931). For example, in his comments on mortality among babies of textile workers, he says:

> Skilled textile workers (Class III) recorded an infant mortality rate of 69.7, significantly above the class average of 57.6, and most of the excess was for deaths occurring within four weeks of birth, the rate being 38.6 per 1000, compared with 29.4 for Class III as a whole. The causes in excess were congenital causes, premature birth and injury at birth . . . The frequent employment of the wives of textile workers in the same occupations as their husbands is probably mainly responsible for this and also for the high rates of neonatal mortality in both III and IV.

No figures are available for stillbirths by occupation of father, but it is reasonable to suppose that increased liability to prematurity and injury at birth among babies of textile workers would entail also an enhanced rate of stillbirths.

It remains to account for the negative influence of D, the measure of close packing of population and size of conurbation. The only possible interpretation seems to be that in the more populous and densely settled conurbations there is a greater quantity and quality of assistance and care available to a woman before, during and immediately after childbirth. Probably there will be a larger proportion of babies born in hospitals and maternity homes. Certainly the marked superiority of Greater London as compared with the rest of the country, shown in Figure 3 – stillbirths about 8.5 per 1000 below the England and Wales figure, and neonatal deaths about six units below – while perhaps partly attributable to relatively greater prosperity, must in the main be ascribed to better medical and social services. In contrast, neonatal mortality among the babies of coalminers, who mainly live in small communities with bad medical and social facilities is exceptionally high. In 1930–2 the figures were 38 per 1000 for coalminers in class III, and 40 for those in classes IV and V, as compared with rates of 29.4, 31.9 and 32.5 for classes III, IV, and V as a whole. In this connection it must be remembered that a large proportion of neonatal deaths, whether ascribed to prematurity or not, occur among premature infants (Crosse, 1945). The chance that a miner's baby will die in its first month is more than 50 per cent higher than the risk to a baby in London of like social class. This gives some idea of the possible reduction of neonatal mortality by improved nutrition and infant care. Such improved conditions might be expected to effect an even bigger reduction in stillbirths. Woolf and Waterhouse tried without success to construct an index measuring

efficiency of maternal and child welfare services. It seems that D can be regarded as fulfilling, though probably not very efficiently, this function, at any rate so far as stillbirths and neonatal deaths are concerned.

The diarrhoea equation is the only one among the cause groups that seems to require a revision of current views on aetiology. All the indices presumably concerned with exposure to infection – H, F, G and D – have substantial positive coefficients, and the two poverty indices – U and P – are credited with a negative influence. Diarrhoea spreads very rapidly among young babies, especially when they are massed in institutions. However, the equation implies that, at equal degrees of exposure to infection, babies in poorer families are less likely than those in better-off homes to succumb to diarrhoea. If this were true, it would explain the high diarrhoea mortality in London. One must reconsider the aetiology of diarrhoea; the various infective conditions lumped under this heading have changed enormously in relative importance in the last few decades. The former epidemics of infantile diarrhoea which flared up in the late summer of hot dry years have now almost ceased, and diarrhoea mortality is very little higher in the summer than in the winter. There was good evidence that the old epidemic diarrhoea was much more deadly to bottle fed than to breast fed babies. The consensus of clinical opinion seems to be that this is still true, but convincing statistically controlled proof is lacking. There is no evidence, either, to suggest that well-to-do babies are less frequently breast fed than those in poorer homes. The indications are rather to the contrary. In view of the precision with which the regression equations for the other cause groups have fitted in with the independent evidence on aetiology, and of the agreement between the equation for diarrhoea and the high mortality in London, it seems that there is a serious case for further investigation.

The next step is to integrate the aetiological picture of stillbirths and infant mortality as suggested by the equations regarded as a whole. In the case of stillbirths, the various social agencies can act on the child only through the mother; and this is largely the case also during the neonatal period. In stillbirths the important influences seem to be: (1) the biological risk, particularly to first births and births to older mothers; (2) the poverty risk (maternal malnutrition); (3) the labour risk (mother working in industry).

The biological risk, denoted by a negative coefficient for G, can be diminished by increasing family size and lowering the age of maternity. As shown by the negative coefficient for D and the contrast between London and the rest of the country, it is also highly amenable to reduction by better social services and obstetric care. Baird (1945) estimates that stillbirth rates can be reduced to 10 per 1000 from the present level of about 40. The scope for improvement in the field of nutrition is shown by wartime experience, a most substantial reduction having been observed which must be attributed to improved feeding of mothers by the virtual abolition of unemployment, the raising of the wage standards of the lowest-paid workers, and the provisions of special dietary supplements. The possibilities are made the more striking by the fact that wartime diets and wage rates still left much to be desired. The labour risk refers to the conditions under which pregnant women worked before the war, mainly in the textile and pottery industries. There is good ground for believing that better antenatal care and cessation of work at an adequate interval before the birth of the child can reduce this risk.

The neonatal risks are similar to those for stillbirths, except that the housing index assumes some importance. This may perhaps be attributed to three aetiological effects: (1) the less efficient care that a baby would be able to receive in bad and overcrowded dwellings; (2) the risk of infection of the child itself; (3) the increased mortality risk to the baby if its mother is ill at the time of birth. The probable existence of such an effect on the child through the mother is indicated by the fact that death-rates attributed to prematurity are higher in winter than in summer, and that neonatal deaths seem to be positively associated with the prevalence of influenza (Registrar-General, Text, 1934).

High stillbirth and neonatal rates are almost certainly associated with high incidence of prematurity. If premature babies, and those full-time infants enfeebled at birth through maternal malnutrition, are more liable than more fortunately born infants to die of infectious diseases in the postnatal period, then part of the crowding and poverty coefficients for the infectious groups of diseases and for postnatal deaths must be assigned to malnutrition of the mother before birth and bad housing in the neonatal period. That adverse conditions prenatally and immediately after birth have a persistent influence in the life of the child long afterwards is shown by a special study made by the Registrar-General (Text, 1934), who found that winter-born children had an excess mortality over the summer-born of 14 per cent in the first year of life and 42 per cent in the second.

Babies who survive the ordeal of birth and the relatively sheltered neonatal period begin to be directly affected by their environment. Crowding in the house (H), especially by other children, whether their own sibs (G) or their neighbours (F), increases their risk of infection. Any good effect associated with better medical and social care in large conurbations is more than neutralized by the action of the large, densely packed herd as an infective reservoir. But they are still subject to the influence of social conditions on their mothers. Not only do they carry the handicap of prematurity or feebleness if their mothers were overworked or malnourished, but they also suffer from past and current maternal malnutrition or illness as these conditions determine the quantity and quality of mother's milk, and whether they shall be breast fed at all. Any social index which is important in stillbirths or neonatal deaths, through its effect directly on the mother, will continue to show a like, though diminishing, effect in the equations for the various categories of postnatal deaths.

In an attempt at an aetiological explanation of the latitude effect Woolf and Waterhouse gave reasons for believing that L, in the equations for infant mortality, is not an expression primarily of climate acting directly on the baby, but rather of the generalized poverty, which increases in England and Wales as one travels north. If L denoted greater influence of infectious disease, one would expect it to have a high coefficient in the equations for POST and for INF, B & P and DIA, and a low one for NEO, CON and OTH. But Table 10 shows that the contrary is the case. The L index has a big effect on neonatal deaths and on congenital and other causes – mainly non-infective conditions – and a small influence on the infantile infections. It is twice as important in the neonatal as in the postnatal period. In the first three months of life (NEO plus 1Q) it increases the mean rate by 3.97. In the successive quarters its contribution is 0.74 and 0.34, fading to zero in the last three months of infancy. This is what one would expect of an index that expressed an aetiological determinant not affecting the baby directly, but acting on it through the mother. Since L is of minor importance to the stillbirth rate, it must be an indication of something connected with birth or neonatal life. When the influence of all the other social indices is discounted there must be an extra hazard connected with being born in the north as compared with the south. This may plausibly be attributed to one or more of the following possibilities:

1 Greater incidence of maternal illness at childbirth, due to more severe climatic conditions and/or lower standard of resistance among women arising from generalized poverty not fully measured by the other indices.
2 Greater unfitness of mothers for child-bearing, attributable to: (a) poorer housing (not measurable by the index of crowding); (b) cumulative effects of female employment before and after marriage; (c) effect of life-long malnutrition, and especially lack of vitamin D

on the reproductive system; (d) migration of healthier women to more prosperous areas, leaving an undue proportion of the less fit.

3 Less efficient care of mother and newborn child, due to bad household facilities, social traditions and maternal efficiency, and/or to inferior medical and social circumstances. In so far as this explanation is true, L can be regarded as supplementing D as a measure of maternal and child care.

A final evaluation of these tentative suggestions cannot be made without special investigation. But, whatever the exact mechanism may be, latitude must be regarded primarily as an index of conditions acting on the baby through the mother. Any direct effect on the baby is probably of secondary importance.

From Tables 10 and 12 one can form an estimate of the relative importance of the various social agencies with respect to the total loss of infant life. The chief indications are as follows:

1 For infant mortality, poverty, presumably mainly malnutrition, contributes about 14.1, bulking rather larger than crowding, which is responsible for about 10.4 out of the difference between the 'better-off' and the mean rate.

2 In stillbirths, however, crowding is of little importance, while poverty adds about 23.0 to the rate.

3 In the IM + STI equation, measuring total reproduction wastage, poverty consequently appears nearly four times as important as housing. Elimination of malnutrition might be expected to reduce the combined mortality rate in county boroughs by about 37 units, and levelling up of housing by about 10.5 units.

4 When the other social indices are allowed for, infant mortality increases with mean family size, the negative effect in the neonatal period being more than counterbalanced by the increased risk of infection during the remainder of the period of infancy. But when infant mortality is combined with stillbirths, the net G effect is negative. If the mean family size could be increased without concomitant aggravation of overcrowding or poverty, one would expect a smaller and not a larger wastage of infant life.

5 The computed total rate at the 'better-off' level is about 52.5, almost equally divided between stillbirths and infant mortality. This is less than half the observed rate of 111.1. More than half the mortality can be regarded as preventable.

It is of interest to inquire how closely the deductions from the equations fit in with wartime experience. The data allow only a very rough comparison; no figures are available for individual municipalities, but only a summary for the whole country. Nor is there any basis for assessing alterations in the social variables. It seems highly probable, however, that the most important change during the war was the levelling up of the standard of nutrition by the virtual abolition of unemployment, the increase in earnings and measures taken by the Ministry of Food. The changes in mortality rates (1938–44) can be compared with those to be expected by the abolition of conditions of extreme poverty, as measured by the index U. The relevant data are shown in Table 14. It will be seen that stillbirth rates fell steadily, neonatal rates rose in 1940 and 1941 but otherwise showed a marked fall, and postnatal rates were more erratic, as would be expected from their dependence on various epidemic periodicities. At the foot of each column is the difference between the rates for 1938 and 1944, compared with the reduction, as shown in Table 10, to be expected by equating the index U to zero. It will be seen that the two figures are remarkably close. However, the figures in Table 10 refer to county boroughs at the average conditions for 1928–38, whereas the figures in Table 14 relate to the whole country during a time of profound social upheaval, so care should be taken in their interpretation. Nevertheless Table 14 does seem to afford some additional evidence of the general validity of the method of analysis used in this paper.

It must be emphasized that these aetiological deductions are not in any sense to be regarded as mathematically demonstrated. The equations show that the mortality of a county borough can be calculated, with a fairly high degree of precision, from the numerical values of its social indices. The interpretation of the equations depends not on mathematical but on social and medical considerations. The explanations sketched out above must be judged as scientific hypotheses, the criteria being:

Their internal consistency in relation to the phenomena of infant mortality.

Their degree of concordance with other independent evidence, and with clinical and social knowledge and experience.

The extent to which they throw light on observations taken from a wider field – as, for example, the pattern of mortality in London.

The extent to which they suggest profitable lines of further investigation, and are confirmed by the results of such researches.

I wish to lay stress on the last of these criteria; many of

Table 14 Stillbirths and infant mortality in England and Wales during the war

Year	Stillbirths	Infant mortality	Neonatal	Postnatal
1938	39.8	52.7	28.3	24.4
1939	39.6	50.6	28.3	22.3
1940	38.6	56.8	29.6	27.2
1941	36.0	60.0	29.0	31.0
1942	34.3	50.6	27.2	23.4
1943	31.0	49.1	25.2	23.9
1944	28.5	45.7	24.5	21.2
Fall since 1938	11.3	7.0	3.8	3.2
Mortality ascribed to U (Table 10)	10.5	8.6	3.4	5.1

the topics touched on call for special *ad hoc* field investigations. It may be claimed that the equations present a consistent aetiological picture; but the full validification of many of the conclusions must await further surveys and inquiries. If the statistical analysis here reported has done nothing more than place the various aetiological problems of infant death into clear perspective, directing attention to aspects amenable to field investigation, it will have been amply worthwhile. Wright and Wright (1942) say that the statistical method 'may be used to test deductively the general applicability of hypotheses based upon field observations, by finding how far inferences made from relatively restricted evidence are supported by statistical findings from larger sources of data.' While fully agreeing with this, I would like to draw attention to the reverse procedure – the function of statistical studies in suggesting profitable topics for field inquiries. It is only by the close interweaving of statistical and field inquiries that a true science of social medicine can be built up. It is hoped that further papers in this series will report the results of field inquiries suggested by the statistical analysis described above.[2]

The balance sheet of infant deaths

It remains to translate the regression equations into terms of actual infant deaths. Woolf and Waterhouse (1945) give detailed reasons for believing such a process is valid, at least to a first approximation, and it will certainly serve to make the meaning of the equations more concrete and vivid. However, in the equations as they stand all the county boroughs have been treated as of equal weight, whatever their population. The equations consequently relate to an imaginary conglomerate consisting of an equal number of babies from each county borough. In order to correct for this, one must use in the computations

the weighted values given in Tables 4 and 12. To do so in detail would involve slight adjustments to all the figures shown in Table 10 but the only change of relevance is in the value of K, the computed mortality rate at the arbitrary 'better-off' level. Weighting makes no material amendment to the results for stillbirths and neonatal deaths. For total infant mortality, the K value is raised by about two units, almost all confined to the postnatal period and to the three zymotic-cause groups, the biggest increase being observed in diarrhoea. Size of population is obviously a social variable that must be taken into account in order to obtain an undistorted picture of the aetiology of deaths from infection, even among the better-off strata. The weighted K figures for cause groups and periods are probably more realistic than the unweighted values. The negative sign for the 4Q equation is reversed, and the very low figures for INF and B & P are raised to a more likely level.

The balance sheet of infant deaths is shown in Table 15. In each category of mortality the total number of deaths in the county boroughs during the eleven-year period is given, rounded off to the nearest hundred, together with the 'unexplained' deaths, the computed number that would have been expected if each social index had been at the 'better-off' level. The difference between the total and the unexplained deaths is divided up according to the calculated influence of the various social agencies. Thus, in the first column relating to total infant mortality, the estimate of lives that would have been saved by the elimination of crowding is 25 700; by elimination of poverty, 32 700; and so on. In the stillbirth column the minus signs indicate that reduction of the size of family and of crowding to the better-off standard, keeping other conditions unchanged, would have been expected to lead to *more* deaths. Out of the 266 300 stillbirths and infant deaths more than half (138 600) are to be regarded as having been preventable by improvement in social

Table 15 Balance sheet of infant deaths, county boroughs, 1928–1938

	Infant mortality	Stillbirths	Total	Neonatal	Postnatal	Congenital causes	Infectious diseases, bronchitis and pneumonia	Diarrhoea	Other causes
Crowding (H & D)	25 700	−1800	23 900	7200	18 500	3500	12 200	8500	1500
Poverty (U & P)	32 700	53 600	86 300	11 500	21 200	14 500	16 100	−6900	9000
Size of family (G)	10 200	−18 800	−8600	−2600	12 800	−300	7700	4700	−1900
Work by mother (F)	16 500	7800	24 300	6300	10 200	7300	6200	2500	500
Latitude (L)	11 900	800	12 700	7900	4000	5600	1900	1300	3100
Total explained	97 000	41 600	138 600	30 300	66 700	30 600	44 100	10 100	12 200
Unexplained	67 400	60 300	127 700	46 600	20 800	46 700	2900	6300	11 500
Total deaths	164 400	101 900	266 300	76 900	87 500	77 300	47 000	16 400	23 700
Per cent explained	59.0	40.8	52.0	39.4	76.2	39.6	93.8	61.6	51.5

conditions, and, of these, 86 300, or more than three-fifths, could have been averted by raising earnings. Over 30 000 neonatal deaths and 66 000 postnatal deaths are calculated to have been preventable, the latter figure including over 44 000 deaths from infectious diseases and bronchitis and pneumonia.

The equations have been used to give an estimate of mortality at one postulated social level – the 'better-off', as defined above. Two other social strata are of special interest – the poorly paid crowded section of the working class, and those living permanently at the level of pre-war unemployment relief. For the first of these, both H and P must be equated to 100 per cent, and U to zero; for the second, H, P and U must each be put at 100 per cent. Plausible values were also chosen for the other indices (F = 0, G = 1.6, D = 80 and L = mean latitude of county boroughs).

The computed mortality rates at these social levels are shown in Table 16, and compared with the 'better-off' figure (weighted K) and the weighted mean for county boroughs. The rates for the crowded poor and the unemployed crowded poor are also shown as percentages of the weighted mean.

It will be seen that the poor have a computed infant mortality rate of 97.8, or 39 per cent, above the mean. Owing to their postulated larger size of family, their expected stillbirth rate is substantially lower than the mean (37.7). Their computed total reproductive loss is 119 per cent of the average. But the unemployed poor show both an infant mortality and a stillbirth rate of double the mean figure. This excess mortality occurs chiefly in the postnatal period and in the infectious and bronchitis and pneumonia cause groups. In the category of other causes, extreme poverty, as measured by U, has

the effect of doubling the computed rate. Bronchitis and pneumonia, and to a lesser extent infectious diseases and congenital causes, also show a material rise with increase in degree of poverty. Table 16 may usefully be compared with Table 4. The highest county borough showed an infant mortality of 97.6, closely similar to the figure for the crowded poor. The lowest rate was 41.9. Since even the most prosperous county borough contains a substantial proportion of crowded, low-paid and unemployed inhabitants, and the most badly off borough has many comparatively prosperous families, the extremes of the rates in individual boroughs cannot be expected to display the full range of mortality risks between the various strata of the population. The ratio of the best to the worst county borough for infant mortality is 2.3; the range between 'better-off' and 'unemployed crowded poor' in Table 16 gives a ratio of 4.9:1. For stillbirths the corresponding figures are: observed ratio among boroughs, 2.1; calculated ratio between social extremes, 3.5. The range of variation shown in Table 16 is of the order of magnitude one would infer from a study of Table 4, and a knowledge of the mixed social composition of all the county boroughs.

The big differences between the computed mortality rates for the 'crowded poor' and the 'unemployed crowded poor' is noteworthy. It indicates that, below a given level, small decreases in income, involving depreciation in the level of nutrition and other human needs, have disproportionately large effects in increasing mortality, and presumably also in adversely affecting the physique and stamina of the survivors. Conversely, any effort at social betterment may be expected to have the greatest effect in reducing mortality and morbidity if it is preferentially applied to raising the standards of the most

Table 16 Estimated mortality rates in crowded poor and unemployed crowded poor strata of population

	'Better-off'	Weighted mean	Crowded poor	Unemployed crowded poor	Percentage of weighted mean	
					Crowded poor	Unemployed crowded poor
IM	28.9	70.4	97.8	141.0	139	200
STI	25.8	43.6	37.7	91.1	86	209
IM + STI	53.7	114.0	135.5	232.1	119	204
CON	20.0	33.1	37.1	52.4	112	159
INF	0.7	4.7	9.4	10.9	201	234
B & P	0.6	15.4	28.9	43.6	187	283
DIA	2.7	7.0	12.8	11.0	182	156
OTH	4.9	10.2	9.6	23.1	94	227
NEO	19.9	32.9	36.6	53.8	111	164
POST	9.0	37.5	61.2	87.2	163	233

unfortunate section of the population. The difference between the last two columns in Table 16 is a sufficient explanation of the dramatic reduction in stillbirth and infant mortality rates during the war, when limited resources were so used as to reduce the pre-war disparity in satisfaction of biological needs among the different income grades of the population.

It is important to bear in mind the limitations of the regression method; any relevant circumstances that affect all places more or less equally cannot enter into the calculations. Since 1900, infant mortality has fallen by about two-thirds, but the relative disparity between the best and the worst places, or between the social classes, has remained remarkably steady. The equations can display how, at one particular period, differences in mortality rates are bound up with variations in social conditions. They cannot directly deal with the effect of the changing social background in lowering the level of mortality for rich and poor alike. The equations indicate that, at any given general level of social progress, the differences in mortality between different strata of the population are largely conditioned by disparities in material environment, and could presumably be diminished by levelling up of social conditions. In this paper an attempt has been made, by comparisons between county boroughs and other types of area, to obtain some estimate of the potency of these general social agencies. It is beyond question that conscious social effort, whether direct as in maternity and child welfare services, or indirect as in universal education, has played a major part in diminishing loss of infant life, and that there is scope for further improvement in the future. But there is also abundant evidence that, at any given time in the past,

variations from the general level of mortality were associated with crowding, malnutrition, industrial employment of women and size of family, with relative effects qualitatively if not quantitatively similar to those obtaining in county boroughs during 1928–38. To reduce infant mortality to the unavoidable minimum it is necessary both to improve the general social, medical and sanitary background and to ensure to each mother and baby the best possible material chance by levelling up social and economic conditions. For the immediate future, it is probable that the equations are a fairly reliable quantitative guide to the degree of reduction in infant deaths to be expected by alteration of this or that feature of the social environment. Similar equations calculated ten or twenty years hence might give different values to the coefficients associated with each social agency. But so long as disparities exist in environment at different social levels, it seems likely that there will continue to be differences in mortality rates bound up with variations in standards of housing, nutrition and other relevant conditions, acting for each category of mortality in the direction indicated by the regression equations.

Notes

1 A section on methods of computation has been omitted here.
2 A discussion of the lack of a suitable test of statistical significance is omitted here.

References

Baird, D. (1945) *J. Obstet. Gynaec. Brit. Emp.*, 52, 217, 339.

Burns, C.M. (1942). *Infant and Maternal Mortality*, Durham.

Charles, E. (1938). Article in *Political Arithmetic*, ed. Hogben, L. London.

Cheeseman, E.A., Martin, W.J., and Russell, W.T. (1939) *J. Hyg.*, Camb., 39, 181.

Crosse, V.M. (1945). *The Premature Baby*, London.

Cruickshank, R. (1945). *Arch. Dis. Childh.*, 20, 145.

Ebbs, J.H., Tisdall, F.F. and Scott, W.A. (1941) *J. Nutrit.*, 22, 515.

Fisher, R.A. (1940) *Ann. Eugen.*, 10, 422.

Halliday, J.L. (1928). *Med. Res. Concl. Sp. Rep. Ser.*, No. 120. London.

Orr, J.B. et al. (1943). *Infant Mortality in Scotland*, HMSO, Edinburgh.

Registrar-General. All references give date to which report refers, not date of publication. Abbreviations: AR, Annual Review; DS, Decennial Supplement (Occupational Mortality); Text, Text Volume of Annual Review.

Spence, J.C. (1933). Annual Report, Min. of Health, 214. London.

Theobald, G.W. (1946) *J. Obstet. Gynaec. Brit. Emp.*, 53, 17.

Woodbury, R.M. (1925). *Causal Factors in Infant Mortality*, Children's Bureau, Washington, DC.

Woolf, B. and Waterhouse, J. (1945) *J. Hyg.*, Camb., 44, 67.

Wright, G.P. and Wright, H.P. (1942) Ibid., 42, 451.

Wright G.P. and Wright H.P. (1945) Ibid., 44, 15.

Young, J. (1945) *Med. Off.*, 74, 119, 127.

Acknowledgement

Woolf, B. (1946) Studies on infant mortality. Part II. Social aetiology of stillbirths and infant deaths in county boroughs of England and Wales. *British Journal of Social Medicine*, 2, 73–125.

4 *Professor Martin Gardner*

Gardner, M.J., Snee, M.P., Hall, A.J., Powell, C.A., Downes, S. and Terrell, J.D. (1990) Results of case–control study of leukaemia and lymphoma among young people near Sellafield nuclear plant in West Cumbria. *British Medical Journal*, 300, 423–9.

INTRODUCTION
Introduction written by Dr Hazel Inskip, MRC Environmental Epidemiology Unit, University of Southampton

Windscale: the Nuclear Laundry, a television programme shown in 1983, gave rise to enormous public concern. It focused on a cluster of childhood leukaemia cases near the Sellafield nuclear plant (formerly known as Windscale) in West Cumbria, and particularly in the neighbouring village of Seascale. The government appointed a committee under the chairmanship of Sir Douglas Black to investigate this issue. The cluster was found to represent a real excess of cases rather than an artefact based on anecdotal evidence. The committee recommended a number of further studies, three of which were undertaken by Gardner and colleagues at the MRC Environmental Epidemiology Unit. Two cohort studies of children born and children attending schools in Seascale[1,2] showed that the excess was confined to those children born in the village. The case–control study of leukaemias and lymphomas in the wider region of West Cumbria was conducted to examine a variety of factors which might explain the excess.

The detailed methods of the case–control study are described in an accompanying paper.[3] In total, 97 cases of leukaemia and lymphoma born in West Cumbria and diagnosed there between 1950 and 1985 under the age of 25 were studied along with 1001 matched controls. Information was collected on possible exposure factors from questionnaires sent to the parents, from hospital records and from records held at the nuclear plant, with interest inevitably focusing on environmental and occupational radiation exposures. The startling result of an association between the father's radiation dose prior to conception of the child and the child's subsequent risk of leukaemia gave rise to a major controversy.

Interpretation of results such as these is not straightforward. The main findings were based on very small numbers, with only four cases of leukaemia having fathers who were in the highest exposure category. Such an association had not been found before in any population studied and there was almost no evidence from animal experiments. Geneticists and radiobiologists argue over the biological plausibility of the findings and epidemiologists are divided as to how they should be interpreted. It may be that some associated exposure is the root cause, of which external radiation exposure is a surrogate measure. Others argue that there is something in the Seascale environment that is to blame, or that the influx of newcomers to the area to work at the plant has brought increased exposure to an infectious agent. Further studies around other nuclear sites where clusters have been observed have given little or no support to the hypothesis.

This paper has featured prominently in a court action brought against British Nuclear Fuels, which operates the Sellafield plant. Many epidemiologists have re-worked the analyses and examined the data collection process. Therefore, this study has received much greater scrutiny than most. Although some aspects of the study have been hotly debated, the association remains.

The concern of the public and in particular of nuclear workers demands an explanation. This study has generated a hypothesis; researchers across many disciplines are attempting to explain or refute it.

References

1 Gardner, M.J., Hall, A.J., Downes, S. and Terrell J.D. (1987) Follow up study of children born elsewhere but attending schools in Seascale, West Cumbria (schools cohort). *British Medical Journal* 295, 819–22.

2 Gardner, M.J., Hall, A.J., Downes, S. and Terrell, J.D. (1987) Follow up study of children born to mothers resident in Seascale, West Cumbria (birth cohort). *British Medical Journal*, 295, 822–7.

3 Gardner, M.J., Hall, A.J., Snee, M.P., Downes, S., Powell, C.A. and Terrell, J.D. (1990) Methods and basic data for case–control study of leukaemia and lymphoma among young people near Sellafield nuclear plant in West Cumbria. *British Medical Journal*, 300, 429–34.

RESULTS OF CASE–CONTROL STUDY OF LEUKAEMIA AND LYMPHOMA AMONG YOUNG PEOPLE NEAR SELLAFIELD NUCLEAR PLANT IN WEST CUMBRIA

Introduction

There has been concern about levels of childhood cancer around nuclear installations in the United Kingdom since 1983, when a Yorkshire Television programme (*Windscale: the Nuclear Laundry*) suggested that there was an excess of leukaemia near Sellafield. Several studies have been carried out since,[1] and the one reported here was a

direct consequence of a recommendation of the Black Committee (of which MJG was a member).[2] This investigation was a case–control study of leukaemia and lymphoma among young people in West Cumbria specifically asking whether known causes or factors associated with the nuclear site might have been responsible for the observed excess.

Methods

The design of the study, methods of data collection and basic information are described in detail in the accompanying paper.[3] Essentially all identified cases of leukaemia and lymphoma among people born in West Cumbria and diagnosed there at ages under 25 during 1950–85 were compared with controls matched by sex and date of birth selected – both unmatched (area controls) and matched (local controls) for civil parish of residence – from the same birth register into which the case's birth was entered. For both types of control up to eight controls were included in the analysis for each case, some of whom were both area and local controls. Comparisons were carried out using data from birth and medical records, from questionnaires to parents, cases and controls, and from employment and radiation records held by British Nuclear Fuels.

The analysis was carried out within the sets of cases and area of local controls, and findings are presented as relative risks with confidence intervals. The results were calculated using conditional logistic regression analysis,[4] which produces estimates of odds ratios that approximate closely to relative risks, with the computer program

Table 1 Numbers of cases and controls with relative risks for leukaemia and non-Hodgkin's lymphoma in children by maternal exposure to abdominal X-rays in pregnancy according to medical records and questionnaires

Source of X-ray information	Type of control	Cases		Controls		Relative risk	95% confidence interval
		Total	No exposed to X-rays	Total	No exposed to X-rays		
Leukaemia							
Medical records	Area	20	3	116	15	1.15	0.31 to 4.28
	Local	20	3	109	13	1.21	0.31 to 4.66
Questionnaire	Area	35	4	116	9	1.74	0.44 to 6.82
	Local	34	4	104	11	1.19	0.33 to 4.31
Leukaemia and non-Hodgkin's lymphoma							
Medical records	Area	28	5	167	25	1.19	0.43 to 3.32
	Local	28	5	153	20	1.34	0.46 to 3.88
Questionnaire	Area	47	5	152	14	1.32	0.43 to 4.08
	Local	45	5	143	15	1.14	0.37 to 3.53

Table 2 Numbers of cases and controls with relative risks for leukaemia and non-Hodgkin's lymphoma in children by some suspected risk factors

Suspected risk factor	Type of control	Cases		Controls		Relative risk	95% confidence interval
		Total	Positive	Total	Positive		
Leukaemia							
Maternal viral infection in	Area	35	2	119	7	1.12	0.22 to 5.67
pregnancy	Local	35	2	103	6	1.23	0.22 to 7.04
Caesarean delivery	Area	20	2	116	8	1.38	0.27 to 6.99
	Local	20	2	109	9	1.17	0.24 to 5.81
Social class[a]	Area	44	9	293	54	1.14	0.50 to 2.60
(birth certificate)	Local	44	9	287	75	0.61	0.25 to 1.47
Social class[a] (questionnaire)	Area	20	5	51	16	0.90	0.24 to 3.34
	Local	19	5	54	21	0.60	0.17 to 2.10
Mother's age	Area	52	32	351	220	0.94	0.51 to 1.72
(≥ 25 v. < 25 years)	Local	52	32	344	213	0.96	0.52 to 1.78
Mother's age	Area	52	4	351	6	4.94	1.11 to 21.85
(≥ 40 v. < 25 years)	Local	52	4	344	8	3.38	0.88 to 13.03
Father's age	Area	46	38	287	220	1.42	0.63 to 3.18
(≥ 25 v. < 25 years)	Local	46	38	276	213	1.43	0.61 to 3.33
Father's age	Area	46	6	287	26	1.87	0.59 to 5.91
(≥ 40 v. < 25 years)	Local	46	6	276	24	2.27	0.66 to 7.76
Birth weight	Area	18	7	99	42	0.88	0.32 to 2.42
(≥ 3.5 v. < 3.5 kg)	Local	18	7	94	41	0.84	0.29 to 2.42
Leukaemia and non-Hodgkin's lymphoma							
Maternal viral infection in	Area	47	2	156	12	0.69	0.15 to 3.24
pregnancy	Local	46	2	144	8	0.94	0.18 to 4.87
Caesarean delivery	Area	28	2	167	15	0.75	0.16 to 3.56
	Local	28	2	153	11	0.95	0.20 to 4.50
Social class[a]	Area	64	14	418	75	1.33	0.68 to 2.59
(birth certificate)	Local	64	14	408	100	0.70	0.33 to 1.49
Social class[a] (questionnaire)	Area	26	7	70	20	1.11	0.34 to 3.64
	Local	25	7	75	30	0.61	0.21 to 1.79
Mother's age	Area	74	47	492	311	0.99	0.60 to 1.65
(≥ 25 v. < 25 years)	Local	74	47	484	305	0.99	0.59 to 1.66
Mother's age	Area	74	7	492	10	5.08	1.66 to 15.53
(≥ 40 v. < 25 years)	Local	74	7	484	12	4.03	1.41 to 11.52
Father's age	Area	66	52	403	318	0.95	0.50 to 1.79
(≥ 25 v. < 25 years)	Local	66	52	389	304	1.00	0.51 to 1.93
Father's age	Area	66	9	403	34	1.51	0.60 to 3.78
(≥ 40 v. < 25 years)	Local	66	9	389	34	1.58	0.60 to 4.16
Birth weight	Area	26	11	149	62	1.01	0.44 to 2.34
(≥ 3.5 v. < 3.5 kg)	Local	26	11	137	64	0.86	0.37 to 2.01

[a] Social class of father at child's birth: I, II, III non-manual v. III manual, IV, V.

EGRET.[5] Unless otherwise stated the relative risks are for presence compared with absence of each factor; where specifically mentioned in tables relative risks are for the first compared with the second grouping, except in ionising radiation dose categories, where the risks are relative to the unexposed group.

Results and comment

Findings are shown for leukaemia alone and for leukaemia and non-Hodgkin's lymphoma combined for area and local controls separately. Because some controls, who were entered closely adjacent to a case in the birth register, were both area and local controls these two analyses by control type were not completely independent statistically – for example, for the 52 leukaemia cases

Table 3 Numbers of cases and controls with relative risks for leukaemia and non-Hodgkin's lymphoma in children by family habit factors from parental questionnaire

Habit factor	Type of control	Cases		Controls		Relative risk	95% confidence interval
		Total	Positive	Total	Positive		
Leukaemia							
Play on beach (more *v.* less	Area	28	13	94	47	0.89	0.37 to 2.17
often than monthly)	Local	28	13	92	57	0.62	0.24 to 1.59
Play on fells (more *v.* less	Area	27	3	77	23	0.29	0.06 to 1.39
often than monthly)	Local	24	3	71	18	0.53	0.14 to 2.07
Eating fish (more *v.* less	Area	29	16	97	49	1.26	0.50 to 3.21
often than weekly)	Local	28	16	93	49	1.16	0.45 to 3.00
Eating shellfish (more *v.* less	Area	15	2	36	1	7.03	0.61 to 80.43
often than weekly)	Local	15	2	29	3	1.11	0.15 to 7.91
Grow own vegetables	Area	35	15	123	54	0.98	0.45 to 2.13
	Local	35	15	112	45	1.07	0.46 to 2.48
Seaweed as fertiliser	Area	11	1	25	1	1.73	0.10 to 30.76
	Local	13	1	25	1	2.00	0.13 to 31.98
Leukaemia and non-Hodgkin's lymphoma							
Play on beach (more *v.* less	Area	40	18	131	61	0.95	0.45 to 2.00
often than monthly)	Local	39	18	131	78	0.66	0.31 to 1.40
Play on fells (more *v.* less	Area	36	4	103	28	0.33	0.09 to 1.21
often than monthly)	Local	32	4	98	31	0.36	0.11 to 1.17
Eating fish (more *v.* less	Area	39	20	126	62	1.03	0.45 to 2.37
often than weekly)	Local	36	19	127	67	0.86	0.38 to 1.98
Eating shellfish (more *v.* less	Area	19	2	44	2	2.99	0.40 to 22.11
often than weekly)	Local	18	2	39	5	0.82	0.14 to 5.01
Grow own vegetables	Area	47	20	161	71	0.99	0.52 to 1.93
	Local	46	20	154	72	0.87	0.42 to 1.81
Seaweed as fertiliser	Area	15	1	30	1	1.73	0.10 to 30.76
	Local	17	1	36	1	2.00	0.13 to 31.98

there were 217 area only controls, 207 local only controls and 140 who were both. Results for non-Hodgkin's lymphoma are presented here only in combination with leukaemia. Numbers of individuals included in the analyses for different factors varied with the availability of data, and the number of case–control sets is given by the total number of cases. Results for Hodgkin's disease are not given in detail as they did not show any important associations with analysed factors in the same way as leukaemia and non-Hodgkin's lymphoma.

Ante-natal X-rays

Table 1 shows relative risks for leukaemia and non-Hodgkin's lymphoma associated with maternal abdominal radiographic examinations according to whether the information was obtained from obstetric records or questionnaire responses. The relative risks ranged from about 1.2 to 1.7, comparable to levels reported in earlier studies. This study was too small for meaningful analysis by number of films or trimester of exposure.

For cases of Hodgkin's disease a report of an abdominal X-ray examination was made for none of the six mothers for whom we located obstetric records and by two of the 12 parents who responded on the questionnaire.

Viral infections and other suspected risk factors

Only one episode of viral infectious illness during pregnancy was recorded in the hospital records examined, so analysis was restricted to data from the questionnaires. Results for any episode of chickenpox, shingles, influenza, measles or rubella are given in Table 2, with no strong finding. Also shown are relative risks, again based on small numbers, for delivery by caesarean section based on information from obstetric records.

Findings are given for social class based on occupation at birth as recorded on each of birth certificates and questionnaires, and the similar results reflect the high level of agreement between the data sources. The table shows relative risks around unity for a broad higher social class category in relation to area controls but lower values for local controls. More detailed analysis did not identify any strong trends by social class.

Relative risks around unity were also found for maternal age at birth of 25 or older compared with under 25 years. For mothers of 40 or older, however, when examined in a comparison of all age groups – that is, < 25, 25–29, 30–34, 35–39 and > 40 years – relative risks were about 4. The latter finding was much less strong for fathers. Birth weight, from obstetric records, showed no particular relation in either the broad categories listed or smaller groups.

For Hodgkin's disease there were no important relationships with any of the above factors including parental ages.

Questionnaire habit factors

Table 3 shows findings based on the behavioural data obtained by questionnaire. The factors included, particularly those for which there were data on substantial numbers of cases, did not show any important relations with leukaemia and non-Hodgkin's lymphoma. Results for playing on the beach are shown in the table with all cases for whom information was available. Children aged under 5 years at diagnosis were less likely because of their illness to have played in the sand, and excluding these cases and their controls made little difference, with the relative risks against area controls for leukaemia alone and combined with non-Hodgkin's lymphoma becoming 0.83 and 1.04 respectively. The relative risks for play on the fells were particularly low.

Analysis by fish eating habits did not indicate any associated risk. For shellfish eating the relative risks were raised compared with area controls but not compared with local controls; the raised relative risks were, however, based on only two exposed cases (both diagnosed before 1980). Restriction of these analyses to cases born during periods when discharges from Sellafield were highest did not show any important differential relative risks. Finally, there was no evidence of any increased risk in conjunction with families growing their own vegetables or using seaweed as a fertiliser.

There were no important relationships of Hodgkin's disease with these factors.

Geography of cases and controls relative to Sellafield

Distances of addresses of cases and controls from Sellafield were calculated by taking the grid reference of the plant to be NY 027 039 as used by the National Radiological Protection Board in its analysis of atmospheric discharges (J. Stather, personal communication). The results given here are for area controls using addresses at birth. Table 4 shows findings in circles of increasing 5 km radiuses moving away from Sellafield, and risks are given relative to the inner circle (which completely contains Seascale and some other smaller villages). All five cases of leukaemia and two of the three cases of non-Hodgkin's lymphoma in the inner circle occurred in children born to parents resident in Seascale. There was a large fall in relative risk in moving to outside the inner circle to levels of about one-third and smaller, with some suggestion also of a decreasing risk with further distance. For leukaemia and non-Hodgkin's lymphoma combined the relative risks away from the inner circle were lower than for leukaemia alone. The relative risk of leukaemia for all children born outside the inner circle was 0.26 (95 per cent confidence interval 0.07 to 1.01) and for leukaemia and non-Hodgkin's lymphoma together it was 0.17 (95 per cent confidence interval 0.05 to 0.53). These latter results also applied when analysis was limited to cases born in the birth registration district containing Sellafield rather than all West Cumbria. None of the 23 cases of Hodgkin's disease in the study had an address at birth within the 5 km radius inner circle. Of the 95 total cases with complete information, 79 (83 per cent) remained in the same 5 km sector from birth to diagnosis.

Father's occupation and employment at Sellafield

Three separate sources of parental occupational information were used: birth certificates, questionnaires, and the computer file of past and present workers at Sellafield. Maternal occupation is generally recorded on a birth certificate only in the absence of paternal occupation, questionnaire data were available for only about half the study members, and relatively few women have worked at Sellafield, so results given here are restricted to father's employment.

Table 5 shows the relative risks for leukaemia and non-Hodgkin's lymphoma associated with various paternal employment categories. These data were taken from birth certificates rather than questionnaires because of the greater completeness of information – for example, data for the 74 fathers of children with leukaemia and non-Hodgkin's lymphoma were available from 64 (86 per cent) birth certificates but only 32 (43 per cent) questionnaires. Results are given for the main industrial groups in West Cumbria which employed more than 5 per cent of control fathers. Raised relative risks were associated with fathers working at Sellafield and in iron and steel, farming and chemicals, with children of coal miners having low

Table 4 Numbers of cases and controls with relative risks for leukaemia and non-Hodgkin's lymphoma in children by distance from Sellafield of residence at birth for area controls

Distance (km)	Leukaemia				Leukaemia and non-Hodgkin's lymphoma			
	Cases (n = 51)	Area controls (n = 350)	Relative risk	95% confidence interval	Cases (n = 73)	Area controls (n = 491)	Relative risk	95% confidence interval
≤ 4	5	14	1		8	16	1	
5–9	5	31	0.35	0.08 to 1.62	6	43	0.21	0.06 to 0.78
10–14	14	117	0.21	0.05 to 0.92	22	160	0.17	0.05 to 0.56
15–19	5	35	0.22	0.04 to 1.22	8	50	0.16	0.04 to 0.67
20–24	9	52	0.22	0.03 to 1.59	11	84	0.07	0.01 to 0.38
25–29	8	60	0.14	0.02 to 0.91	12	100	0.06	0.01 to 0.31
≥ 30	5	35	0.17	0.02 to 1.88	6	38	0.11	0.02 to 0.80

relative risks but based on small numbers. Similar results were found using the questionnaire data and when examining employment on the questionnaire at conception rather than birth, although then relative risks were somewhat higher in relation to Sellafield and farming than those shown in Table 5.

For Hodgkin's disease the relative risks associated with fathers working at Sellafield according to data from birth certificates were low – for example, for local controls the relative risk was 0.71 (95 per cent confidence interval 0.08 to 6.03). The result was based on only one positive case, since, although we had records that four fathers altogether were Sellafield workers, for three this employment occurred after the birth of their children.

Radiation dosimetry at Sellafield

Table 6 shows relative risks for leukaemia and non-Hodgkin's lymphoma in children associated with their fathers' employment and exposure to ionising radiation obtained through linkage with the Sellafield workforce file. As well as analysing the total radiation dose recorded before conception (taken as nine months before birth) we looked at that during the immediately preceding six months, since it has been suggested that this is the most sensitive period for the induction of transmissible genetic damage.[6] The six monthly doses were estimated proportionally from the recorded annual doses of the father and the date of birth of his child.

For paternal employment at the plant relative risks were higher for leukaemia alone than for leukaemia and non-Hodgkin's lymphoma combined and were higher for employment at conception than at any other time. Relative risks for leukaemia and non-Hodgkin's lymphoma were higher for fathers with a radiation dose record at conception than for those with a radiation dose record at any time before conception or diagnosis. The highest relative risks – of the order of sixfold – were for fathers with total radiation doses of 100 mSv or greater before the date of their child's conception or doses of 10 mSv or greater during the six months before conception. Figures for all the control fathers in this study indicated that about 9 per cent of the workforce had accumulated preconceptual doses over 100 mSv and about 13 per cent had doses over 10 mSv during the six months before conception.

The results shown in Table 6 relate to all fathers in the study for whom we could make a definite positive or negative linkage to the Sellafield file. The same analysis limited to fathers positively linked to the Sellafield file showed similar relations to ionising radiation dose but with larger relative risks in the highest categories. For example, there was a relative risk of 17.2 for leukaemia compared with area controls in children of fathers with total radiation doses before conception of 100 mSv or more with a 95 per cent confidence interval of 1.1 to 278, the wide interval reflecting that the analysis was based on a total of 11 case–control sets rather than 46 as in the table.

For cases of Hodgkin's disease none of the four fathers employed at Sellafield had a record of occupational radiation exposure before their child's conception.

Seascale

Earlier studies have concentrated on the geographical excess of childhood leukaemia in the neighbourhood of the Sellafield plant. This excess was found in Seascale particularly and was based on around five cases compared with fewer than one expected, depending on

Table 5 Numbers of cases and controls with relative risks for leukaemia and non-Hodgkin's lymphoma in children by paternal occupation and industry recorded on birth certificates

Father's occupation/ industry	Type of control	Cases	Controls	Relative risk	95% confidence interval
Leukaemia					
Total	Area	46	286		
	Local	46	277		
Sellafield	Area	9	29	2.82	1.07 to 7.40
	Local	9	41	2.03	0.69 to 5.93
Coal mining	Area	2	33	0.37	0.09 to 1.61
	Local	2	31	0.35	0.08 to 1.60
Iron and steel	Area	5	18	1.84	0.60 to 5.60
	Local	5	16	2.36	0.71 to 7.78
Farming	Area	5	19	1.98	0.66 to 5.96
	Local	5	11	2.63	0.77 to 8.95
Chemicals	Area	5	25	1.39	0.49 to 3.97
	Local	5	23	1.58	0.52 to 4.84
Leukaemia and non-Hodgkin's lymphoma					
Total	Area	64	393		
	Local	64	383		
Sellafield	Area	10	38	2.02	0.87 to 4.67
	Local	10	54	1.32	0.51 to 3.43
Coal mining	Area	5	53	0.51	0.19 to 1.39
	Local	5	53	0.46	0.16 to 1.30
Iron and steel	Area	9	31	2.06	0.88 to 4.82
	Local	9	25	3.20	1.23 to 8.28
Farming	Area	6	27	1.54	0.57 to 4.11
	Local	6	16	2.15	0.71 to 6.51
Chemicals	Area	7	27	1.90	0.75 to 4.78
	Local	7	25	2.15	0.80 to 5.77

which age group and calendar period were reported. A pertinent question is to what degree this excess may be explained statistically by the demonstrated relationship with paternal radiation dose during employment.

Three of the five Seascale cases in this study were among the four cases of leukaemia with fathers in the highest total radiation dose group (Table 6), with doses of 102 mSv (over about 7 years' employment), 162 mSv (about 6 years) and 188 mSv (about 7 years). The one case in the intermediate group was also from Seascale, with a paternal total dose of 97 mSv (over about 13 years). The fifth Seascale leukaemia case was not, however, linked with the Sellafield computer file owing to our being unable to trace a date of birth for his father, although we know that the father worked at Sellafield from the child's birth certificate and the mother's questionnaire. Thus, we know that three of the five Seascale cases had fathers whose accumulated preconceptual radiation dose was in the group with an estimated sixfold to eightfold relative risk of leukaemia and the father of the fourth was in the group just below the cut off value used. These five

Seascale leukaemia cases were precisely those in the inner circle of Table 4, where the risk was highest.

If the exposure of the father to ionising radiation was the cause of leukaemia in the children then the reported geographical excess could effectively be explained on this basis. If, alternatively, the fact of living in Seascale itself were responsible for the excess then it would not be expected that three of the four fathers linked to the Sellafield workforce file would have a total radiation dose before conception in the highest category, whereas 16 out of 20 fathers of the local controls for these four cases (also born to mothers resident in Seascale) had a radiation record with only one in the highest category (the other four had not been employed at Sellafield). Moreover, in no father of the 20 local controls was their total pre-conception dose as high as in the father of their related case. For fathers of the area controls the corresponding figures were 9 out of 27 with a radiation record but none in the highest category (17 of the other 18 had not been employed at Sellafield), and all the total preconception doses of the fathers of the 27 area controls were lower

Table 6 Numbers of cases and controls with relative risks for leukaemia and non-Hodgkin's lymphoma in children by timing of paternal employment and external ionising radiation dosimetry at Sellafield

Father's employment/radiation group	Type of control	Cases	Controls	Relative risk	95% confidence interval
Leukaemia					
Total	Area	46	288		
	Local	46	276		
Employed					
Before conception	Area	9	36	1.97	0.82 to 4.78
	Local	9	45	1.39	0.53 to 3.65
At conception	Area	8	25	2.79	1.04 to 7.52
	Local	8	32	2.07	0.69 to 6.14
At birth	Area	8	27	2.51	0.95 to 6.67
	Local	8	33	1.92	0.66 to 5.56
Before diagnosis	Area	9	53	1.17	0.49 to 2.76
	Local	9	58	0.89	0.36 to 2.18
Ever	Area	12	65	1.35	0.61 to 2.96
	Local	12	65	1.22	0.54 to 2.74
Dose record					
Before conception	Area	8	35	1.71	0.68 to 4.26
	Local	8	40	1.40	0.50 to 3.94
At conception	Area	8	24	3.07	1.09 to 8.65
	Local	8	30	2.43	0.80 to 7.41
Before diagnosis	Area	8	48	1.11	0.45 to 2.72
	Local	8	54	0.81	0.31 to 2.10
Total dose before conception					
1–49 mSv	Area	3	19	1.12	0.31 to 4.05
	Local	3	26	0.77	0.20 to 3.00
50–99 mSv	Area	1	11	0.69	0.08 to 5.73
	Local	1	11	0.78	0.08 to 7.73
≥ 100 mSv	Area	4	5	6.24	1.51 to 25.76
	Local	4	3	8.38	1.35 to 51.99
Dose during 6 months before conception					
1–4 mSv	Area	3	18	1.30	0.32 to 5.34
	Local	3	24	1.10	0.25 to 4.91
5–9 mSv	Area	1	3	3.54	0.32 to 38.88
	Local	1	3	3.04	0.28 to 32.61
≥ 10 mSv	Area	4	5	7.17	1.69 to 30.44
	Local	4	3	8.21	1.62 to 41.73
Leukaemia and non-Hodgkin's lymphoma					
Total	Area	66	404		
	Local	66	389		
Employed					
Before conception	Area	11	47	1.77	0.82 to 3.85
	Local	11	62	1.08	0.47 to 2.52
At conception	Area	10	34	2.44	1.04 to 5.71
	Local	10	46	1.48	0.59 to 3.75
At birth	Area	10	37	2.14	0.93 to 4.92
	Local	10	50	1.26	0.48 to 3.28
Before diagnosis	Area	11	72	0.97	0.46 to 2.03
	Local	11	83	0.64	0.28 to 1.45
Ever	Area	14	88	1.01	0.51 to 2.02
	Local	14	93	0.81	0.39 to 1.69
Dose record					
Before conception	Area	10	45	1.63	0.73 to 3.64
	Local	10	58	1.00	0.40 to 2.51
At conception	Area	10	32	2.71	1.12 to 6.60
	Local	10	45	1.58	0.60 to 4.18
Before diagnosis	Area	10	66	0.95	0.44 to 2.05
	Local	10	78	0.60	0.25 to 1.41
Total dose before conception					
1–49 mSv	Area	4	27	1.06	0.35 to 3.21
	Local	4	41	0.53	0.16 to 1.78
50–99 mSv	Area	2	13	1.16	0.24 to 5.46
	Local	2	14	0.95	0.17 to 5.28
≥ 100 mSv	Area	4	5	6.42	1.57 to 26.32
	Local	4	3	8.30	1.36 to 50.56
Dose during 6 months before conception					
1–4 mSv	Area	5	22	1.80	0.59 to 5.53
	Local	5	33	0.97	0.28 to 3.41
5–9 mSv	Area	1	4	2.41	0.25 to 23.43
	Local	1	7	1.12	0.13 to 9.93
≥ 10 mSv	Area	4	8	4.33	1.16 to 16.12
	Local	4	5	5.01	1.13 to 22.24

Table 7 Numbers of Seascale leukaemia cases and their controls by paternal employment and total external ionising radiation dose at Sellafield before their child's conception

Paternal employment/ preconceptual radiation dose at Sellafield	Cases	Controls	
		Local	Area
Not employed	0	4	17
No dose record	0	0	1
1–49 mSv	0	8	6
50–99 mSv	1	7	3
⩾ 100 mSv	3	1	0
Total	4	20	27

One Seascale case (and associated controls) is omitted from this table owing to lack of information on the father (see text). The 20 local controls, as the four cases, were all born to mothers resident in Seascale but only four of the 27 area controls.

than those of the father of their related case. These comparisons are shown in Table 7 and graphically in Figure 1, where case 1 was in the intermediate dose category of Table 6 and cases 2, 3 and 4 in the highest category. Similar results were found for radiation dose during the six months before conception, except that two of the 18 fathers of the total of 43 controls with a radiation record during this period had higher doses than the father of their associated case. Two mothers of the five leukaemia cases had been employed at Sellafield; neither worked there at the time of conception of their child, but one had experienced previous exposure to radiation (of 26 mSv) at the plant.

None of the 23 cases of Hodgkin's disease had an address at birth in Seascale.

Discussion

The main finding of this study is that the recorded external dose of whole body ionising radiation to fathers during their employment at Sellafield is associated with the development of leukaemia among their children. Since radiation badge recording will reflect gonadal dose we interpret this finding to suggest an effect of the radiation exposure on germ cells producing a mutation in sperm that may be leukaemogenic in subsequent offspring. Other explanations may be possible, such as exposure to internally incorporated radionuclides or other concomitant exposures in the workplace: it has not been possible to examine the first of these so far, and the second seems unlikely (see below). Additionally, contamination of the

home with radioactive or other material through occupational exposure may be relevant, although there is no evidence to support this.

The results suggest highest risks in those with the highest accumulated ionising radiation doses before conception, either over their total duration of exposure or during the preceding six months. For both periods of exposure the same four cases of leukaemia were in the highest groups, three of them in children born in Seascale, and none were lymphomas. We have not yet examined any other duration of exposure period. Comparison of the relative size of various calculated risks associated with fathers' being employed or having a radiation record at Sellafield either at any time or before the diagnosis of their children's illness supports the relevance of preconceptual exposure.

Other factors that we examined indicated smaller relations with leukaemia. Some of those were expected, such as antenatal exposure to X-rays, but the high relative risk in mothers aged over 40 was at least twice that previously reported.[7] This was not due to an excess of Down's syndrome as none of the cases in our study born to mothers in this age group had trisomy 21. The question arises whether any of these other factors explain the relation with paternal radiation dose. The one well

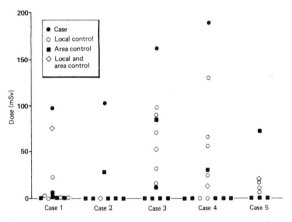

Fig. 1 Total external ionising radiation dose during employment at Sellafield before the child's conception in fathers of Seascale leukaemia cases and in fathers of their controls (case 5 not linked to Sellafield workforce file). The different numbers of controls for each case are due to loss from the study of original controls who had moved from Seascale before their case's diagnosis and varying success in identifying fathers and obtaining information to attempt their linkage to the Sellafield file. The local and local and area controls were born to mothers resident in Seascale at the time (as were the five cases); the area controls were born outside Seascale but resident in the same birth registration district.

established cause of childhood leukaemia, exposure *in utero* to X-rays, is considered to have a relative risk of around 1.5 and to be responsible alone for some 5 per cent of cases. This level of increase is not sufficient to explain the observed relative risks for the highest occupational radiation doses. Moreover, each mother of the four cases in the highest exposure category reported on her questionnaire that she had not had an abdominal X-ray examination during pregnancy, although we could trace the hospital record of only one mother to verify this information. The high risk found in mothers aged over 40 was also not an explanation since only one of the four cases in the highest radiation dose group was born to a mother of this age, as was one of three in the lowest group. Neither of these two cases born to mothers aged 40 or over with paternal radiation exposure at Sellafield was born in Seascale.

Of the four cases of leukaemia in the highest radiation dose group three were acute lymphatic leukaemia. The father of the non-Seascale case in this group had a total preconceptual dose of 370 mSv (over about 10 years). On their children's birth certificates two of the fathers were described as process workers, one as an analytical chemist and the other as a fitter's mate. Although we have not yet examined jobs in detail, these various occupations do not suggest common non-radiation exposures that might be relevant to these findings. We are limited in the identification of individual cases that we can give both from our own ethical considerations and also from our undertakings to the British Medical Association ethical committee and British Nuclear Fuels.

The results for non-Hodgkin's lymphoma, for which the number of cases was much smaller, were less suggestive than for leukaemia. However, one of the two Seascale cases in this study had a father with a total preconceptual radiation dose of 97 mSv (during about 15 years' employment), higher than all 11 related control fathers, of whom six had a radiation record before their child's conception. The father of the other case was not employed at Sellafield. There were no cases of Hodgkin's disease with paternal ionising radiation dose records at Sellafield before their conception nor among Seascale children; this lack of association with radiation exposure is as could be expected and strengthens the findings in this paper.

One of the weaknesses of this study might be considered to be the relatively low quality information on potential confounding factors, such as antenatal exposure to X-rays and infectious illnesses in the mother during pregnancy. Nevertheless, the strength of the observed finding, together with the mothers of the relevant cases not reporting having had an abdominal X-ray examination, would suggest that the imperfections

in measuring confounders of lower and uncertain risk are not detrimental. Additionally the potential for low quality data on children playing on the beach and families' seafood eating habits, for example, is acknowledged, but this would be a more serious criticism if there had been a trend for positive answers by parents of cases. We recognise also the possibility of bias from the absence of information on some factors for a number of cases and controls, but this is due to the unavailability of old records and our failure to trace parents as well as to parents' failures to respond to the questionnaire. Also this absence of data did not greatly affect what seems to be the important risk variable.

These findings support the hypothesis, incorporated as part of this study, that exposure of fathers to ionising radiation before conception is related to the development of leukaemia in their offspring. The observed finding (the first of its kind with human data), however, is stronger than could have been expected from past knowledge, although relevant studies have largely not been undertaken. In a study of the offspring of 7387 men irradiated to an estimated mean dose of 492 mSv as a result of exposure to atomic bombs in Japan there was no excess of leukaemia (5 cases observed, 5.2 expected).[8] Nevertheless, the radiation doses in Hiroshima and Nagasaki were instantaneous compared with accumulated over years in the Sellafield workers; the different dose rates may be important.

Studies of high doses (360–5040 mSv) in mice have, none the less, indicated that paternal (as well as maternal) exposure to X-rays induces heritable tumours in their first and second generation progeny, the tumours mainly being in the lung (papillary adenomas) but including lymphocytic leukaemia as well as leading to an increase in anomalies.[9] It was suggested that this effect might operate through germ line mutations, and the finding lends biological plausibility to the pathway suggested here.

Further data relevant to the results shown here are expected from two other British case–control studies currently in progress. These are in areas around other nuclear installations where excesses of childhood leukaemia in particular, but also of other childhood cancers in one instance, have been reported – Dounreay in Caithness and Aldermaston and Burghfield in Berkshire.[10,11] In the latter report the raised incidence in the neighbourhood was much less than around Sellafield or Dounreay (as it has also been much less around other nuclear plants[1]), but this would be expected if the results reported here are applicable since there is no dominant settlement of workers equivalent to Seascale or Thurso. The occupational radiation doses, however, have been somewhat less at these two establishments than at Sellafield. Consideration is currently being given to setting up cohort studies to examine the incidence of cancer among the offspring of nuclear plant workers, as well as other radiation workers, and these are also relevant to provide support or otherwise for the findings shown in this paper.[10,11]

The results here are of interest in relation to those in the cohort studies of Seascale children.[12,13] These showed increased rates of leukaemia and total cancer among children born in Seascale (6 observed cases compared with 0.6 expected and 12 compared with 2.8 respectively) but not among children moving in after birth and attending the local schools (0 compared with 0.6 and 4 compared with 4.0 respectively). If there is a causal role for radiation operating through paternal occupational exposure these very different findings among children born in Seascale and those attending school there are as would be expected, apart possibly from the fact that some at least of the Seascale immigrants came from other nuclear establishments. It seems important now not only to extend the cohort studies in time forward from 1983 and backwards before 1950, which is currently being done, but also to carry out for all parents of children born in Seascale a similar linkage exercise as in this study with the Sellafield workforce file and radiation dose records. Additionally, we are planning to examine recent cases diagnosed in the Seascale area in the same manner as in this study. Furthermore, data on internally incorporated radionuclides will be analysed when these become available. Possibly men with high external doses also have high internal exposure. Certainly some degree of correlation between cumulative radiation dose and monitoring for possible internal contamination by specific radionuclides, including plutonium and tritium, was found among workers at United Kingdom Atomic Energy Authority establishments and the Atomic Weapons Establishment.[14,15]

One of the considerations made at the time of the Black Inquiry was that the levels of radioactive discharges from Sellafield to atmosphere and sea were too low to account for the number of excess cases of leukaemia being observed in the Seascale area.[2] This was based on the relatively small additional contribution from Sellafield to total radiation exposure from natural background, medical and other sources. This conclusion would be supported by the results in this study for playing on the beach and eating seafood. The findings here in relation to occupational radiation exposure of the father suggest a totally different pathway and do not conflict with the reasoning. These results also make other alternative hypotheses that have been proposed unlikely to be the explanations – for example, that epidemics of common infections produce a leukaemic response by mixing of populations[16] and that areas chosen as nuclear sites, existing or potential, share unrecognised risk factors.[17]

The range of total preconceptual external radiation doses of fathers in this study was from 0 to 383 mSv, the worker with the highest dose being employed over seven years. The range of estimated radiation doses during the six months before conception was 0 to 31 mSv. An annual dose limit of 50 mSv for radiation workers was recommended in 1965 by the International Commission on Radiological Protection,[18] and this figure still operates in the United Kingdom, although in 1987 the National Radiological Protection Board recommended a reduction to 15 mSv per year.[19] During 1987 in the United Kingdom some 1100 workers received annual doses above 15 mSv from artificial sources; most of these worked in nuclear fuel processing, with fewer than 10 being, for example, health professionals.[20]

If the associations reported in this paper are causal they need to be explored further to help determine which period of exposure may be most relevant. Although the two measures we have examined this far are highly correlated and show similar relations, there is a more convincing trend of increasing relative risks of leukaemia for paternal radiation dose during the six months preceding conception than for total exposure (Table 6). The findings here contrast with those in the mortality follow up of Sellafield radiation workers themselves, among whom there were no excess deaths from leukaemia and only a limited suggestion of an association of death from leukaemia with dose of ionising radiation when considering a lag period of 15 years.[21] However, if these results have causal significance then they are of much importance to radiological protection of potential parents and their children.

References

1 Gardner, M.J. Review of reported increases of childhood cancer rates in the vicinity of nuclear installations in the UK. *J. R. Statist. Soc. (A)* 1989: 152; 307–25.

2 Black, D. *Investigation of the possible increased incidence of cancer in West Cumbria*. London: HMSO, 1984.

3 Gardner, M.J., Hall, A.J., Snee, M.P., Downes, S., Powell, C.A., Terrell, J.D. Methods and basic data of case–control study of leukaemia and lymphoma among young people near Sellafield nuclear plant in West Cumbria. *Br. Med. J.* 1990: 300; 429–34.

4 Breslow, N.E., Day, N.E. *Statistical methods in cancer research*. Vol 1. *The analysis of case–control studies*. Lyon: International Agency for Research on Cancer, 1980: Chapters V and VII.

5 Anonymous. EGRET. Seattle: Statistics and Epidemiology Research Corporation, 1989.

6 Hall, E.J. *Radiobiology for the radiologist*. Philadelphia: Harper and Row, 1978: Chapter 19.

7 Doll, R. The epidemiology of childhood leukaemia. *J. R. Statist. Soc. (A)* 1989: 152; 341–51.

8 Ishimaru, T., Ichimaru, M., Mikami, M. *Leukaemia incidence among individuals exposed in utero, children of atomic bomb survivors and their controls, Hiroshima and Nagasaki, 1945–79*. Hiroshima: Radiation Effects Research Foundation, 1981. (RERF Technical Report 11–81.)

9 Nomura, T. Parental exposure to X-rays and chemicals induces heritable tumours and anomalies in mice. *Nature* 1982: 296; 575–7.

10 Committee on Medical Aspects of Radiation in the Environment. *Investigation of the possible increased incidence of leukaemia in young people near Dounreay Nuclear Establishment, Caithness, Scotland*. London: HMSO, 1988.

11 Committee on Medical Aspects of Radiation in the Environment. *Report on the incidence of childhood cancer in the West Berkshire and North Hampshire area, in which are situated the Atomic Weapons Research Establishment, Aldermaston and the Royal Ordnance Factory, Burghfield*. London: HMSO, 1989.

12 Gardner, M.J., Hall, A.J., Downes, S., Terrell, J.D. Follow up study of children born to mothers resident in Seascale, West Cumbria (birth cohort). *Br. Med. J.* 1987: 295; 822–7.

13 Gardner, M.J., Hall, A.J., Downes, S., Terrell, J.D. Follow up study of children born elsewhere but attending school in Seascale, West Cumbria (birth cohort). *Br. Med. J.* 1987: 295; 819–22.

14 Beral, V., Inskip, H., Fraser, P., Booth, M., Coleman, D., Rose, G. Mortality of employees of the United Kingdom Atomic Energy Authority, 1946–1979. *Br. Med. J.* 1985: 291; 440–7.

15 Beral, V., Fraser, P., Carpenter, L., Booth, M., Brown, A., Rose, G. Mortality of employees of the Atomic Weapons Establishment, 1951–82. *Br. Med. J.* 1988: 297; 757–70.

16 Kinlen, L.J. The relevance of population mixing to the aetiology of childhood leukaemia. In: Crosbie W.A., Gittrus J.H., eds, *Medical response to effects of ionising radiation*. London: Elsevier, 1989: 272–8.

17 Cook-Mozaffari, P., Darby, S., Doll, R. Cancer near potential sites of nuclear installations. *Lancet* 1989: ii; 1145–7.

18 International Commission on Radiological Protection. *Recommendations of the International Commission on Radiological Protection*. Oxford: Pergamon Press, 1966. (ICRP Publication Number 9.)

19 National Radiological Protection Board. *Interim guidance on the implications of recent revisions of risk estimates and the ICRP 1987 Como statement*. London: HMSO, 1987: 4. (NRPB-G59.)

20 National Radiological Protection Board. *Radiation exposure of the UK population – 1988 review*. London: HMSO, 1989–86 (NRPB-R227).

21 Smith, P.G., Douglas, A.J. Mortality of workers at the Sellafield plant of British Nuclear Fuels. *Br. Med. J.* 1986: 293; 845–54.

Acknowledgement

Gardner, M.J., Snee, M.P., Hall, A.J., Powell, C.A., Downes, S. and Terrell, J.D. (1990) Results of case–control study of leukaemia and lymphoma among young people near Sellafield nuclear plant in West Cumbria. *British Medical Journal*, 1990: 300; 423–9.

Case, R.A.M., Hosker, M.E., McDonald, D.B., Pearson, J.T. (1954) Tumours of the urinary bladder in workmen engaged in the manufacture and use of certain dyestuff intermediates in the British chemical industries. Part 1. The role of aniline, benzidine, alpha-naphthylamine, and beta-naphthylamine. *British Journal of Industrial Medicine*, 11, 75–104.

INTRODUCTION
Introduction written by Dr David Coggan, MRC Environmental Epidemiology Unit, University of Southampton

Many of the established causes of human cancer are industrial chemicals. This partly reflects the large number of toxic substances handled in industry, and also the relative ease with which people's occupational histories can be ascertained for epidemiological investigation. The hazard of bladder cancer in the dyestuffs industry was one of the first to be recognized. As early as 1895, Rehn reported an apparent excess of the tumour in men making magenta, and by the time Robert Case and his colleagues began their study, there was general agreement that one of the chemicals used in the industry, β-naphthylamine, was a bladder carcinogen. However, it was unclear whether other substances also contributed to the hazard, and how far the problem had been controlled by improvements in plant design during the 1940s.

Case's investigation went a long way towards answering these questions. He used various analytical techniques, but most notable is the comparison which he made between mortality in dye manufacturers and in the general population. With help from the industry he was able to compile an almost complete list of men who had been employed for six months or longer at 21 participating companies since 1920, and who had worked with at least one of four suspect chemicals. From their ages and the dates when they had started employment, he calculated that between three and five of these men would have been expected to die with mention of bladder tumour on the death certificate, assuming that they experienced the same rates of disease as the national population. In contrast, searches of company, hospital and death records revealed that at least 127 such cases had actually occurred – a more than 25-fold excess.

This retrospective cohort study served as a model for later investigations. Techniques have now been refined to allow more precise calculation of expected numbers of cancer cases, taking into account the exact period for which each subject is followed up. However, the approach is essentially that devised by Case.

Case's report is also remarkable for the clarity with which possible sources of error are identified and evaluated. These include potential biases in the identification of the study population and incomplete enumeration of bladder cancer cases. The study demonstrates how useful conclusions can be drawn from imperfect data, provided they are interpreted with care.

One variable not discussed is smoking. This is because smoking was not known at the time to be a cause of bladder tumour. However, with hindsight we can be confident that a confounding effect of smoking would not come near explaining risks of the magnitude that were found.

The main conclusions of the study were that β-naphthylamine was the most potent bladder carcinogen among the substances examined, and that aniline did not appear to cause bladder cancer. Contact with benzidine and α-naphthylamine carried an increased risk, but this could have been due, at least in part, to their contamination by β-naphthylamine. Risk was lower in men who had joined the industry most recently, but was still elevated as compared with the general population.

As a consequence of these findings working practices were modified further to eliminate the use of products containing β-naphthylamine, and bladder cancer was declared a prescribed industrial disease in dyestuff workers for the purposes of compensation. Screening programmes were introduced in an attempt to detect and treat bladder tumours at an early stage in workers who had been placed at increased risk by earlier contact with the carcinogen.

TUMOURS OF THE URINARY BLADDER IN WORKMEN ENGAGED IN THE MANUFACTURE AND USE OF CERTAIN DYESTUFF INTERMEDIATES IN THE BRITISH CHEMICAL INDUSTRIES
Abridged by Dr Alison Rylands

The scope of the report

The genesis, history, and achievements of the Association of British Chemical Manufacturers' research scheme for the investigation of tumour of the urinary bladder in a section of the chemical industry have recently been described in some detail by the Association (1953). The present paper is the result of a five-year field survey of the problem conducted in the factories of, and among the workpeople employed by, a group of interested member firms of the Association which had contributed towards the cost of the research. Part I has been written in two sections: the one, in narrative form, is the report proper and does not presuppose any detailed medical or statistical knowledge on the part of the reader; the other is an appendix where some of the statistical manipulations to which the data have been subjected are set out in full.[1]

It was laid down in the terms of reference that the function of the field survey was to establish whether the manufacture or use of aniline, benzidine, α-naphthylamine or β-naphthylamine could be shown to produce tumours of the urinary bladder in men so engaged. Accordingly, the scope of this report has been limited to this topic, with but minor digressions to consider other possible causative substances. Furthermore, many medical aspects of the problem have been ignored or simplified. Both cancer of the bladder and papilloma of the bladder have been considered as an entity, after a purely statistical investigation to see that they could be so considered, and treatment has been ignored.

Historical

In 1895 the German surgeon Rehn reported what he considered to be an undue incidence of bladder tumours in a group of men employed in the manufacture of fuchsine (magenta), and he concluded that aniline was the most suspicious of the substances used in this process. From this supposition the term 'aniline tumour of the bladder' stemmed, and has since become current in medical textbooks. Since this time there have been numerous reports from Great Britain, Germany, Japan, Switzerland, France, Italy and America on this topic, and unanimity of opinion has been reached only about β-naphthylamine, which has been generally accepted as a cause of human bladder cancer. α-Naphthylamine has been suggested as a possible cause by some authorities, and strenuously denied this status by others. Those who believe that α-naphthylamine is dangerous seem to have tacitly accepted that the substance acts because it always contains a small proportion of β-naphthylamine. Benzidine has also been a subject of controversy, and, though American opinion on the whole seems to favour the theory that this substance is not a cause of bladder tumour, the opposite view seems to be held in Europe. There never appears to have been much evidence to implicate aniline as such, although the original observations on the manufacture of magenta were certainly valid.

Hueper, Wiley and Wolfe (1938) conclusively showed that β-naphthylamine, in its commercially available form, caused bladder tumours in dogs, and Bonser (1943) confirmed these observations using a partially purified product. No convincing evidence of induction of bladder tumours by aniline, α-naphthylamine or benzidine in dogs or other animals has yet been produced although Baker (1950) claims bladder tumours in mice from 3,3'-dihydroxy-4,4'-diaminodiphenyl which he considered to be a metabolite of benzidine; and Spitz, Maguigan and Dobriner (1950) have induced tumours in other situations with benzidine itself. The evidence that pure β-naphthylamine or one of its metabolites are the only active carcinogens concerned in the production of tumours by this substance is not yet completely convincing, despite the work of Bonser, Clayson and Jull (1951), who induced bladder tumours in mice by implanting paraffin wax pellets containing 2-amino–1-naphthol into the bladder, since Case and Pearson (1952) have demonstrated carcinogenic impurities in commercial β-naphthylamine and in what had previously been considered as 'pure' β-naphthylamine. For the purposes of this report, therefore, the terms aniline, benzidine and naphthylamine will mean these substances as encountered in industrial practice, and will not mean these substances as pure chemicals in the sense that an organic chemist might use such a term.

Goldblatt (1947) and Müller (1949) have reviewed the risk in industry at length, and Bonser (1947) has discussed the experimental aspects of the problem.

Sources of information

The following sources of information have been available.

Cases of bladder tumour in the industry

This is found in cases reported by firms; cases found in hospital records and confirmed by firms; cases found in hospital records and confirmed by the patient or near relative; cases found from an examination of death certificates where the chemical industry was mentioned as the occupation of the deceased; cases found from a cross-check between a nominal roll of persons known to be at risk and all the names collected by the means listed above; cases found in coroners' records.

The populations at risk

The firms participating in the scheme were asked to provide a nominal roll of all workers known to have had any contact with aniline, benzidine, α-naphthylamine or β-naphthylamine, stating the age of the worker and the dates between which he was exposed to these substances. Twenty-one firms complied with this request to the best of their ability, and a reasonably complete nominal roll from 1920 was compiled.

Natural history of the incidence of the disease in males in general population

All death certificates mentioning bladder tumour for males dying in England and Wales between the years 1921 and 1949 were available. Many hospitals collaborated by allowing the use of their records for recent years.

Processes and local conditions

All the participating firms cooperated by allowing complete facilities to inspect processes, and by collecting works-history data of cases known to have occurred in their factories.

Many other firms, members of the ABCM but not participating in the scheme, helped by giving information about ex-employees who developed bladder tumour.

The nature of the problem

Tumour of the urinary bladder occurs in both sexes in the general population. It is more frequent in males (about 2.5 males to 1 female) and is predominantly a disease appearing in the later years of life. Only 14 per cent of all adult male deaths in England and Wales from the disease occur before the age of 55. Although the disease may be divided roughly into papilloma and cancer of the bladder, death certificates show that at death 88 per cent of

the deaths from bladder tumour are attributed to cancer and 12 per cent to papilloma or benign tumour. This figure applies to all male deaths in England and Wales. In the cases found in the chemical industry this proportion is 94 per cent cancer and 6 per cent papilloma. This difference is of no statistical significance; in other words, there is no special tendency for industrial tumours to be either more or less predominantly papilloma than non-industrial ones, as judged from death certificate data. The disorder, tumour of the bladder, must be regarded as a killing disease; only 20 per cent of all cases found by this survey in the dyestuffs industry survived more than ten years from the first recognition of the disease. Since, as will be shown later, the age of onset of the industrial form of the disease depends almost entirely on the age of entry into the relevant occupations, this high case mortality is serious. All patients who develop bladder tumour are not, of course, eventually certified as having a bladder tumour at death. Out of 819 cases notified by hospitals and known to be dead, 666 (81.3 per cent) had a mention of bladder tumour on the death certificate.

Results

In all, by 1 February 1952, 455 cases of bladder tumour had been found in the British chemical industry. Four hundred and forty-four of these cases were found in and after 1921, the first year in which death certificates were available for a systematic search. Of the 341 cases occurring in employees of the member firms participating in the scheme, 298 (87.4 per cent) had had contact with benzidine, β-naphthylamine, or α-naphthylamine, and only 32 (9.4 per cent) were known not to have had such contact. It is necessary, as a starting point, to assess whether or not these 341 cases are more than could reasonably be expected by chance, on the assumption that the industry is exposed to only the same risk of developing bladder tumour as the general population. To do this it is necessary to form an estimate of the number of cases expected on this assumption, and this requires a knowledge of the population at risk. The nominal roll provides such knowledge in some detail, and of the 311 cases which had had contact with aniline, benzidine, β-naphthylamine, or α-naphthylamine, 262 were persons whose names appeared on the nominal roll. This figure of 311 consists of 298 cases with contact with benzidine, α-naphthylamine, or β-naphthylamine, four with contact with aniline only, and nine with contact only with magenta.

A qualification for the nominal roll was that the persons must have been employed in the chemical industry for more than six months, though not necessarily in contact with the suspected substances. This limit was imposed because many firms did not provide records of men with shorter employment times, and, where such records were provided, a very large proportion of men worked for only a week or so. It was felt that these men would contain a high percentage of migrant types, whom it would not be possible to trace. The nominal roll used contains records of 4622 men, who entered the industry at different times and at different ages.

Now it is not possible to estimate the number of cases of bladder tumour that would be expected from the 4622 men if no special risk were attached to their work, but it is possible to form a reasonable estimate of the number of death certificates mentioning tumour of the bladder which would be expected on this assumption (Case, 1953a, b). This expected number is between three and five for the 4622 men, all due allowance being made for the age of the men and their date of entry into the work with the four substances mentioned; and the number of death certificates mentioning tumour of the bladder found among the 262 cases whose names appear on the nominal roll was 127. There is therefore no doubt that a risk of dying of tumour of the bladder exists among that group of people who have had contact with aniline, benzidine, β-naphthylamine, or α-naphthylamine. In this group, that is those men who are known to have had contact with any of the four substances named and have been employed in the chemical industry for more than six months, even though their period of contact with any of the four substances was not necessarily six months, the data indicate that the overall risk of dying of bladder tumour is approximately 30 times that of the general population.

The localization of the risk within the industry

It is now necessary to examine this group more carefully to see where the risk lies, and to see which of the specific substances mentioned can be implicated and which exonerated as causative agents. It seems very unlikely that the employees of the 21 participating firms could fairly be regarded as having equal chances of exposure to the suspected substances, but statistical analysis is hampered because no actual measure of exposure exists. It was therefore decided to consider the nominal roll in three sections, an arbitrary classification being made as follows.

Group I. The nominal roll of those firms which manufacture any one or more of the substances, aniline, benzidine, α-naphthylamine, β-naphthylamine; it will of course consist of men exposed in both manufacture and use, since these firms also use these substances. This group consists of 3198 men.

Group II. The nominal roll of those firms which use but do not manufacture any of these substances, excluding those firms whose use is confined to the purification of the substances for sale as fine chemicals. This group consists of 1275 men.

Group III. The nominal roll of those firms which only purify any of these substances: this group consists of 149 men.

The distribution of the 311 cases of bladder tumour which had had contact with one or more of these four substances, with the number of death certificates mentioning tumour of the bladder expected and found, is shown for each group in Table 1 (rank 9), and it is apparent that Groups I and II have an undoubted occupational risk of dying with bladder tumour. The one death in Group III is suspicious considering the low expectation of such an event.

It is convenient here to depart from a logical sequence of development, and to discuss an indication the justification for which will be dealt with more fully later. This is that the age of death was 51 in the one dead case in Group III, and that the age of onset was 29 in the other case. Both these ages are low compared with the most frequent age of death (65 to 70 years) or onset (60 to 70 years) found for bladder tumour in the general population and this fact lends weight to the suspicion that an occupational risk is operating.

Thus we may say that the occupational hazard at work is most intense in Group I, less so, but still definitely present in Group II, and probably still operating in Group III.

The localization of the risk to particular substances

It is now necessary to consider the evidence for the implication of each of these substances as the cause of bladder tumour, again using the death certificate criterion since this is the most precise measure available.

Aniline

This is considered separately as a special case, since, as will be shown, the effect of the substance is different from that of the remaining three substances.

When the compilation of the nominal roll by member firms was first requested, the possible importance of

Table 1 The number of death certificates expected if no special risk were operating and the number of cases and death certificates found for the various exposure classes

Rank	Class	Group	Total no. of cases found	Cases on nominal roll			Cases on nominal roll where death certificate mentions bladder tumour	Expected no. of such cases	% of expected no. derived from incomplete data	Significance of difference	P
				Total	Alive	Dead					
1	Aniline without magenta contact	I	4	4	2[a]	2[a]	1	0.30	35.8	None	>0.1
		II	0	0	0	0	0	0.23		None	>0.1
		III	0	0	0	0	0	0.01		None	>0.1
		All	4	4	2[a]	2[a]	1	0.54		None	>0.1
2	Aniline with possible magenta contact	I	8	5	3	2	2	0.30	15.6	Suspicious	0.025
		II	1	1	0	1	1	0.05		None	>0.1
		III	0	0	0	0	0	0.00		None	>0.9
		All	9	6	3	3	3	0.35		Significant	<0.02
3	All aniline	I	12	9	5[a]	4[a]	3	0.60	20.3	Suspicious	0.025
		II	1	1	0	1	1	0.28		None	<0.1
		III	0	0	0	0	0	0.01		None	<0.1
		All	13	10	5[a]	5[a]	4	0.89		Suspicious	0.025
4	Benzidine	I	38	34	21	13	10	0.54	3.7	Very high	<0.001
		II	0	0	0	0	0	0.17		None	>0.1
		III	0	0	0	0	0	0.01		None	>0.1
		All	38	34	21	13	10	0.72		Very high	<0.001
5	α-Naphthylamine	I	28	19	13	6	6	0.66	3.2	High	0.005
		II	0	0	0	0	0	0.04		None	>0.1
		III	0	0	0	0	0	0.00		None	>0.9
		All	28	19	13	6	6	0.70		High	<0.005
6	β-Naphthylamine	I	59	55	28	27	26	0.30	4.1	Very high	<0.001
		II	0	0	0	0	0	0.00		None	>0.9
		III	0	0	0	0	0	0.00		None	>0.9
		All	59	55	28	27	26	0.30		Very high	<0.001
7	Mixed exposures	I	162	135	50	85	75	1.15	13.5	Very high	<0.001
		II	9	7	0	7	5	0.32		High	<0.005
		III	2	2	1	1	1	0.006		Significant	0.005
		All	173	144	51	93	81	1.48		Very high	<0.001
8	All classes, excluding aniline	I	287	243	112	131	117	2.65	7.3	Very high	<0.001
		II	9	7	0	7	5	0.53		High	<0.005
		III	2	2	1	1	1	0.02		Suspicious	0.025
		All	298	252	113	139	123	3.20		Very high	<0.001
9	All classes	I	299	252	117	135	120	3.25	9.3	Very high	<0.001
		II	10	8	0	8	6	0.81		High	<0.005
		III	2	2	1	1	1	0.03		Suspicious	0.025
		All	311	262	118	144	127	4.09		Very high	<0.001

[a] Also manufacturer of auramine.

magenta was not realized, but all manufacturers of magenta are automatically qualified for the nominal roll in virtue of the fact that they must handle aniline, and it is possible to divide the aniline nominal roll into two sections: (1) that derived from firms where it is known that magenta is not manufactured; (2) that derived from firms where it is known that magenta is manufactured. Only a small proportion of the names on the second list will have been exposed to the manufacture of magenta. Ranks 1, 2, and 3 of Table 1 show the tumour cases and the expectation of death certificates from the aniline nominal roll divided in this way for the three groups of firms. It can be seen from these figures that there is not a sufficient excess of certificates found over certificates expected to warrant saying that aniline, as manufactured or used between 1915 and 1950, is a cause of bladder tumour.

Table 2 Job analysis

Job	Manufacture (M) or use (U)	Group I					Group II	Group III	Total all groups
		Benzidine	α-Naphthylamine	β-Naphthylamine	Mixed	Total group I			
Scientific staff	M	0	0	0	0	0 ⎱ 2	0	0	0 ⎱ 4
	U	0	0	0	2	2 ⎰	0	2	4 ⎰
Foremen	M	2	1	5	5	14 ⎱ 21	0	0	14 ⎱ 21
	U	0	1	1	6	7 ⎰	0	0	7 ⎰
Processmen, pressmen, filtermen, labourers	M	25	17	37	56	135 ⎱ 224	0	0	135 ⎱ 226
	U	8	5	9	67	89 ⎰	2	0	91 ⎰
Stillmen not included in above	M	1	2	0	1	4 ⎱ 4	0	0	4 ⎱ 6
	U	0	0	0	0	0 ⎰	2	0	2 ⎰
Weighmen	M	0	0	0	0	0 ⎱ 2	0	0	0 ⎱ 2
	U	0	0	0	2	2 ⎰	0	0	⎰
Dryers and ovenmen	M	0	0	1	0	1 ⎱ 12	0	0	1 ⎱ 12
	U	2	2	2	5	11 ⎰	0	0	11 ⎰
Grinders	M	0	0	0	1	1 ⎱ 7	0	0	1 ⎱ 11
	U	0	0	0	6	6 ⎰	4	0	10 ⎰
Maintenance men, plumbers, and fitters	M	0	0	0	0	0 ⎱ 12	0	0	0 ⎱ 13
	U	0	0	4	8	12 ⎰	1	0	13 ⎰
Coopers and cask washers	M	0	0	0	0	0 ⎱ 3	0	0	0 ⎱ 3
	U	0	0	0	3	3 ⎰	0	0	3 ⎰
Total	M	28	20	42	63	153 ⎱ 287	0	0	153 ⎱ 298
	U	10	8	17	99	134 ⎰	9	2	145 ⎰
Overall total		38	28	59	162	287	9	2	298

Two other points require mention. (1) While, as the figures stand, there is only just enough excess of death certificates found over death certificates expected to be statistically significant in the magenta group, the whole picture is more strongly suggestive that magenta may be dangerous, since it is known that the nominal roll for the magenta group is much too large. (2) Two of the four cases occurring in the aniline group are also concerned with the manufacture of auramine, and there is some reason, as will be seen later, to suspect this substance.

Thus aniline, on present evidence, does not appear to be a cause of bladder tumour. If this conclusion is accepted for the purposes of this analysis, then men who have had contact with aniline and one other of the three substances benzidine, α-naphthylamine or β-naphthylamine, can now be allocated to contact with that other substance only.

α-Naphthylamine, β-naphthylamine, and benzidine.

The remainder of the 311 cases which had had contact with one of the four substances mentioned above can be subdivided into the following exposure classes: (1) those who have had contact with benzidine only of the three substances; (2) those who have had contact with α-naphthylamine only of the three substances; (3) those who have had contact with β-naphthylamine only of the three substances; (4) those who have had a mixed contact with two or more of the three substances.

Ranks 4 to 8 of Table 1 show the tumour cases, the number with bladder tumour death certificates and the number of death certificates expected if no special risk existed for these exposure classes and for the three groups of firms. These data show that benzidine, α-naphthylamine, and β-naphthylamine are associated with an increased death certification rate from tumour of the bladder. It will also be seen that only 2.6 per cent of all the cases with bladder tumour death certificates would be expected to be of natural occurrence. If this ratio is even approximately valid for the remainder, it means that the whole group of cases can be considered as consisting of virtually only occupational tumours, and accordingly will be so considered.

It is necessary to examine the works history of the cases to see what types of job give rise to this risk. The nominal roll does not give full occupational details, so that differential rates cannot be obtained. The job-analysis of the 298 cases which had contact with one or more of the three substances under consideration is set out in Table 2 for each exposure class of substance and for each group of firms, and an inspection of Table 2 shows that the substances benzidine, α-naphthylamine, and β-naphthylamine can cause bladder tumour in workers engaged in either the manufacture or use of the material, and that the risk spreads through a wide variety of methods of coming into contact with the substances. A multiplicity of processes is covered by the jobs mentioned in the table.

It is necessary to consider the characteristics of occupational tumours of the bladder in order that the course of events may be understood. The methods of determining the factors at work are technical, and the factors largely interdependent. It is therefore difficult to develop the argument in a strictly logical sequence; some of the characteristics will be used before their meaning is discussed and, in general, the technical process of arriving at the characteristics will be dealt with in the statistical appendix. In these statistical procedures, unless otherwise stated, only the cases derived from Group I α- or β-naphthylamine, benzidine or mixed contacts will be used. This is to avoid using a heterogeneous group, and to provide a standard measure of risk. The number of cases in the other two groups is too small to allow statistical conclusions to be drawn about the characteristics of induced tumours, but the cases can be used for comparison with Group I (see Table 7).

The first characteristics to be considered will be the age at which the tumours appear and the length of time which elapses between the first exposure to risk and the recognition of the tumour. These will be termed the age of onset and the induction period respectively. The age at which naturally occurring tumours appear in the general population is required, but, since there is not enough information available to form a reliable estimate for the whole country, this cannot be determined at present. However, the age at death for all males in England and Wales whose death certificates mention bladder tumour can be determined for any year from 1921 to 1949, and therefore these figures are compared with the age at death of the 137 cases from Group I whose death certificates mention tumour of the bladder. (These cases are not all derived from the nominal roll.)

These 137 cases from firms in Group I died of bladder tumour at an earlier age than would be expected from the data relating to England and Wales, the most frequent age of death in the occupational group (50 to 55 years) being 15 years earlier than the most frequent age (65 to 70 years) in the general population. Thus the occupational hazard produces not only an increased number of deaths from bladder tumour, but also death from this complaint at an earlier age.

It now becomes pertinent to enquire whether this earlier age at death from bladder tumour is due first to a more limited survival time from the outset of the disorder; secondly to a selectively greater susceptibility to the disorder in younger men; and thirdly to a relationship between the age at exposure to risk and the age at onset; or whether some combination of these factors is at work. The first of these hypotheses cannot be tested directly by comparison with survival times since proper hospital records have not been available for a long enough period. An approximate answer can be given by comparing the age at onset of a group of chemical workers with the age at onset of a group of 750 male cases of bladder tumour reported from the Birmingham hospitals between 1936 and 1951. This comparison shows clearly that the movement to lower age groups is still very marked, the most frequent age of onset of the chemical workers in firms in Group I (40 to 50 years) being 20 years earlier than the most frequent age of onset for Birmingham males (60 to 70 years). It is thus apparent that the earlier age at death is not due to a more limited survival time.

The second hypothesis was tested by calculating the number of cases that would be expected from persons entering any of the hazardous occupations (exposure to benzidine, α-naphthylamine, or β-naphthylamine) in the different age groups at the time of entry, on the assumption that this played no part in the production of tumours, and comparing the expected number with the number actually found, and these figures are shown in Table 3. It is shown that an older age of entry into risk increases somewhat the chance of developing a tumour, and

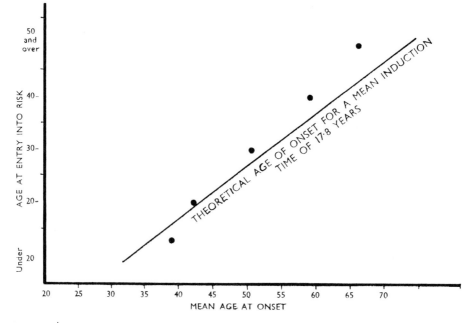

Fig. 1   Age at entry and age at onset.

therefore the earlier age of onset is not due to an increased susceptibility of younger persons.

The third hypothesis was tested by plotting the average age of onset against the age at entry in age groups. The result of this calculation is shown in Figure 1. This shows that the age of onset is dependent almost entirely upon the age of entry, the induction period being nearly constant. The lack of complete agreement shown can be accounted for by the increasing loss of men who might otherwise develop bladder tumours by death from other causes in the older age groups. For all practical purposes, the younger a man is when he enters risk, the younger will he be when he gets a tumour, and the most common time to develop a tumour will be between 15 and 20 years after starting work in the dangerous environment.

The apparent constancy of the average time from first exposure to development of a tumour for each age group of entry into risk suggested that the induction time should be studied further. Accordingly, the induction times of all cases in each exposure class were examined, and the average time and the scatter around it determined. The values are benzidine exposures 16 (SD 5) years, α-naphthylamine exposures 22 (SD 6) years, β-naphthylamine exposures 16 (SD 6) years, mixed exposures 18 (SD 7) years, and the mean for the combined series 18 (SD 7) years. The mean induction time for benzidine and β-naphthylamine is the same, but there is a real difference

Table 3   Number of expected cases if age at entry had no effect on incidence and number found

Age at entry	Expected no. of cases allowing for death from all causes at 1931 rates	Tumours found
Under 20	22	13
20–29	109	90
30–39	74	75
40–49	29	52
50–59	5	8
60 and over	0	0
Total	239	238
Unknown	–	5
Total		243

$\chi^2 = 27.6$, $n = 4$, $P < 0.001$.

between this time and that for α-naphthylamine, where the mean time is six years (37.5 per cent) longer. The spread of the induction times for all the cases pooled together suggests that while the most frequent induction time is between 15 and 20 years from exposure, tumours can develop within five years or after 45 years from the first entry into risk. This is of practical importance because

Table 4 The effect of manufacturing or use on the induction time

Induction time (years)	Under 5	5–9	10–14	15–19	20–29	Over 30	Mean and SD
Cases found in the manufacturing group	2	18	38	47	35	9	18.18 ± 8.5
Cases in user group calculated for a group of equal size	3	14	35	43	43	11	17.63 ± 7.3

The dotted line indicates groups combined together in carrying out the χ^2 test. Difference of distribution: $\chi^2 = 4.09$, $n = 4$, $P = 0.4$. Difference of means: $\chi^2 = 0.55$, $t = 0.72$, $P = 0.4$.

it means that it is possible for a case of bladder tumour to be of occupational origin even if the induction time is very short or very long.

It is necessary to see whether the variation in induction time is an expression of the dose of the noxious material encountered. If it is such an expression, then men receiving a smaller dose should tend to get tumours after a longer interval, and men receiving a larger dose after a shorter interval. No direct measure of the dosage received is available but it is reasonable to suppose that the length of exposure will be some sort of indication of the amount of the substance encountered. However, there will obviously be a number of patients who have worked in the hazardous environment until the onset of the disorder, and here of course the length of exposure and the induction time will be identical. There will also be a number of men where the induction time exceeds the exposure time. In all, there are 281 cases in Group I where both the exposure and induction times are known. These 281 cases were subdivided into groups according to the length of the two times. The number of cases in each group that would be expected if the exposure time did not affect the induction time has been calculated. The method of calculation is discussed in the appendix. There is no trend to suggest that there is an association between short exposure times and long induction times, or vice versa, and the deviations from the expectation are no more than could be reasonably attributed to chance variations of sampling.

Another more approximate measure of the severity of exposure might be the supposition that manufacturers of a substance will be more heavily exposed than users. If this is so and if the severity of exposure did affect the induction time, then the manufacturers should show a preponderance of shorter induction times and a shorter mean induction time. Table 4 shows the number of cases in each group of induction times that would be expected in users if severity of exposure had no effect, and if there were equal numbers of users and manufacturers, and also

the number actually found. The observed differences are no greater than could easily occur by chance. The mean induction time of the manufacturing group (17.7 years) does not differ from that of the using group (18.3 years) by more than might occur by chance. Thus it may be concluded that the severity of exposure, as judged by these methods, has no effect on the induction time of the disorder. The mean induction time in Groups II and III combined, where, as will be shown later, the risk is much smaller, does not differ materially from these figures. It would therefore appear that this mean induction time is characteristic of the particular substance concerned, and not dependent on the severity of the exposure. The fact that, within the terms chosen for the analysis, these factors are independent makes it possible to use the observed distribution of the induction times as a basis for calculating the expected appearance of tumours, and the underlying principle of the subsequent analysis rests upon this independence.

Another implication of the independence is that the difference of the mean induction times for α-naphthylamine and β-naphthylamine suggests that the β-naphthylamine content of the α-isomer may not be the sole active agent, unless α-naphthylamine exerts a delaying action on the rate of development of β-naphthylamine tumours.

Severity of the incidence in population at risk at different times

It is necessary to consider how the incidence in the population at risk varies at different times, and what factors influence this variation. Accordingly the nominal roll for Group I was divided into groups who started work in the hazardous occupations in the years 1910–19, 1920–4, 1925–9, and so on in five-year groups to 1945–9. Each group was further subdivided into the length of time which the man remained in the occupation. This subdivision was carried out for each class of

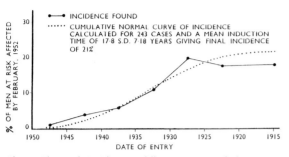

Fig. 2 The crude incidence at different times: pooled exposures in 243 cases of Group I.

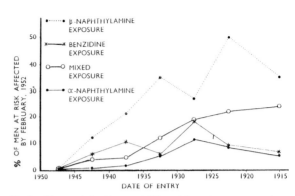

Fig. 3 The crude incidence at different times by exposure class.

benzidine exposure, α-naphthylamine exposure, β-naphthylamine exposure and mixed exposure, and also for all these exposures pooled together. The cases derived from the nominal roll were arranged in similar subdivisions, so that the percentage incidence arising from each subdivision could be calculated. Figure 2 shows the percentage of the population in each group according to the date of starting developing bladder tumour, irrespective of the date of tumour development, age at entry or length of service. This figure is calculated from the pooled classes. It is seen that as the date of starting gets earlier the percentage of the population affected gets larger, until a steady level of just under 20 per cent of the original population being affected is reached. It becomes necessary to find out which factors other than the induction times are responsible for the shape of the graph. It might be that in earlier times exposures were greater and protective methods less good; it might be that men were exposed for longer periods in earlier years, or it might be that some combination of these factors is at work. It is also necessary to see whether each of the three substances produces a similar or dissimilar severity of incidence. Figure 3 shows a graph for each of the four classes of exposure that were combined in Figure 2. Although these graphs show obvious dissimilarity, a consideration of this must be postponed until the effect of the length of exposure has been evaluated.

There is already a suggestion that the severity of exposure affects the number of cases that will be found, since relatively fewer cases occurred among the employees of Group II and III firms. The length of exposure may, as said before, be regarded as some measure of the severity of exposure. The graphs already considered (Figures 2 and 3) did not take any account of the length of exposure in each date group of entry into work. They may thus be regarded as being calculated from the mean effective exposure, which is defined as the length of time

of exposure necessary for the particular class of exposure to produce the average risk for that class of exposure.

The number of cases of tumour occurring in each grouped length of exposure class, using the groupings shown, was found, and the figures expressed as a percentage of those expected if the length of exposure had no effect, i.e. the figure for the mean effective exposure is called 100 per cent. The results of these calculations are shown for each class of exposure in Figure 4. From this it can be seen that the length of exposure has in all classes a profound effect on the number of cases produced, and that the mean effective exposure is reached after a varying exposure time. It is also shown that the risk of developing a tumour increases to a maximum and then decreases for men who have been employed for a long time. This strongly suggests that for a given level of risk, where risk is the sum total of all factors causing bladder tumour, there are members of the population being considered who are susceptible to the disorder and members who are not. Altering the level of risk will alter the relative proportions of these two groups, and it is probable that a high enough level would produce a 100 per cent affected group and a low enough level an almost unaffected group. The fall in the severity of incidence after long exposure times means that most of the persons who will be affected have already contracted tumours, and so have been removed from the figures available for calculation. This apparent immunity is a statistical concept. It may be due to the fact that the population at risk consists of some who really have little or no contact with the substance concerned; that some of the men acquire a 'knowledge', either conscious or unconscious, that enables them to avoid risk; that inherently in themselves they possess a resistance; or that more than one of these factors is at work.

Whatever the actual explanation of the graph, from a practical aspect it means that exposures of less than one

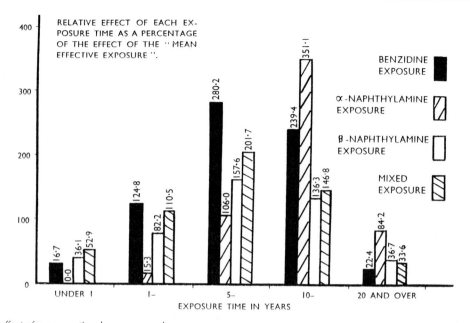

RELATIVE EFFECT OF EACH EX-
POSURE TIME AS A PERCENTAGE
OF THE EFFECT OF THE "MEAN
EFFECTIVE EXPOSURE".

BENZIDINE EXPOSURE

α-NAPHTHYLAMINE EXPOSURE

β-NAPHTHYLAMINE EXPOSURE

MIXED EXPOSURE

EXPOSURE TIME IN YEARS

Fig. 4 The effect of exposure time by exposure class.

year to benzidine, β-naphthylamine and mixed exposures have already produced sufficient effect to make it impracticable to attempt to obviate the risk solely by reducing the employment time. α-Naphthylamine appears to require a longer exposure for equivalent effect, but too much reliance should not be placed on the low incidence found at very short exposures, since the number of cases available for study is very small, and therefore the conclusions tend to be unreliable.

Applying this knowledge of the effect of the exposure time on the number of tumours produced, it becomes possible to represent graphically the tumour incidence that would occur at different times if all the exposures had been of the same length, namely of the mean effective exposure. In this way the number of tumours that would have occurred in the nominal roll for each class of substance had the men been exposed for the mean effective exposure to a standard substance that has a mean potency can be calculated, and is shown in Table 5. (A standard substance is defined as a hypothetical substance whose activity in the production of bladder tumours represents the average activity of the substances actually met with by the men at standard risk, and a mean potency as the average measure of the power of the standard substance, with exposure of the mean effective exposure time to produce tumours in a population at risk of known size observed from the date of entry into risk after 1910 until 1952.) A comparison of these numbers

with the numbers actually found gives a measure of the relative potency of each individual compound expressed as a percentage of the mean potency; where the relative potency is defined as the average measure of the power, expressed as a percentage of the mean potency, of a specified class of exposure, with exposure for the mean effective exposure time for that class of exposure, to produce tumours in a population at risk of known size, observed from the date of entry into risk after 1910 until 1952.

Statistical tests show that this relationship between the substances held true generally over the period between 1915 and 1950. Thus it can be said that, under the exposure conditions obtaining in the Group I firms between these dates, β-naphthylamine has been the most potent cause of bladder tumour, followed by mixed exposures, then by benzidine, with α-naphthylamine the least potent of these substances. β-Naphthylamine has been about five times as potent as α-naphthylamine, and three times as potent as benzidine.

However, the differing mean induction times for the different substances suggest that this may underestimate the relative potency of the substances with the longer induction times. Therefore a measure, called the 'ultimate relative potency', has been calculated and is necessary to express what these relationships would be when all the expected cases at the mean risk have developed, on the assumption that men die of all causes at 1931 rates. This

Table 5 Effect of the exposure class

Exposure class	Benzidine	α-Naphthylamine	β-Naphthylamine	Mixed exposures
No. of cases expected	47.0	46.9	25.5	124.0
No. of cases found	34	19	55	135
Relative potency (%)	72	41	216	109
Ultimate relative potency (%)	68	58	185	127

measure is defined as the measure of the power, expressed as a percentage of the ultimate mean potency, of a specified class of exposure, with exposure for the mean effective time for that class of exposure, to produce tumours of the bladder in a population at risk of known size observed until all have died, on the assumption that death from all causes acts at the 1931 rate for males in England and Wales. These ultimate relative potencies are also shown in Table 5. It can now be seen that the relative potencies of α-naphthylamine and mixed exposures have been underestimated and that of β-naphthylamine overestimated by the relative potency figures.

Effect of changing conditions and altered techniques on the incidence at different times

The only factors so far investigated that affect the final incidence of tumours are the type of substance encountered and the length of exposure. Figure 5 shows what the result would be if all the men had been exposed to each exposure class for the mean effective exposure time, and, by the use of the potency factors, if all the men were working at the mean potency. This removes chance influences due to the number of men working on a particular substance at a given time, and to different movements of labour that may take place at different times. The incidence in the population at risk entering the relevant occupations at different dates increases, slowly at first, then more sharply, and then again slowly, with the passage of time since starting work. The highest figure reached is about 24 per cent, and a time will come when the final incidence is reached since deaths from all causes will leave no more men in the original population to be affected.

The data that have been collected about the induction times make it possible to calculate a graph of the way in which the incidence figures would behave if it is assumed that the 'danger-value' of exposure for a given time is constant between 1915 and 1950; in other words, that any alterations of plant and process have been without effect, and if it is further assumed that deaths from all

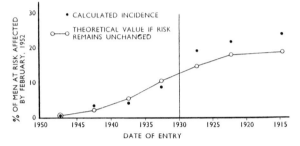

Fig. 5 The incidence at different times calculated from the mean effective exposure time and the mean potency in 243 cases of Group I.

causes affect the men at the rates found in the male population of England and Wales for 1931, this date being the nearest to the centre of the period being considered for which such information is available. Figure 5 shows this curve as well as the values that were actually found.

Alterations of plant and technique which might be expected to have affected the risk were made first in about 1935, and developed progressively with additional impetus after 1945. Since it has already been shown that the full effect of exposure is not experienced until after an exposure time of more than five years, the men entering between 1930 and 1935 may be expected to benefit to some extent by any reduction of risk that has taken place between 1935 and 1940. If, therefore, this graph is considered as consisting of two groups of men, those entering before 1930 and those entering after 1930, it can be seen that the theoretical line underestimates the risk in the earlier period, and overestimates the risk in the later period. Statistical tests show that this difference of estimate is slightly more than could reasonably be expected to occur by chance. The analysis of the figures reveals that the mean post-1930 risk is about 66 per cent of the mean pre-1930 risk, but it is safer to limit this conclusion more generally to stating that the risk is reduced just significantly. It is not possible yet to say that this improvement is progressive, since cases which may

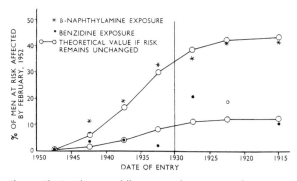

Fig. 6 The incidence at different times by exposure class.

be expected to occur in men who entered after 1945 would be very few, and the results of improvements inaugurated then are not yet assessable.

How individual classes of exposure follow the type of theoretical curve in Figures 6 and 7

Figures 6 and 7 show the theoretical expected incidence for the four exposure classes calculated on the assumptions that the risk remained constant throughout the whole period, and that the death rate from all causes was at the 1931 figure. The incidences actually found are also shown. An analysis of these curves shows that the mean post-1930 risks for benzidine and for mixed exposures are reduced by more than could be expected from chance sampling variations (to 39 and 67 per cent of the pre-1930 risk respectively) and also that the mean post-1930 risks for α-naphthylamine and β-naphthylamine have risen, being 118 per cent of the pre-1930 risk in each case, but this difference does not exceed what

might be attributed to chance sampling variations. The slight total diminution of risk shown in Figure 5 is derived from the benzidine and mixed exposures classes, though any quantitative estimate of the change should also be treated with reserve.

The theoretical graphs for the mean risk over the whole period conform reasonably closely to the curve that has been found for the exposure classes α-naphthylamine, β-naphthylamine, and (apart from the diminution of risk since 1930 already noted) mixed exposures. In the case of benzidine the scatter of the observed values around the theoretical graph will be seen to be greater. Detailed histories of changes in industrial technique are not available for all firms or for all of the exposure classes, but 68 per cent of the benzidine cases are contributed by one firm, and were engaged in the manufacture of this substance. Scott (1952) has given a historical summary of the manufacture of benzidine by that concern.

Total expected number of cases from the nominal roll in Group I only

The type of graph shown to fit the observed incidences of bladder tumour in the various classes (see Figures 6 and 7) makes it possible to calculate the numbers of cases that will be expected to occur on the assumptions that the death rate from other causes remains at the 1931 level, that none of the men on the nominal roll received further exposure after the end of 1950, and that the cases occur at the mean risk for the pre- and post-1930 periods for the men who entered at these times. By assuming in this way that conditions have remained static, it is practicable to obtain an indication of the number of cases which may still be expected in the population here considered, but since conditions have not in fact remained static the

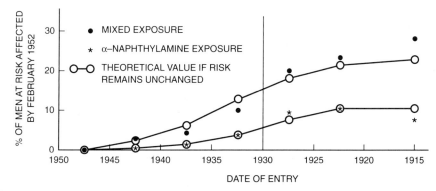

Fig. 7 The incidence at different times by exposure class.

Table 6 Number of cases expected from Group I

Exposure class	Total no. of cases expected	No. of cases already found	Further cases to be expected
Benzidine	58	34	24
α-Naphthylamine	70	19	51
β-Naphthylamine	93	55	38
Mixed exposures	265	135	130
Total	486	243	243

Table 7 Severity of risk in Groups II and III firms compared with risk in Group I firms

Group under consideration	No. of cases expected	No. of cases found	Potency of risk as % of Group I risk
Group II	48.7	7	14.4
Group III	4.1	2	48.7
Groups II and III combined	52.8	9	17.0

figures obtained are only a rough measure of the problems to be faced. They are shown in Table 6.

Another measure of the severities of the risks in each exposure class and in the general population

In considering the risk involved in exposure to the three substances benzidine, α-naphthylamine, and β-naphthylamine, only patients who were dead, and where death certificates mentioning bladder tumour had been issued, could be used in determining the risk. It is now possible to devise another measure which will utilize the information from all the cases on the Group I nominal roll. This measure is the final incidence, after allowing for deaths from all causes at the 1931 rate, that will be reached for each class of exposure, and the comparison is with the final incidence for the general population. This can be calculated from the final incidence of death certification with mention of bladder tumour, together with the percentage certification with mention of bladder tumour of the cases in the hospital survey. The final incidence of death certification with mention of bladder tumour used is the figure for 1931 (0.56 per cent) for men entering at age 34, this being the average age of entry for the period investigated. From this we find that the final incidence of cases of bladder tumour in the male general population is 0.70 per cent, while the final incidences for benzidine, α-naphthylamine, β-naphthylamine and mixed exposures in Group I are 13, 11, 43 and 23 per cent respectively.

This confirms the previous test and further provides a rough estimate of the severity of the hazard, the benzidine hazard being 19 times, the α-naphthylamine hazard 16 times, the β-naphthylamine 61 times and the hazard from mixed exposures 33 times as great as that in the general population. In addition to the increased number of cases found, the occupational cases occur at a much earlier age than the non-occupational ones.

The severity of the risk in Groups II and III firms

From the foregoing it is possible to calculate the number of cases that would have been expected from the nominal rolls of Group II and Group III firms if the risk were the same as in Group I, and to compare this expectation with the number of cases found whose names appear on the nominal rolls as having had contact with benzidine, α-naphthylamine, or β-naphthylamine. These figures are shown in Table 7. Both Group II and Group III firms have a lesser risk than Group I firms but the risk in Group III firms is not as small as was suggested by the figures derived from death certificates only.

These figures also offer an additional means of testing the hypothesis that the mean induction time is not dependent on the severity of exposure. If it were, the mean induction time for these nine mixed exposure cases in the combined two groups should be longer than for the mixed exposure cases in Group I, and longer than the α-naphthylamine cases also. In fact, the mean induction time (21 SD 9 years) is not materially different from that of mixed exposure cases in Group I (18.3 SD 7, $P = 0.25$), and is shorter, though not materially so, than that of the α-naphthylamine cases from Group I firms (22.5 SD 7, $P = 0.55$).

Discussion

In general, each result has been discussed as it was achieved. Therefore no further discussion of the foregoing is needed. Certain general topics are, however, raised, and these are dealt with below.

It does not fall within the scope of this report to suggest alterations in industrial practice. However, it might not be out of place to make some suggestions for future investigation of the risk, so that changes due to better industrial practice can be assessed at an early date.

First, it is apparent that an accurate picture of what is happening can be obtained only from a study of both the population at risk and the cases derived from this population. Therefore it is important that accurate records of men employed should be kept, and their age, date of starting work and occupational history noted. It would be desirable if records of causes of death of employees or past employees were also kept. It would then be possible for a firm concerned to make an estimate of the number of cases that might occur by the ordinary risk of the disease and the observed number, and so see what processes came under suspicion. The methods for doing this are set out and discussed elsewhere (Case, 1953b) and could be used by either the medical officer or the personnel management department.

Secondly, the number of cases that may be expected in the future makes early diagnosis important. The work of Crabbe (1952) using exfoliative cytology suggests that this method appears to offer advantages over older techniques. It might therefore be advisable to consider how far such a method could be applied in the dyestuffs industry generally.

Thirdly, it would seem desirable at this stage to emphasize the need for more experimental work. If trace substances in intermediates play any part in the production of tumours, a possibility suggested by Case and Pearson (1952) and the unpublished work of Case (1948–52), quite different protective measures may be needed from those that would be required to prevent contact with the intermediates themselves. A prerequisite of protection is a knowledge of the forces against which protection is required.

Summary and conclusions

This statistical survey demonstrates that contact with benzidine, α-naphthylamine and β-naphthylamine in either manufacture or use causes many more bladder tumours in workmen so exposed than would appear if no special risk was operating. Furthermore, both the onset of and death from these occupational tumours takes place at a much earlier age than in non-occupational cases.

There is no evidence that aniline causes an increased number of bladder tumours in men who manufacture or handle it. There is, however, some evidence to suggest that the manufacture of magenta and auramine may cause tumours.

There is some evidence that work in the chemical industry which does not involve contact with any of these substances may cause earlier deaths from bladder tumour than occur in the general population, although figures are

not available to measure whether a greater number of tumours is produced than would occur in the general population.

β-Naphthylamine has been the most potent cause of occupational bladder tumour between 1915 and 1951. In those firms which manufacture aniline, benzidine, α-naphthylamine or β-naphthylamine, the ratios of the potencies of β-naphthylamine, mixed exposures, benzidine, and α-naphthylamine in manufacture or use have been respectively 5.2, 2.7, 1.7 and 1.0. However, when all the cases expected from this group have appeared, this ratio should change to 3.8, 2.0, 1.2 and 1.0. This difference of ratio is due to the different times required for the tumours to become manifest.

The tumours appear after an induction period of an average length of 16 years for β-naphthylamine and benzidine and 22 years for α-naphthylamine. However, tumours may appear in less than two years from the first exposure or after more than 45 years from first exposure. Thus the length of time between the first exposure and the development of a tumour should not be considered as a bar to recognizing the tumour as being of industrial origin.

The average induction time is not appreciably influenced by the severity or duration of the exposure. It therefore appears to be a characteristic of the causal agent. This suggests that it is possible that the β-naphthylamine content of α-naphthylamine is not the sole causative agent in the latter substance unless it is assumed that α-naphthylamine could retard the production of β-naphthylamine tumours.

In the largest group available for study, that is the group of firms which manufacture aniline, benzidine and either α- or β-naphthylamine, the final proportion of all workers employed for more than six months who had any contact, in the manufacture or use, with the latter three of these substances was about 20 per cent.

Calculations suggest that, in the absence of any further exposure after 1951, this group of 2466 men, which has already given rise to 243 cases, may be expected to produce a further 243 cases, making 486 cases in all. This calculation indicates only an approximate expectation, since many relevant conditions may be expected to have altered.

In other words, in this section of the chemical industry (Group I) one in ten of the men exposed in the way defined above between 1915 and 1950 has already developed bladder tumour, and this figure may be expected to reach one in five before all the men are dead from all causes. The severity of the risk seems to have been mitigated slightly for men employed since 1930, and the data suggest that this comes from a diminution of risk in persons exposed to benzidine and mixed exposures. However, the risk is still such that taking the average post-1930 values, one in six of all men employed in contact with any of these substances may be expected to develop a tumour, whereas, before 1930, one in four would be expected to do so. Since these data were collected, the manufacture of β-naphthylamine has been abandoned in Great Britain, and major alterations in techniques of manufacture and handling of α-naphthylamine have been introduced.

The actual risk of developing a tumour is influenced to a small extent by the age at which a man starts work in a hazardous occupation, there being a slightly increased susceptibility in older men. For all practical purposes, however, the age at which he is likely to develop a tumour, if he does so, is almost entirely dependent on the age at which he starts, being on the average 18 years later.

The length of exposure to a hazardous environment affects the chances of a man developing a tumour, but exposures of less than one year to β-naphthylamine, benzidine or mixed exposures carry a definite risk. α-Naphthylamine requires a longer exposure to produce an equivalent effect but too much reliance should not be placed on the absence of any cases with under one year's exposure, since the number of cases that could be expected if a risk is present is very small.

The use of sulphates or hydrochlorides instead of bases does not remove the risk, but there is evidence to suggest that the manufacture of benzidine sulphate followed by conversion to the base may be less hazardous than the direct isolation of the base.

Note

1 For the purpose of this book the full statistical discussion has been abridged. For the full analysis and discussion see the original paper.

References

Association of British Chemical Manufacturers (1953) *Papilloma of the Bladder in the Chemical Industry*. London.

Baker, K. (1950) *Acta Un. int. cancer.*, 7, 46.

Bonser, G. M. (1943) *J. Path. Bact.*, 55, 1.

Bonser, G.M. (1947) *Brit. Med. Bull.*, 4, 379.

Bonser, G.M., Clayson, D.B. and Jull, J.W. (1951) *Lancet,* 2, 286.

Case, R.A.M. (1953a) *Brit. J. Prev. Soc. Med.*, 7, 14.

Case, R.A.M. (1953b) *British Journal of Industrial Medicine*, 10, 114.

Case, R.A.M. and Pearson, J. T. (1952) IIè Congrès international de Biochimie, Paris, 1952. *Résumé des Communications*, 464.

Crabbe, J.G.S. (1952) *Brit. Med. J.*, 2, 1072.

General Register Office (1924) Census of England and Wales, 1921. Occupations. HMSO, London.

General Register Office (1934) Census of England and Wales, 1931. Occupation Tables. HMSO, London.

General Register Office (1952) Census 1951 Great Britain. One per cent sample tables. Part HMSO, London.

Goldblatt, M.W. (1947) *Brit. Med. Bull.*, 4, 405.

Hueper, W.C., Wiley, F.H. and Wolfe, H.D. (1938) *J. Industr. Hyg.*, 20, 46.

Müller, A. (1949) *Schweiz. Med. Wschr.*, 79, 445.

Padley, R. (1951) City of Birmingham Central Statistical Office, Annual Abstracts of Statistics, No. 1 (1931–1949) p. 7.

Registrar General (1945) The Registrar General's Decennial Supplement, England and Wales, 1931, Part 1, Life Tables, p. 48. HMSO, London.

Rehn, L. (1895) *Arch. Klin. Chir.*, 50, 588.

Scott, T.S. (1952) *British Journal of Industrial Medicine*, 9, 127.

Spitz, S., Maguigan, W.H. and Dobriner, K. (1950) *Cancer*, 3, 789.

Statutory Instrument No. 1740 (1953) HMSO, London.

'Student' (1908) *Biometrika*, 6, 1.

Yates, F. (1934) *J. Roy. Statist. Soc.*, Suppl., 1, 217.

Acknowledgement

Case, R.A.M., Hosker, M.E., McDonald, B.E. and Pearson, J.T. (1954) Tumours of the urinary bladder in workmen engaged in the manufacture and use of certain dyestuff intermediates in the British chemical industries. Part 1. The role of aniline, benzidine, alpha-naphthylamine, and beta-naphthylamine. *British Journal of Industrial Medicine*, 11, 75–104.

5   *Professor Walter Holland*

Holland, W.W. (1963) **The reduction of observer variability in the measurement of blood pressure.** *Epidemiology Reports on Research and Teaching 1962.* **Coordinating editor J. Pemberton. Oxford: Oxford University Press, 271–81.**

Fairbairn, A.S. and Reid, D.D. (1958) **Air pollution and other local factors in respiratory disease.** *British Journal of Preventive and Social Medicine,* **12, 94–103.**

INTRODUCTION

In the late 1950s there was great argument between two 'schools' on the distribution of blood pressure. Platt and his colleagues believed that blood pressure was bimodally distributed. Pickering and his colleagues believed that blood pressure followed a continuous distribution skewed to the right. This obviously had major implications both for aetiology and for methods of treatment. If Pickering was right then there was no absolute cut-off point at which treatment had to be instituted for high levels of blood pressure, whereas with Platt's hypothesis it was obvious that all individuals above a certain level needed treatment.

A number of studies were undertaken by a variety of epidemiologists at that time to test these two hypotheses. We were involved in investigations of the aetiology of cardiovascular and chronic respiratory disease in Donald Reid and Bradford Hill's department at the London School of Hygiene. We observed that there were problems in the recording of blood pressure; for example, there was a great over-representation of zeros in the recording of blood pressure, and clinical teaching recommended that one recorded to the nearest 0 or 5, even though 5 is not recorded on any measuring instrument! We thus devised a simple machine, together with Heinz Wolff of the National Institute of Medical Research, which consisted of three mercury columns that were not visible to the observer while blood pressure was being measured. One pressed a button at the various end points. In a survey, three observers used both the normal

sphygmomanometer to record blood pressure and the new method, in random order. This demonstrated that if one used the new 'blind' method the concentration of noughts disappeared and similarly we were able to demonstrate that, when using a normal sphygmomanometer, the population was put into two discrete groups, i.e. confirming Platt's hypothesis, whereas when the blind method of recording was used a normal distribution was shown in that population. Thus, this demonstrated quite nicely that methods of recording were influenced by the observer and that they were important in the measurement of characteristics in epidemiological population studies.

The paper 'Air pollution and other local factors in respiratory disease' by Fairbairn and Reid has been chosen because it is the best example that I know where routinely available information has been used to explore a hypothesis in an imaginative, innovative way.

As a result of the 1952 London smog episode a number of groups began work on both the acute and chronic effects of air pollution. Although the London smog episode was clearly associated with a large number of excess deaths, little, if any, evidence was available that this type of air pollution could cause a prolonged health effect. Reid and his group at the London School of Hygiene began a variety of studies to try to disentangle the relationship between air pollution and other social factors on the aetiology of chronic respiratory disease.

This paper is probably the best example of how such a study can be done. As a measure of level of air pollution the authors used a fog index since no routine methods of

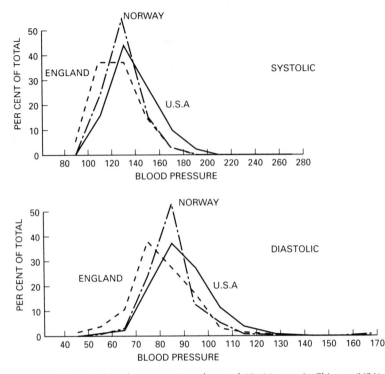

Fig. 1 Distribution of systolic and diastolic blood pressures in males aged 40–64 years in Chicago (USA), Bergen (Norway) and London (England).

measurement of pollution were available at that time. Using this index they then undertook a variety of analyses to determine the association between fog occurrence, disease and a number of other social variables. They were able to show that, for bronchitis, fog was the most important and consistent association whereas this was not true for other conditions, such as cancer of the lung, pulmonary tuberculosis or influenza.

To explore this hypothesis further, they then used routinely available sickness absence data, sickness disability data and premature retirement data from an occupational group undertaking the same work in all parts of the country – Post Office workers. They were able to show that the associations shown through mortality analyses were also present for morbidity analyses and they were then able further to disentangle social and environmental factors by examining the records of individuals of approximately the same social standing who were exposed and not exposed. The Post Office clerks, who sorted the mail, had almost the same pay rates as the postmen who delivered the mail. As they showed, it was only the postmen who had an excess of bronchitis and pneumonia with differing levels of air pollution, and this

was not true for colds or for influenza in the same consistent way.

The paper is also exceptional in that it emphasizes the importance of consistency of patterns observed and was able to disentangle the different effects of air pollution from other features of urban life on respiratory disease and mortality.

THE REDUCTION OF OBSERVER VARIABILITY IN THE MEASUREMENT OF BLOOD PRESSURE

Introduction

The distribution of blood pressure in a population is of interest and may be of importance in explaining the level of mortality from cardiovascular disease in a population. Figure 1 illustrates the distribution of blood pressures in three somewhat similar working groups of men aged

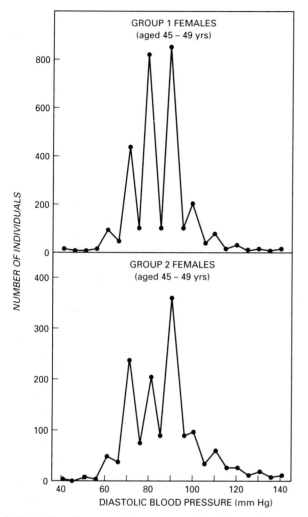

Fig. 2 Diastolic pressure in two groups of females aged 45–49 years.

40–64 in England, Norway and America. As can be seen there is some disparity in the distribution of blood pressures in these three groups. The question arises whether this difference is a true one or whether it merely reflects differences between observers in their technique of measurement. It is therefore important to assess the consistent differences between observers in blood pressure recording and to develop a method of measurement which reduces or abolishes them.

Drawbacks of sphygmomanometers

The disadvantages of measuring blood pressure using the conventional sphygmomanometer are as follows.

Errors due to unconscious digit preference

In any measurement in which numbers are recorded, different individual preference for one or more final digits is always found. This is particularly marked when judgement is difficult, e.g. observing a moving column of mercury; but is also present in any other method of recording, and is unavoidable. In recording blood pressure to the nearest 0 or 5 preference becomes very marked, usually with under-recording of the digit 5 as shown in Figure 2. Recording to the nearest even number, which is the only other alternative, does not eliminate the preference for multiples of ten.

Bias for or against certain figures

Every medical student is taught to regard certain readings of blood pressure as normal, e.g. 120/80, and others as being at the lower limit of abnormality, e.g. 150/100. This idea of a limit may cause apparently borderline readings to be concentrated at or away from these conventional normal or abnormal figures.

Confusion of auditory and visual indicators

In recording blood pressure in the usual way, the sounds are listened to and the falling column of mercury usually begins to oscillate. If one is relying entirely on sound cues, one may discount the first sound as an artifact. It is easy to over-compensate for this by recording the reading as that at which the column of mercury began to oscillate. Thus the appearance of oscillation may actually be recorded instead of the appearance of sound.

Forgetting the observed figure before it is written down

This may be important when recording a large number of readings, as in a field survey.

Variation in rate of cuff inflation and deflation

Inflating the cuff slowly will give rise to venous engorgement which may raise arterial pressure or alter the appearance and quality of the Korotkow sounds. Deflating the cuff quickly may mean that the appearance of sound will occur at too low a pressure.

A method of reducing the sources of variation in taking blood pressure

In view of these difficulties, which may give rise to wide variations between observers, we have developed a new

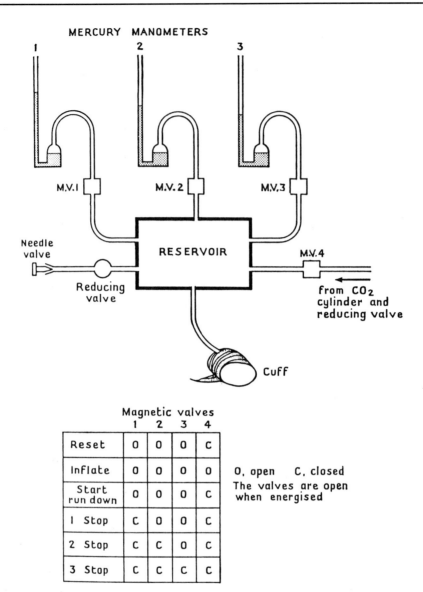

Fig. 3 Diagram of the apparatus.

apparatus. The original mechanical model was developed by Dr G. A. Rose of our Department, while Mr H. G. Wolff of the Medical Research Council Bio-engineering Laboratory and I are responsible for this present development.

A schematic diagram of the instrument is shown in Figure 3. It consists essentially of three standard mercury manometers connected to a gas reservoir. Each manometer can be isolated from the reservoir by a separate magnetic valve to a CO_2 cylinder fitted with a reducing

valve set to supply gas at approximately 4 1b. per in.^{2}. The output is connected to a standard blood pressure cuff.

When the instrument is prepared for use, the valves (MV 1, 2, 3) leading to the manometers are open, and the inflation valve (MV 4) is closed. On inflating the cuff (by pressing the 'inflate' switch on the control panel), MV 4 is opened and the pressure in the reservoir and cuff rises to about 250 mmHg. At the same time the mercury in all three manometers rises to this level. The 'start run down'

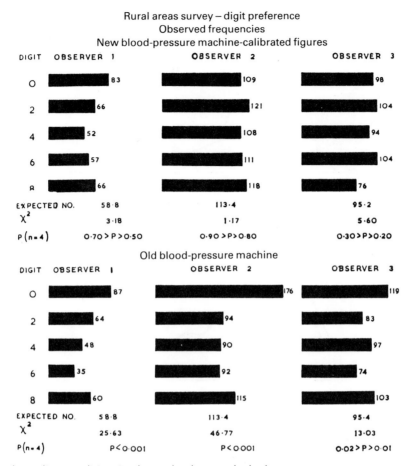

Fig. 4   Frequency of recording even digits using the usual and new methods of measurement.

switch is then operated, MV 4 closes, and gas escapes through the needle valve so that the pressure in the system falls. The rate of decline of pressure (normally 2 mmHg/sec.) is made independent of system pressure by the reducing valve which keeps the pressure upstream from the needle valve constant at about 50 mmHg until the system pressure approaches this value.

As the pressure in the cuff drops, the Korotkow sounds appear at the systolic pressure and the 1 'stop' switch is operated, which closes MV 1; the mercury in the associated manometer, now isolated from the reservoir, ceases to fall. Similarly when switches 2 'stop' and 3 'stop' are operated when the sounds fade and when they disappear, the corresponding valves arrest the mercury in the other two manometers.

The manometers are housed in a box equipped with a microswitch which is operated only when the door is firmly closed. This is connected in such a manner that should the door be opened before the 3 'stop' switch has been operated, two of the manometer valves open again and no reading can be made. For the same reason no readings can be taken with the door open. In this way bias from visual clues is removed.

The instruments have an arbitrary scale over a range of 185 mmHg. The origin of this scale can be adjusted; 2.7 units of the scale are approximately equivalent to 1 mmHg. Calibration is carried out by connecting a cuff to both the instrument and a conventional mercury manometer and inflating the cuff to different levels. Thus the readings are recorded without knowing where 'critical levels' of pressure lie.

By these means, the observer is prevented from exercising any personal bias during the period of blood pressure measurement.

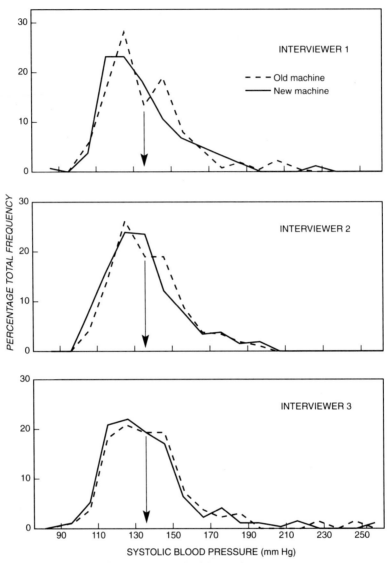

Fig. 5   Frequency of distribution of readings of systolic pressure by different observers.

Testing the new instrument

During a survey

In a study of the prevalence of cardio-respiratory disease in a working group of 446 men aged 40–64 in three country towns in England, the blood pressure of each man interviewed was taken by both the usual and the new method by one of three observers. The blood pressure was always taken at the same point during the course of the examination. The order in which the instruments were used was randomized – if a man was born on an odd date, the usual method was used first, and vice versa.

Results

Digit preference

Figure 4 shows the frequency of recording even digits using the usual method of blood pressure measurement and that obtained on the new machine after conversion of the scale readings to the corresponding values in mmHg.

Table 1 Mean and standard deviations of the blood pressures of a group of Post Office drivers aged 40–64 in English country towns by observer, measured by usual and new methods

Pressure	Observer 1		Observer 2		Observer 3	
	Usual	New	Usual	New	Usual	New
Systolic	135.00	133.47	135.79	133.89	135.57	133.62
	±20.00	±21.22	±18.30	±19.14	±21.61	±11.51
Diastolic 1	86.63	88.37	87.06	87.12	83.11	81.84
	±12.89	±18.50	±10.08	±12.75	±11.37	±11.90
Diastolic 2	82.96	82.45	82.78	82.62	79.40	78.58
	±12.10	±15.28	±9.80	±11.81	±11.99	±10.79
No. of men examined	98		189		159	

Each of the three observers showed significant digit preference when using the usual method (particularly for 0) but this was markedly reduced with the new method.

Bias at certain levels

Figure 5 illustrates the frequency distribution of readings of the systolic pressure by different observers in the group examined. Each of the three interviewers obtained a bimodal frequency distribution of the *systolic* blood pressure when using the usual instrument. The dip in the curve occurs at the same point with each interviewer (135 mmHg). With the new method there is no bimodality in the frequency distribution.

The frequency distributions of *diastolic 2* blood pressure, where the end-point is clear, showed little difference with the two methods of measuring blood pressure. No bimodality was found with either method.

Mean blood pressures of a group by the two methods

The subjects were not allocated at random to the observers so that 'between' observer comparisons cannot be made. It will be seen in Table 1 that each observer recorded a lower *systolic* blood pressure with the new machine, the difference being of the order of 0.95–1.90 mmHg. This is to be expected, since with the new instrument the 'stop' switch cannot be pressed until two or three beats have been heard. In the usual method of taking blood pressure visual allowance for missing the first few beats is often made. The standard deviations of the readings obtained by the two methods are essentially the same in each observer, except observer 3, whose standard deviation was lower with the new instrument.

The mean *diastolic* 1 pressures recorded by the two methods were similar, varying from being 1.74 mmHg higher to 1.26 mmHg lower. The standard deviation of the readings of each observer increased with the new method.

The mean *diastolic 2* pressures recorded by the two methods also differed little, the mean values obtained with the new method being consistently lower, by 0.16–0.82 mmHg. This would also be expected for the same reasons as for the *systolic* pressure.

Testing 'between' observer variation

This was determined in an experiment in which each observer measured, according to a randomized and balanced experimental plan, the blood pressure of each of a number of subjects on one occasion by each method.

The blood pressure of seven normal subjects was measured once by each of five observers (public health doctors) by each method in a prescribed random order. The results are given in Table 2.

For *systolic* blood pressure there is little difference in the 'between subject' mean square (variance). This indicates that, with both methods, the same order of differences between subjects is recorded. The 'between observer' variance is, however, much less with the new than with the old method, showing a reduction of variation between the observers.

For *diastolic* 1 there is again little difference 'between subjects' in the two methods, but there is some increase in the 'between observer' variance. This is to be expected since with the old method, when one is in doubt, one tends to make a reading near the conventional expectation, which may thus reduce 'between observer' variation. On the other hand, for *diastolic 2* the clearer end-point has reduced observer variance.

Table 2 Blood pressure measured by usual and new methods on each of 7 normal subjects by 5 observers (analysis of variance of results)

Source of variance	Usual method			New method		
	DF	Mean square	Variance ratio	DF	Mean square	Variance ratio
Systolic						
Between observers	4	113.5	2.0	4	49.2	1.5
Between subjects	6	455.3	8.1	6	508.2	15.1
Residual	24	56.4		24	33.7	
Diastolic 1						
Between observers	4	45.0	1.6	4	61.7	0.97
Between subjects	6	228.5	8.1	6	229.0	3.6
Residual	24	28.3		24	63.8	
Diastolic 2						
Between observers	4	96.5	3.8	4	23.2	0.7
Between subjects	6	152.3	6.0	6	235.2	6.8
Residual	24	25.3		24	34.5	

Discussion

The main advantages of the new method of taking blood pressure are that the apparatus ensures an entirely uniform means of inflating and deflating the cuff, and that it eliminates any possibility of subjective bias in the assessment of the end-points. This is of particular importance in epidemiological studies in which large numbers of individuals may be examined by many observers. It may also be of use in therapeutic tests in which it is necessary to make repeated measurements of the blood pressure, and in which both conscious and unconscious bias may affect the results.

The effect of digit preference on recording numerical readings is diminished by use of stationary columns of mercury and an arbitrary scale. Elimination of visual judgement of end-points eliminated bimodality in the frequency distribution of *systolic* blood pressures recorded in a survey, by three observers, of men aged 40–64 years which is thus shown to be artificial. The mean blood pressures of the various groups examined with the new method do not differ by more than 1.9 mmHg. from those obtained with the usual method.

In comparing the levels of blood pressure of groups of individuals the mean and standard deviation of the mean of the group are somewhat crude expressions of the characteristics of the group. The precise form or shape of the frequency distribution of the pressures in the group examined is of greater importance. The new machine may enable these to be obtained more accurately without distortion by subjective bias.

Errors due to kinking of the rubber tubing connecting manometer and cuffs, and to dirt at the top of the manometer preventing smooth fall of the mercury column must be avoided by scrupulous technique and maintenance. Errors due to the emotional effect of observer on subject cannot, of course, be removed by any instrumental device. They may be an important source of difference between observers in field surveys.

Acknowledgement

Holland, W.W. (1963) The reduction of observer variability in the measurement of blood pressure. *Epidemiology Reports on Research and Teaching 1962*. Coordinating editor J. Pemberton. Oxford: Oxford University Press 271–81.

Reprinted by permission of Oxford University Press.

AIR POLLUTION AND OTHER LOCAL FACTORS IN RESPIRATORY DISEASE

The mortal risks of acute episodes such as the London smog of December 1952 are well recognized, but the

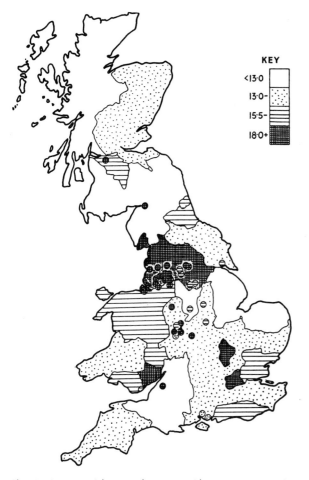

KEY

<13·0

13·0-

15·5-

18·0+

Fig. 1 Average sick rate of postmen (days per man-year), 1947–1953, in the counties of England, Wales and Scotland (large county boroughs shown separately).

insidious effects of lesser but more continuous atmospheric pollution are less clearly understood. Contrasts in bronchitic mortality between Great Britain and Scandinavia, and between town and country in the United Kingdom, strongly suggest that such effects are important. Uncovering the aetiology of a slowly progressive disease like chronic bronchitis involves the study of its evolution from trivial illness to ultimate death and its relation to other respiratory diseases. As a step towards this, we have used the sickness absence experience of British civil servants to supplement the usual mortality data available from the Registrar General's publications.

The British Civil Service offers considerable advantages as a population for epidemiological study. Numbering some 600 000, it has standard conditions of sick pay and superannuation and contains large groups, uniform in

pay and job, widely distributed throughout the United Kingdom. The individual sickness absence records, giving the dates of onset and return to work and the certified diagnosis, are available for the whole of an employee's service and are afterwards retained for 10 years. They present a unique opportunity both for longitudinal studies of the natural history of disease and for the more usual cross-sectional study of current morbidity experience. The potential value of these data is evident in Figure 1, which shows the distribution of the average time lost through sickness absence by postmen in different parts of the United Kingdom. This morbidity pattern again suggests the hazards to health of urban life which are so clearly implied by the urban–rural contrast in bronchitis mortality.

The limitations of such material must, however, be emphasized. Any occupational group is selected both by the individual's choice of career and by the employer's policy of recruitment and discharge. In the Civil Service such policy may vary between different occupations and at different periods. The effect of changes in retirement policy on sickness rates in the Post Office from 1891 to 1946 has been shown by Roberts (1948). Moreover, some illnesses may incapacitate, whether temporarily or permanently, those in arduous occupations but not those doing light indoor work. Sickness rates should thus be used with caution as measures of relative occupational risk or trends in morbidity. In ascribing importance to the different sickness rates of postmen and indoor workers, we have therefore looked for changes in difference with age, locality or diagnosis. No secular comparison of sick rates has been made. On the other hand, uniform medical standards of recruitment and ill-health retirement are applied by the Civil Service Commission and the Treasury Medical Service over the whole country, and comparisons by locality are largely free from bias due to staff selection as well as from that due to pay and job.

In this study respiratory mortality in the middle-aged population at large is first correlated with measures of air pollution, population density and domestic overcrowding, in different areas of the United Kingdom. Wastage and sickness rates among civil servants are then related to the same indices in the same areas. There follows a more detailed analysis of morbidity among the same civil servants at different ages and in areas with contrasting degrees of air pollution.

Fog index of presumptive air pollution

While the acute effects of air pollution can be shown by time relationships, the study of its long-term effects

Table 1 Areas of United Kingdom ranked according to increasing values of fog index, in four groups of approximately equal population

Group	Area
I	1 NORTHUMBERLAND, CUMBERLAND, WESTMORLAND, YORKS (N.R.), Carlisle
	2 ALL WALES and MONMOUTHSHIRE (*except* Cardiff)
	3 ALL SCOTLAND (*except* Glasgow, LANARKSHIRE, and RENFREWSHIRE)
	4 Southampton
	5 GLOUCESTERSHIRE, WILTS, SOMERSET, DEVON, CORNWALL, Gloucester, Exeter, Bath
	6 Bristol
	7 MIDDLESEX
	8 CHESHIRE, LANCS, Barrow, Blackpool, Southport, Chester
	9 Plymouth
II	10 BUCKS, OXON, BERKS, HANTS, DORSET, Oxford, Reading, Bournemouth
	11 SURREY, KENT, SUSSEX, Brighton, Eastbourne, Hastings, Canterbury
	12 NORTHAMPTONSHIRE, Northampton
	13 STAFFS, SHROPSHIRE, HEREFORD, WORCS, WARWICKS, Burton-on-Trent, Worcester
	14 Portsmouth
	15 Preston, Blackburn, Burnley
	16 NORFOLK, Ely, HUNTS, CAMBS, SUFFOLK, ESSEX, HERTS, BEDS, Norwich, Gt Yarmouth, Ipswich, Southend, Cambridge
	17 Middlesbrough, Darlington, Sunderland, West Hartlepool, DURHAM
	18 YORKS (W.R.), YORKS, (E.R.), Doncaster, York
	19 Coventry
	20 Cardiff
III	21 Glasgow, LANARKS, RENFREWSHIRE
	22 Leicester
	23 Leeds
	24 DERBYSHIRE, NOTTS, LINCS, RUTLAND, LEICS, Lincoln, Grimsby
	25 Newcastle, Tynemouth, Gateshead, South Shields
	26 Bradford
	27 Hull
	28 Manchester, Salford, Stockport
	29 Liverpool, Birkenhead, Wallasey, Bootle
	30 Rochdale, Oldham, Bury, Bolton
	31 Stoke-on-Trent
	32 Halifax, Huddersfield, Dewsbury, Wakefield
	33 St Helens, Wigan, Warrington
	34 Birmingham, Smethwick, Dudley, Walsall, West Bromwich, Wolverhampton
IV	35 London, East Ham, West Ham, Croydon
	36 Nottingham, Derby
	37 Sheffield, Rotherham, Barnsley

usually depends on local contrasts in death and sickness in areas with different atmospheric conditions. Such comparisons have been hampered by the scarcity of stations for measuring air pollutants. Even now, these are largely confined to the more heavily polluted areas. Pemberton and Goldberg (1954), who correlated bronchitis mortality in the county boroughs of England and Wales with measurements of sulphur dioxide and smoke concentration, could obtain such data for only 37 of them. Daly (1954) calculated an index, based on fuel consumption, for all 83 county boroughs of England and Wales. Because our sickness absence data related to the whole country, we needed a still more comprehensive index, which we based on the results of a survey of visibility made in the winters of 1936–7 and 1937–8 (Durst, 1940). In this survey, about 1000 volunteers stationed in both town and country observed whether, at 9 a.m. each morning, objects could be seen at a distance of 200 yards, 1100 yards or 1¼ miles. For each station the index of visibility used was the percentage of occasions on which an object at 1100 yards was invisible. (The use of alternative ranges makes no material difference to the results.) For an area we took as an index the unweighted average of such frequencies.

Since the concentration of pollutants can increase without visible fog or smoke, visibility is only an indirect measure of atmospheric pollution. Unpolluted mist can occur; but this is mostly in the less populated hilly and coastal districts where it disperses quickly. These local exceptions have little effect on the values of the index for such grouped areas as were used in this study. Durst states that poor visibility is more closely associated with air pollution in winter when these observations were made. The consistency of the index between the two years of the survey and its high correlation with recent measures of sulphur dioxide and with Daly's index of fuel consumption in areas where these were available warrant the assumption that the index is a useful guide to local levels of air pollution.

Selection of areas

The United Kingdom was divided into the 37 areas listed in Table 1, each consisting of one or more administrative districts. Grouping was designed to avoid, as far as possible, sampling fluctuations due to a small Civil Service population or to scarcity of fog measuring stations. At the same time the aim was to combine only fairly homogeneous districts. Neighbouring administrative counties, for example, might form a rural area which excluded any large county borough within it. The more urban areas were generally single county boroughs or larger conurbations. On the other hand, the areas had to be large enough to correspond with the location code used to indicate the place of work in the Civil Service Staff Record. Areas such as Nos 2, 3 and 16 were thus unavoidably larger than would seem appropriate.

Indices of population density and domestic overcrowding

Respiratory disease is likely to be affected, independently of fog, by other urban characteristics. So that the effects of two of the major factors could be taken into account we calculated from the 1951 Census data indices for each area of population density and domestic overcrowding: the number of persons per acre and the percentage of persons living more than two to a room.

Mortality study

From the Annual Reviews of the Registrars General for England and Wales and Scotland, the number of deaths in

Table 2 Detailed diagnostic categories used in mortality study

Diagnosis	International List code number
Bronchitis	500–502
Pneumonia	490–493
Influenza	480–483
Tuberculosis of respiratory system	001–008
Malignant neoplasm of trachea, lung and bronchus (England and Wales only)	162, 163

the 37 areas for each sex at ages 45–64 from 1948 to 1954 have been extracted and related to the corresponding 1951 Census populations. The diagnostic categories include the main certified causes of respiratory death: bronchitis, pneumonia, pulmonary tuberculosis, and cancer of the lung. Details of these are shown in Table 2. Influenza was included, although the deaths are few, so that its pattern could be compared with that of sickness absence from the same certified cause.

The independent associations between the mortality rates and the indices of pollution, population density and domestic overcrowding have been expressed by second order product-moment correlation coefficients which allowed for variation in the other two factors. Any skew distributions were brought to approximate normality by transformations of the general type $\log(a + x)$, where the value of a was chosen to bring the median of the distribution to the mid-point of the range (Table 3).

The association of *bronchitis* mortality with the fog index in both sexes is highly significant; with population density and domestic overcrowding, it falls below the 5 per cent significance level.

Male *pneumonia* mortality is significantly correlated with fog and population density; for females, however, the coefficients, although ranked in the same order as for males, are not significantly high.

Because there are so few certified deaths, any relationship between *influenza* mortality and the other indices may be obscured; but the ranking of the coefficients is similar in both sexes and the correlations are greatest with fog.

Fog bears no direct relationship to *pulmonary tuberculosis* mortality, which shows a significant relationship in each sex to domestic overcrowding. Death in both sexes from *pulmonary tuberculosis* and *cancer of the lung* shows high associations with population density. Neither male nor female *lung cancer* death rates show any relation to fog or domestic overcrowding.

103

Table 3 Correlation of respiratory mortality at ages 45–64 with indices of air pollution, population density and domestic overcrowding in 37 areas of the United Kingdom

Diagnosis	Sex	Fog index	Persons per acre	Per cent persons more than two per room
Bronchitis	M	+0.60[b]	+0.25	+0.28
	F	+0.57[b]	+0.07	+0.27
Pneumonia	M	+0.51[b]	+0.46[b]	+0.15
	F	+0.33	+0.28	+0.26
Influenza	M	+0.23	−0.01	+0.06
	F	+0.33	−0.09	+0.04
Pulmonary tuberculosis	M	+0.02	+0.65[b]	+0.49[b]
	F	−0.16	+0.48[b]	+0.39[a]
Cancer of the lung[c]	M	+0.18	+0.71[b]	+0.23
	F	+0.23	+0.59[b]	−0.03

Product-moment correlation coefficients, allowing for variation in the other two factors.
[a] Significant at 5 per cent level. [b] Significant at 1 per cent level. [c] England and Wales only (35 areas).

Table 4 Correlation of 'total sickness' and 'bronchitis wastage' rates in postmen with indices of air pollution, population density and domestic overcrowding in 37 areas of the United Kingdom

Rate	Fog index	Persons per acre	Per cent persons more than two per room
Total sickness	+0.36[a]	+0.39[a]	+0.13
Bronchitis wastage	+0.41[a]	−0.03	+0.02

Product-moment correlation coefficients, allowing for variation in the other two factors.
[a] Significant at 5 per cent level.

Use of routinely collected Post Office data

All 412 Postal Head Offices in the United Kingdom render an annual return showing the number of staff and the number of days lost through sickness absence in different grades. Through the kindness of the Deputy Treasury Medical Adviser, Dr M. C. W. Long, and the Post Office authorities, we were provided with these data for the years 1948–54. These allowed the calculation of 'total sickness' rates for postmen grouped according to their place of work. As in the Deputy Treasury Medical Adviser's Annual Report, these rates are expressed as the number of days lost per person per year. Dr Long also gave us access to Treasury Medical Service registers, from which were extracted particulars of all postmen dying in the service or prematurely retired between 1950 and 1954 because of bronchitis. By dividing the sum of deaths

and retirements by the populations of postmen given in the annual returns, 'bronchitis wastage' rates were derived for each of the 37 areas. The age distribution of postmen hardly differed between areas, and the rates were not standardized for age. These 'total sickness' and 'bronchitis wastage' rates were correlated, in the same way as the mortality rates, with the same environmental indices. The results are shown in Table 4.

The most serious index of bronchitic morbidity, given by the *bronchitis wastage*, is, like the mortality rate, significantly correlated only with fog. *Total sickness* shows significant associations with both fog and population density.

Sample survey of Civil Service sickness absence

More detailed information on age and diagnosis is available from a sample survey of sickness absence incurred in the Civil Service during 1946–53. The sickness records of all permanent civil servants born on the nineteenth day of any month who had served at any time during that period provided a quasi-random sample of about 3 per cent. For mechanical sorting, the particulars of each absence ending during the eight years (diagnosis, and dates of onset and return to work) were punched on a card, together with the officer's grade, age, place of work and other personal details.

To study differences between men doing indoor and outdoor work, and between men and women doing the same work, we took three large sections of the Civil Service: postmen, male clerical and executive staff, and single female clerical and executive staff. For brevity the

Table 5 Sample survey of Civil Service sickness absence: populations by age and occupational group (man-years)

Age group (years)	Occupational group		
	Postmen	Indoor males	Indoor females
15–24	1530	2005	3208
25–34	2336	7064	3361
35–44	3017	4613	2446
45–54	3987	8629	2030
55–59	1394	4170	500

last two groups are referred to as 'indoor males' and 'indoor females'. The total man-years of service for these populations available from the sample are shown in Table 5. Because of social factors affecting the absence pattern of married women, a better sex comparison is obtained by using the data for single women only. We have also excluded staff of 60 years old and over; because of the option of retirement at that age with immediate payment of pension, those who remain are a selected group.

For these three populations the sample survey provided attack rates averaged over the eight years for all absences certified as due to the main categories of respiratory illness. These categories, chosen to give rates based on reasonable numbers, are shown in Table 6. It may be noted that they differ from those of the mortality study. Diseases such as cancer of the lung and pulmonary tuberculosis cause few spells of sickness absence; conversely, very few deaths are certified as due to upper respiratory disease and comparatively few from influenza. Moreover, the same diagnosis which appears in certificates of both death and sickness absence may indicate illness that is different in kind as well as degree. Thus deaths from influenza are due chiefly to its pulmonary complications, while sickness absence generally relates to the uncomplicated initial illness.

In four areas, the sample populations were too small for

analysis in this detail. Correlation coefficients were again calculated with the same indices but only in the remaining 33 areas. As in the case of postmen, age-standardization was unnecessary for indoor males, but for indoor females we used a standardized ratio of the observed attack rate in each area to that expected in the same population at total sample survey age–sex specific rates. The results are shown in Table 7.

Variability due to the rather small numbers of staff sampled in each may have reduced the number of significant results, and these respiratory attack rates are more usefully studied in the section that follows.

The only formally significant relationships are those of *influenza* with domestic overcrowding in both male populations. Despite this, the pattern of these coefficients can with advantage be compared with previous results. The association of *bronchitis and pneumonia* absence with fog approaches significance in all three populations, repeating at a lower level the significant relationship to fog of bronchitis wastage and death. *Colds and sore throats* present no features of interest.

Analysis of morbidity sample data by age and presumptive air pollution

For the more detailed analysis of morbidity in relation to air pollution, age, sex and job, the 37 areas were ranked according to the level of the fog index and divided into quartiles with nearly equal populations as shown in Table 1. Within each of the pollution groups of areas age-specific attack rates were calculated for the same diagnostic categories in each Civil Service population. To show the trend of sickness in relation to air pollution, age-standardized attack rates were calculated by averaging these age-specific rates within each pollution group. Conversely, averaging the age-specific rates over the four pollution groups gave the age-trend in morbidity after allowing for differences between these groups in their age structure.

Table 6 Sample survey of Civil Service absence: detailed diagnostic categories used in study of respiratory attack rates

	Diagnosis	International List code number
1 Lower respiratory group	Bronchitis	500–502
	Pneumonia	490–493
2 Upper respiratory group	Acute nasopharyngitis (common cold)	470
	Acute pharyngitis, tonsillitis, etc.	472, 473, 510
	Diseases of the ear and mastoid process	390–398
3 Influenza		480–483

Table 7 Sample survey of Civil Service sickness absence: correlation of respiratory attack rates in three occupational groups with indices of fog, population density and domestic overcrowding in 33 areas of the United Kingdom

Diagnosis	Occupational group	Fog index	Persons per acre	Per cent persons more than two per room
Bronchitis and pneumonia	Postmen	+0.32	+0.30	+0.14
	Indoor males	+0.29	−0.15	0.00
	Indoor females	+0.36	−0.18	+0.10
Colds, sore throats, etc	Postmen	+0.24	+0.05	+0.10
	Indoor males	−0.31	+0.29	−0.02
	Indoor females	−0.24	+0.28	−0.29
Influenza	Postmen	+0.12	+0.26	+0.43[a]
	Indoor males	−0.32	+0.21	+0.42[a]
	Indoor females	0.00	+0.18	−0.12

Product-moment correlation coefficients, allowing for variation in the other two factors.
[a] Significant at 5 per cent level.

Table 8 Sample survey of Civil Service sickness absence: local fog frequency and respiratory disease incidence

Diagnosis	Occupational group	Fog group			
		I	II	III	IV
Bronchitis and pneumonia	Postmen	40	53	115	122
	Indoor males	32	41	47	39
	Indoor females	37	49	51	52
Colds, sore throats, etc	Postmen	75	84	113	171
	Indoor males	53	51	63	64
	Indoor females	77	109	98	115
Influenza	Postmen	131	124	197	184
	Indoor males	88	81	90	102
	Indoor females	90	122	105	102

Age-standardization attack rates per 1000 man-years.

Table 8 and Figure 2 show the age-standardized attack rates for each diagnostic category plotted against the logarithm of the median fog index in each pollution group.

Table 9 and Figure 3 show attack rates in the same populations, standardized for the fog index, in five age groups from 15 to 59 years.

Bronchitis and pneumonia attack rates in postmen and indoor males are closely similar in fog Groups I and II; but there is a wide gap between the attack rates for postmen and indoor males in the more foggy districts. The attack rate for indoor males, unlike that for postmen, shows no rise with age until 35–44 years. It then rises in parallel with that for postmen. Indoor males thus have about the same attack rate as postmen 20 years younger. There is little difference between indoor males and females in any pollution or age group; the slight female excess in early life and male excess after age 45 is barely significant.

For *colds, sore throats, etc.* the rate for postmen diverges from that for indoor males with increasing pollution and the gap widens relatively and absolutely from fog Group I to IV. In contrast to that for bronchitis and pneumonia, however, the attack rate in both occupations is highest at 15–24 years and decreases progressively with age. The curve is steeper in postmen and the absolute and relative gap between the two rates progressively decreases. There is an indoor female excess over indoor males at all ages but especially before 35 years.

The *influenza* attack rate shows a difference between postmen and indoor males, which is unaffected by age but is relatively large in fog Groups III and IV. There is no important difference between indoor males and females.

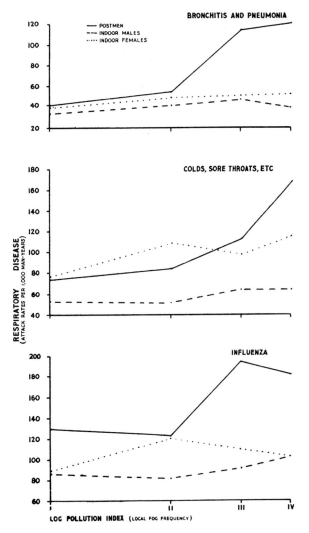

Fig. 2 Local fog frequency and respiratory disease incidence, by occupation.

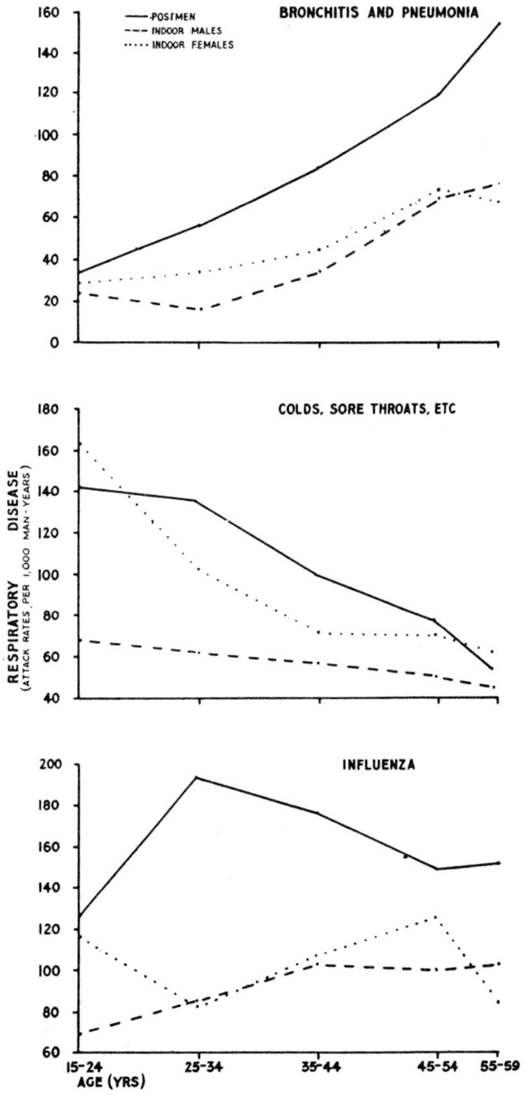

Fig. 3 Respiratory disease incidence, by age and occupation.

Discussion

The prime interest in this study lay in the effects of air pollution and other features of urban life on respiratory disease and mortality. The interpretation of the results largely depends on the consistency of the patterns observed. From each source of data has come evidence on the relevance of air pollution to respiratory disease. Severe chronic bronchitis, causing disablement or death among postmen or death among middle-aged men and women in different parts of the country, is, for example, specifically related to the frequency of winter fog in the

same areas. Pneumonia mortality among males is significantly and independently associated with fog frequency as well as with population density. The death rates in both sexes from influenza, so commonly lethal in bronchitics, are associated, although not significantly, with fog rather than with the other local indices. Sickness absences from bronchitis and pneumonia among all grades of staff also bear a consistent, though not a technically significant, relation to fog. Among postmen working out of doors in areas of high presumptive air pollution, the bronchitis and pneumonia absence rate is much higher than among

Table 9 Sample survey of Civil Service sickness absence: respiratory disease incidence by age

Diagnosis	Occupational group	Age group (years)				
		15–24	25–34	35–44	45–54	55–59
Bronchitis and pneumonia	Postmen	34	58	83	120	154
	Indoor males	24	18	33	67	76
	Indoor females	30	33	42	74	65
Colds, sore throats, etc	Postmen	143	138	110	79	56
	Indoor males	69	61	57	51	45
	Indoor females	164	104	74	73	65
Influenza	Postmen	126	193	176	147	149
	Indoor males	71	85	103	98	99
	Indoor females	118	83	108	124	78

Attack rates per 1000 man-years standardized for local fog frequency.

male indoor staff. Colds and sore throats show the same selective incidence in postmen in these more polluted areas. The steady rise with age in the bronchitic absence rate among postmen contrasts with an increase in male indoor workers which occurs only after the age of 45. The complementary age trends in upper and lower respiratory disease, which suggest more frequent chest complications with advancing age, are especially marked among postmen. All these findings are consistent with a specific effect on outdoor staff of exposure to fog and, presumably, to air pollution. This seems reasonable, for not only may outdoor levels of pollution be greater but the physical demands of the postman's round increase the amount of such air inhaled. Early duty may also expose him to morning peaks in the concentration of pollutants (Department of Scientific and Industrial Research, 1955).

On the other hand, the independent relation of these rates to population density may well result from variation in morale and sickness absence in general with the size of the working group (Acton Society Trust, 1953). Morale may be better in the small rural offices where the contact between management and staff can be more personal. Similarly, a peak at the menopausal age in all female sickness absence rates is of a general nature and not restricted to any particular diagnostic category.

An urban excess in respiratory disease could be due to increased opportunities for infective contact. The higher influenza attack rates among male staff in areas with much domestic overcrowding, like the corresponding death rates from pulmonary tuberculosis, emphasize the importance of cross-infection in respiratory morbidity. The absence of such a correlation among single female staff may be explained by the lesser risk of their contact with infection from school children in the home.

Increased opportunities for cross-infection outside the home might be suggested by the correlation between population density and mortality from pulmonary tuberculosis and pneumonia. On the other hand, the corresponding correlation for cancer of the lung can hardly have the same basis. Neither pulmonary tuberculosis nor lung cancer is directly related to local fog frequency. No support is therefore given to the suggestion of Stocks and Campbell (1955) that air pollution contributes appreciably to the genesis of lung cancer. Lowe (1956) found that the notification rate for pulmonary tuberculosis among older subjects of both sexes was related to smoking frequency, which suggests that this is the urban factor common to middle-age mortality both from this disease and from cancer of the lung. Although, according to a recent report, the current urban–rural gradient in cigarette smoking is small (Todd, 1957), it may have been greater in previous decades.

Smoking could also explain the relationship between male pneumonia mortality and population density, particularly in view of the possible diagnostic confusion with lung cancer. No evidence on the effect of smoking on the incidence of bronchitis emerges from this study. The urban–rural gradient in bronchitic mortality or serious morbidity can be explained by local variations in fog frequency. The excess of bronchitic morbidity in indoor male staff over 45 years of age compared with their female colleagues, which might be attributable to smoking (Oswald and Medvei, 1955), is small, though consistent with previous findings (Reid, 1956; Higgins, 1957) and with the excessive male mortality in later life. But without further information, the relevance of smoking to bronchitis in the occupational groups surveyed cannot be assessed.

Summary

Respiratory sickness and death rates obtained from various sources have been related to indices of air pollution and other urban characteristics in different areas of the United Kingdom.

Sickness absence data, derived from a survey among civil servants, allowed comparisons between outdoor postmen and indoor male office workers, and between men and women doing the same work in the same indoor environment. Attack rates from four major types of respiratory illness have been calculated in these groups for 37 urban and rural areas of the United Kingdom. From routinely collected data on the experience of postmen, the rates for death and permanent disablement from chronic bronchitis and the total time lost through sickness have been calculated for the same areas.

These Civil Service data have been collated with death rates from bronchitis, pneumonia, pulmonary tuberculosis, cancer of the lung and influenza among the general middle-aged population (45–64 years) of both sexes in these 37 areas over the same period. Both mortality and morbidity rates have been correlated with three indices of local environment: frequency of fog, number of persons per acre and percentage of persons living more than two to a room.

The trends with age and with fog frequency in the respiratory attack rates have also been examined.

Analysis of the material suggests that, apart from general influences affecting sickness absence, such as group morale or the 'menopausal peak', environmental factors influence the distribution of respiratory disease in the populations surveyed. Severe bronchitis causing permanent disablement and death among postmen exposed by their job to atmospheric conditions is uniquely related to the frequency of fog, and, presumably, to the level of air pollution. These rates in a group whose job and pay are uniform throughout the country run parallel to local bronchitis death rates in middle age. Variations in the latter are not related to population density or to domestic overcrowding, and may thus result from a specific effect of air pollution on respiratory disease.

The high incidence of influenza morbidity and tuberculosis mortality in areas with much domestic overcrowding emphasizes the importance of cross-infection in the home. Some of the excessive urban mortality from pulmonary tuberculosis and pneumonia may also be due to increased opportunities for infection; but the singular association of lung cancer mortality with population density and not with the fog index of air pollution suggests that urban–rural differences in smoking habits may have affected the risk of death from three major causes of respiratory mortality: lung cancer, pulmonary tuberculosis and, perhaps, pneumonia. The relevance of smoking habits to bronchitis could not be assessed from the available data.

References

Acton Society Trust (1953). *Size and Morale*.

Daly, C. (1954) *Brit. Med. J.*, 2, 687.

Department of Scientific and Industrial Research (1955). *The Investigation of Atmospheric Pollution*.

Durst, C.S. (1940). *Winter Fog and Mist Investigations in the British Isles 1930–7*. Met Office Mem.

Higgins, I.T. (1957). *Brit. Med. J.*, 2, 1198.

Lowe, C.R. (1956). *Ibid.*, 2, 1081.

Oswald, N.E. and Medvei, V.C. (1955). *Lancet*, 2, 843.

Pemberton, J. and Goldberg, C. (1954). *Brit. Med. J.*, 2, 567.

Reid, D. (1956). *Proc. Roy. Soc. Med.*, 49, 767.

Roberts, C. (1948). *Monthly Bull. Minist. Hlth.*, 7, 189.

Stocks, P. and Campbell, J.M. (1955). *Brit. Med. J.*, 2, 923.

Todd, G.F. (1957). Tobacco Manufacturers' Standing Committee, Research Papers. *No. 1: Statistics of Smoking*.

Acknowledgement

Fairbairn, A.S. and Reid, D.D. (1958). Air pollution and other local factors in respiratory disease. *British Journal of Preventive and Social Medicine*, 12, 94–103.

6 Professor John Last

Morris, J.N. (1955) Uses of epidemiology. *British Medical Journal*, 13 August, 305–401.

Last, J.M. (1963) The iceberg: 'Completing the clinical picture' in general practice. *The Lancet*, 6 July, 28–31.

INTRODUCTION

In the middle and late 1950s, I was a general practitioner in Adelaide, Australia; I began to recognize different ways my patients reacted to sickness, pregnancy and the difficulties of child-rearing. Sensing that their cultural origins might have something to do with the differences, I started to classify and count the problems I was seeing. When I talked about this with the professor of medicine in Adelaide, he described what I was doing as epidemiology. I think that was the first time I ever heard this word. Then I read 'The uses of epidemiology' in the *British Medical Journal*, and my life was transformed. I realized what exciting prospects there were in a rigorously numerical approach to studying the problems of sickness and health in populations. The process of gaining new insights into ways to combine a medical training with concern about the disorders and dysfunctions of industrial civilization was, for me, an exhilarating experience that remains as fresh now as it was 35 years ago.

But I get ahead of my story. Having read this mind-expanding paper by J. N. Morris, I had to find a way to apprentice myself to him. And so, a couple of years later, I did. The MRC Social Medicine Research Unit was then located on the second floor of a building behind the London Hospital Medical College. My stay there as a visiting fellow was a rich learning experience. Jerry Morris taught me more in a few precious months than I had learnt in my whole life up to that time. Above all, I learnt the value of making maximum use of existing data. I learnt how to examine these data from new and unusual directions, in ways that not only could lead to fresh

scientific inferences but also could be used to generate and even test hypotheses. In the *BMJ* article, and in the elaborations of the same themes in the first and subsequent editions of the famous book that grew out of the article, Jerry Morris defined seven uses of epidemiology and posed provocative questions suggested by examining the data. The most rewarding of the many things I did as a visiting fellow in the Social Medicine Research Unit was revising and refining tables and figures from the first edition of *Uses of Epidemiology*, helping Jerry Morris to produce more powerful and persuasive arguments that would strengthen the second edition.

As I worked on the sources of the data for a table that appears on page 122 of the second edition of *Uses of Epidemiology*, showing activity in a typical general practice, it struck me that there was a story here worth expanding into a modest paper. I discussed it with Jerry, who agreed and encouraged me to go ahead with it. I had met the late Robbie (Sir Theodore) Fox, editor of the *Lancet*, and told him what I was doing when he invited me to lunch with him at the Atheneum. After I returned to Australia, Robbie Fox came out there to collect material for the article he wrote on the Antipodes, and I showed him a near-final text of the paper. He asked me to send it to him when it was ready, and this I duly did. He made only one change in the manuscript I sent him: I had.called it 'Completing the clinical picture in general practice'. In his letter accepting it for publication, he suggested calling the paper 'The iceberg'.

And so the term was born. Mindful of the needs of indexers, I asked to keep the subtitle, but I needn't have bothered. The iceberg has become part of the lore and language of epidemiology.

'Completing the clinical picture' has other applications, but its greatest utility is probably in primary care. It is an excellent way to evaluate the process and the outcome of health care, simply by comparing the observed numbers of cases with the numbers that would be expected if the distribution were the same as in a population in which both numerators and denominator are known, and that has been carefully studied in relation to the disease or condition for which that piece of 'the iceberg' is required. Many have used the method, including some of the pioneers who have made modern general practice into a respectable branch of clinical and epidemiological science. 'The iceberg' has become part of contemporary medical culture.

Looking back over the progress of epidemiology since late in the nineteenth century, I am struck by the way that epidemiological discoveries have contributed to improving the human condition. The most important of these discoveries – including several made in the Social Medicine Research Unit – have been disseminated by the media, become part of general knowledge and popular culture; and this knowledge has shaped social values and health-related behaviour. Thus ideas about personal hygiene and about sanitation in the late nineteenth and early twentieth centuries, and ideas about smoking, exercise and diet in the second half of the twentieth century, are known to everybody, are integral to our belief systems – and all of us benefit as a result.

What of the future? Health for all remains a mirage; as we solve one health problem, others appear over the horizon to threaten us. At the end of the twentieth and the beginning of the twenty-first centuries, we face greater threats to health, even to life itself on our dangerously polluted planet, than any in previous human history. Values and behaviour that might lead to sustainable development are slowly emerging among better educated members of society. Epidemiological knowledge could influence the spread of values and behaviour that would be healthier than current ones, for the Earth and everybody on it. This kind of knowledge can come from environmental epidemiology, an emerging science that we must encourage entrants to the field to explore and expand.

USES OF EPIDEMIOLOGY

Until about 1900 death rates in middle age were high and worsening (Figure 1a), but about the turn of the century sanitary reform began to show results in this age group.

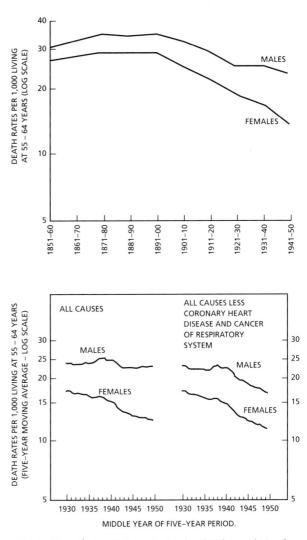

Fig. 1 Mortality in middle age England and Wales. a, during the past 100 years, all causes. b, 1928–1953.

Mortality rates for both men and women began to fall, and they continued to fall fairly sharply until the 1920s. Then something happened. Female mortality maintained its downward course; but the reduction of male mortality slackened and almost stopped. One result of this is that death rates for these men, which were about 10 per cent higher than for women a hundred years ago, and about 33 per cent higher after the First World War, are now 90 per cent higher. What happened?

As we now know, many strange things were happening, and are reflected, in the vital statistics of the interwar years. The most important was the emergence from obscurity of three diseases, particularly affecting males, and very common in middle age: duodenal ulcer, cancer of the bronchus and 'coronary thrombosis'. The first of these is mainly important as a cause of morbidity; the other two are now major causes of death, killing annually over 20 000 middle-aged men. Figure 1b shows the figures for 1928–53, and the contribution of these two diseases to the course of mortality: the trend among men is very different without them.

Figure 1 illustrates one use of epidemiology – in historical study. But first let me explain that what I am speaking of is the study of health and disease of populations and groups, the epidemiology of which Farr, Snow and Goldberger are the masters. By contrast with clinical medicine the unit of study in epidemiology is the group, not the individual: deaths, or any other event, are studied only if information can be obtained, or inferred, about the group in which the events occurred. The clinician deals with *cases*. The epidemiologist deals with cases *in their population*. They may start with a population and seek out the cases in it; or start with cases and refer them back to a population, or what can be taken to represent a population. But always the epidemiologist ends up with some estimate of cases/population. In consequence questions can sometimes be asked which the clinician may also ask, and get better or different information in reply. Sometimes they can ask questions that cannot be asked in clinical work at all. They can, for example, calculate the rates of occurrence, or frequency, of phenomena in the population – such as the deaths, from all and from particular causes, per 1000 aged 55–64, a hundred years ago and now, to make possible the kind of comparison shown in Figure 1.

In this paper I am considering epidemiology as a procedure for finding things out, of asking questions, and of getting answers that raise further questions – that is, as a *method* – and I will have less time to consider the *results*, the information, obtained in reply. I shall confine myself to the non-infectious diseases, and try to illustrate them mostly from investigations carried out from the Social Medicine Research Unit, or with material worked up in that unit. Seven 'uses' of epidemiology are described – different ways of looking at epidemiological data, or applications of the method.

Historical

Historical statements made in medicine are of two broad kinds. The first describe the *decline* of infections, for example, and of nutritional deficiencies, and the main

trends are usually very obvious. The others raise problems about the possible *increase* of various disorders, which is quite another matter. The questions usually put ('Have disk syndromes become commoner?' for example) are bedeviled by uncertainty about diagnosis and nomenclature in the past, and the lack of quantitative estimates of frequency at any time: How many cases occurred annually per 1000 men, aged x, in the 1930s and in the early 1950s? In such problems as the frequency of psychoneuroses, historical questions, which are often asked, are hopeless of direct answer; but even in disorders like leukaemia, urinary cancer or cerebral tumour, subarachnoid haemorrhage, dissecting aneurysm and the collagen diseases, it is exceedingly difficult to estimate how much a recent apparent increase reflects a *true* increase of disease, and how much it is the product merely of better recognition and greater availability of diagnostic services, etc. Such questions are clearly important because the role of environmental factors in aetiology, and of recent social change which may be associated with the increase, arises. As a result of a great deal of work, the increase of duodenal ulcer, cancer of the bronchus and coronary heart disease must now be accepted as a working hypothesis and guide to environmental study.

History in the making

Epidemiology may further be defined as the *study of health and disease of populations in relation to their environment and ways of living*. In a society that is changing as rapidly as our own, epidemiology has an important duty to observe contemporary social movements for their impact on the health of the population, and to try to assess where we are making progress and where falling back – an activity in line with the classic descriptions of famine and pestilence, of the relations of health and disease to social dislocations, wars and crises. What are the public health implications of the 1000 extra motor-vehicles a day; the modern distribution of poverty so different from the 1930s; the sophistication of foods; the rising consumption of sugar, our astonishing taste for sweets; the derationing of fats; more smoking in women; more married women going out to work; less physical activity in work and more bodily sloth generally; multiple chemical and physical exposures, known and potentially hazardous; the prodigious increase of medical treatments; the 11-plus examination; still increasing urbanization and sub-urbanization; the rapid creation of new towns; smokeless zones (still with sulphur); the building of new power stations? And what can we learn from other indicators of community health: crime, for example – the ups and downs of juvenile delinquency, and the apparent increase of sex crimes and of crimes of violence during a period when so much other crime is decreasing?

Some of these questions are being studied, some cannot yet be framed in scientific terms; but parts at least of some could be better tackled than they are. And there are even more fundamental problems in our society; perhaps epidemiology, with its concern for woods rather than trees, its special ability to isolate major characteristics for study, can simplify the issues and usefully raise some bold questions about these, too. Indices of health are available, and their quality is improving, although many more are needed, particularly in 'mental health'.

Looking ahead

For many the main interest of history is the light it can throw on the future. Vital statistics is better placed than most disciplines to forecast – for example, the whole population of old people of the second half of the century are already born and are leading their lives under the conditions we know. Figure 1a can therefore be projected ahead, if only with wide margins of confidence. What seems to be keeping the male death rate even as moderately satisfactory as it is now is the balancing of those diseases which are increasing (such as 'coronary thrombosis') by those which are declining (tuberculosis and other infections). If the infectious diseases begin to reach some minimum before the *modern* epidemics are brought under control, or if their decline is halted, and if the large group of conditions which are relatively static (cancer of the stomach, cerebrovascular disease, etc.) do not show improvements in the meanwhile, the overall middle-aged male death rate will actually begin to rise. One consequence of this would be that the population of old people in the future will consist more and more of solitary old women (whatever the increasing popularity of marriage during recent years). The current trend of mortality in middle-aged males is the most striking feature of Western vital statistics. Very interestingly – another kind of epidemiological comparison – the situation is better in Scandinavia than in the English-speaking world, as illustrated by figures like these:

Mortality per 1000 aged 55–64 from all causes (mean of rates for separate countries, latest available year)

	Males	Females
Scotland, England and Wales, Canada, USA, New Zealand, Australia	22.3	12.9
Norway, Sweden, Denmark	13.9	10.5

Searching questions need to be asked in this kind of situation. A first 'reconnaissance' suggests that there is no simple answer – all these populations, for example, have high living standards and nutritional levels.

Community diagnosis

Epidemiology provides the facts about community health; it describes the nature and relative size of the problems to be dealt with, and 'maps' are produced of such scales as are required or possible. Results are sometimes surprising – at any rate in contrast with the type of problem of which there is general awareness and concern in the public health movement. Over 10 per cent of sickness absence in male industrial workers in 1951 was ascribed to 'bronchitis' (16 million days). 'Psychological' disorders accounted for more than 13 million days; gastric and duodenal ailments for over 11 million, 'rheumatism and arthritis' for over 11 million. [15]

Usually, however, we are concerned with the distribution of phenomena, and not merely their totals. Such distributions are firstly in terms of age and sex (race or colour, where applicable), economic status, and so on. Table 1 is an example of a social-economic distribution in relation to primigravidae in Aberdeen. It shows some interesting similarities, as in nutrition, and the remarkable differences that still remain between the social classes in 'capital' goods like housing and education (in these early days of the Welfare State). There is a wide range of reproductive performance in this relatively homogeneous town. Such demonstration of inequalities between groups is a standard function of epidemiology, and it can be put to many uses – for example, in the same field as Table 1, to identify *'vulnerable groups'* meriting special attention by health services (Figure 2).

The individual's chances

The risks to the individual – or at any rate their order of magnitude – of suffering an accident as a schoolboy cyclist or an elderly pedestrian, of developing leukaemia for a radiologist, of producing malformation from rubella or breast cancer from chronic mastitis, can be estimated only if the experience of whole populations of individuals is known and the relevant averages can thus be calculated. Figure 3 uses the method of the life-table, an easy and rather neglected technique, to give a rough idea of the 'risks' the average male in England and Wales now runs during his middle age, and it complements the picture of Figure 1. It is in the light of something like a

Table 1 First reproductive 'cycle' in a Scottish city

Findings in married women	Social class of husband		
	I & II	III	IV & V
Physique of women – height			
Per cent 5ft 1 in. (155 cm.) or smaller	12	24	28
Intelligence[a]			
Per cent above average on matrix test	80	42	26
Education			
Per cent leaving school over minimum age	56	14	3
Housing			
Per cent living more than 2 per room	2	7	15
Family budget[a,b]			
Average weekly income (after compulsory deductions)	150s.	129s.	119s.
Nutrition[a]			
Calcium intake (mg/day)	1219	1071	868
Animal protein intake (g/day)	48.6	44.0	40.4
Reproduction			
Per cent under 20 years old	2	11	17
Per cent 30 years old or over	22	10	7
Per cent pre-nuptial conceptions	15	24	37
Per cent babies 5½ lb. (2.5 kg) or less at birth	4	8	10
Child care			
Per cent fully breast-feeding at 3 months[a]	60	37	29
Per cent 'potting' regularly at end of first month[a]	72	49	28

This table deals with local married primigravidae 'booked' for the Aberdeen Maternity Hospital, 1948–52; and includes 85–90 per cent of all who were eligible. Data are for periods varying from one year (818 cases) to five years (4365 cases). Social classes I and II include the professions and business; class III are the skilled workers; IV and V the semi-skilled and unskilled workers.

[a] Items are for samples of the total.

[b] Clerical workers in social class III are included with classes I and II for Family Budget only. For other reasons, also, the sample of classes I and II for Budgets was not altogether satisfactory.

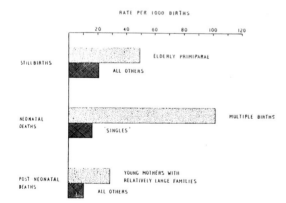

Fig. 2 Three groups with particularly high foetal and infant mortality rates, England and Wales, 1949.

one-in-eight chance of suffering from coronary heart disease, or one-in-ten from peptic ulcer, that the use of such terms as 'epidemic' have their warrant. About 33 per cent of men reaching 35 now die before they reach 65, compared with just over 20 per cent of women. This approach is likely to become increasingly useful as forward-looking 'prospective' studies are initiated, for example, to try to learn something about the differences made to middle-age mortality by different ways of living.

Operational research

The study of community health services – how they are working, what needs they are serving and how well, what they ought to be doing – is a slowly developing branch of social medicine little speeded by the wartime successes in rather different fields. Table 2 gives a few examples of simple analyses, using epidemiological methods, and the kind of questions (rather than answers) that emerge.

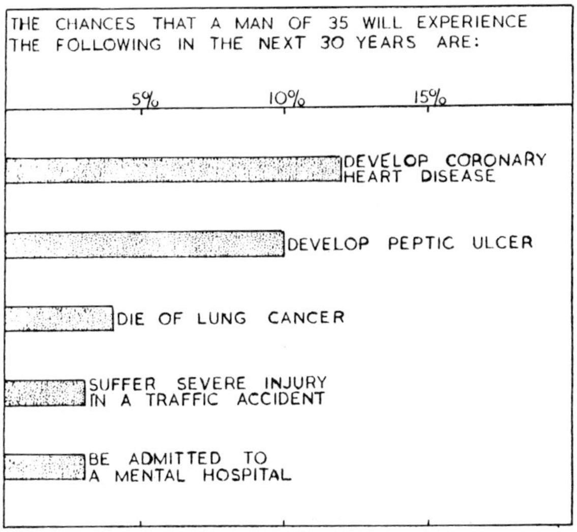

THE CHANCES THAT A MAN OF 35 WILL EXPERIENCE
THE FOLLOWING IN THE NEXT 30 YEARS ARE:

Fig. 3 The middle-aged man's risks today, England and Wales, rough estimates.

Why has the introduction of the National Health Service, in which for the first time every child has, or can have, a general practitioner, made so little difference to the school health service (Table 2A)? What are the appropriate roles today of school doctor and GP? How much 'family medicine' can the general practitioner do if the children are treated elsewhere?

Is there enough 'serious' medicine to maintain keen clinical interest in general practice; how is the work divided between 'serious' and other problems (Table 2B)?

Since most attendances at these large and representative industrial medical officers' clinics (Table 2C) seem to be for 'industrial' reasons, who, it may be asked, does the industrial medicine in the great majority of factories and other work-places where there is little or no industrial health service? What are the different elements in industrial medicine (carried out on the shop floor as well as in the clinic), and what is their relative importance, so that priorities for early advance can be planned?

The diabetes figures (Table 2D) show that social classes I and II did much better with the introduction of insulin than classes IV and V (this is seen throughout 'young' diabetes). How are the benefits of anticoagulants being distributed today, or of the new cardiac surgery? Differences are, I fancy, more likely to be regional and local than related to 'social class'. And tonsillectomy? Is Glover's fantastic tale[10] still true today? Do children in Leeds, Leicester and Exeter still run three times the risk of losing their tonsils as do the children of Manchester, Bradford and Gloucester? (And do these differences affect

Table 2 Working of health services
A   Treatment of minor ailments by school health service, before and after the National Health Service

Year	No. of pupils	No. of defects treated at school clinics
1947	5 034 275	1 190 754
1952–3	6 088 000	1 154 467

B   'Serious' clinical medicine in a general practice, during one year, 1949–50

Age	Frequency of serious problems per 100 persons	Proportion these formed of all the doctor's work with age group (%)
0–14	22	20
15–44	23	34
45–64	41	55
65+	83	76
All ages	32	43

C   Functions of occupational health service, 1951, analysis of sample attendances at 12 industrial medical officers' clinics

No. of attendances in year	1952
Proportion for 'occupational reasons'	79%
Proportion for 'non-occupational reasons'	21%

D   Impact of a new therapy, death rates per million from diabetes at 20–35 years of age, males

Social class	1921–3	1930–
I and II	64	26
III	50	25
IV and V	46	35

the children who most need to have their tonsils removed?) In how many other examples of medical, obstetric or dental care would such *community* comparisons stimulate fresh *clinical* thinking?

Housing policy, pursuing the figures in Table 1, evidently does not mean in the comparatively prosperous city of Aberdeen, little affected by bombing, that young

115

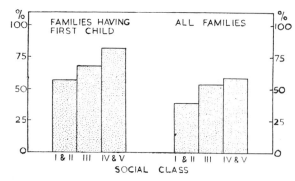

Fig. 4 Proportion of families living in shared houses or flats, Aberdeen, 1951.

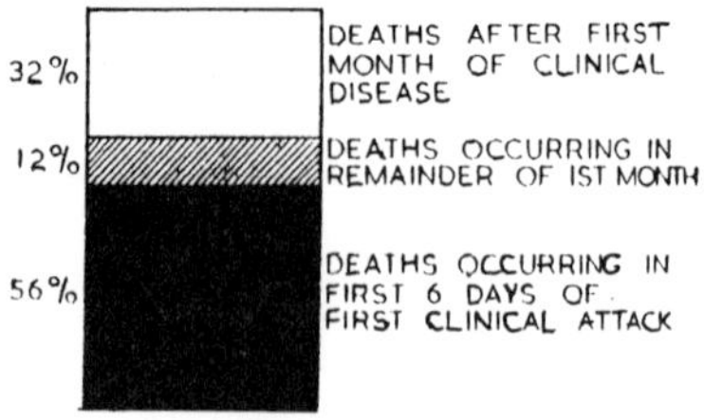

Fig. 5 Deaths from coronary heart disease during middle age: relation to first clinical attack, male medical practitioners, 40–64 years, 1940–1952 (there were 136 deaths in 13 years).

people of any social class are finding it at all easy to start a home of their own (Figure 4). Half of all families in 1951 were sharing dwellings. These housing figures are an illustration of the value of trying to base 'operational research' about social services on populations: the idea of the *human needs* the services are and should be meeting at once becomes important. (Not that the assessment of 'needs' is at all easy: so often 'demand' is revealed – created? – by supply. However, in the health services – school, maternity and child welfare, appointed factory doctor – which were established to meet needs that certainly have since changed and may have lessened, a reassessment of the present situation is urgent. My private notion is that the Central Health Services Council might be armed with a research secretariat; otherwise I see no prospect of having enough 'operational research' carried out.)

Completing the clinical picture

The most obvious example of this function is the contribution of the epidemiological method in determining the sex and age incidence of disease. The calculation of accurate age-specific rates showing, for instance, that cancer of the ovary, and possibly of the breast, reach peak frequency late in middle age is of course a help in understanding these conditions, as are the relations with parity. But it is possible to go further. Epidemiology, being by definition concerned with all ascertainable cases in a population, often produces *different* pictures of disease from those derived only from hospitals, for example. Thus half or more of the deaths of men from coronary heart disease in middle age (56 per cent here) seem to occur in the first few days of the first clinical attack of 'coronary thrombosis' (Figure 5). A quite incomplete picture of

coronary heart disease must result if many of these cases are excluded. But often these deaths are 'sudden', known only to the general practitioner and the coroner's pathologist. Special efforts are therefore needed to discover them, and dependent on the success of such efforts, so may any picture presented of the prognosis in this disease, of survival and of the results of new treatments be very considerably modified.

The same is probably true at the other end of the spectrum: to get an idea of how much there is of mild ischaemic heart disease, minor and maybe atypical, reliance cannot be placed on the cases that happen to turn up in a particular practice or out-patient department, but an inclusive and extensive study is needed. (This principle is made use of in 'screening' surveys to detect early subclinical disease. Thus detected, as in diabetes, progression may be halted, and the surveys are thus a measure of control or prevention.)

In brief, studies of the natural history of disease will be more complete and correctly proportioned if based on all the cases satisfying specified diagnostic criteria occurring in a defined population. Pneumoconiosis, byssinosis, rheumatoid arthritis and nutritional disorders such as anaemia come to mind in this context.[6,13,27]

Identification of syndromes

This use again relates directly to clinical medicine. Broad descriptive clinical and pathological categories often include very different elements. Their different statistical distribution, and their different behaviour among the population, may make it possible to distinguish such elements from each other, and thus help to identify characteristic syndromes. Consider the mortality from 'peptic ulcer' in 1921–3 (Figure 6). Clearly there were at least two conditions to be studied – conditions with possibly different causes. My own main interest in this field is in trying to disentangle coronary heart disease from

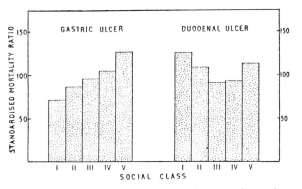

Fig. 6 Social class differences in 'peptic ulcer' mortality, males, England and Wales, 1921–1923.

coronary atheroma, by study of their different distributions in the population today, and their different histories in the past 40 years.[17] Table 3 illustrates again from cardiovascular disease. The common lumping together of coronary and cerebrovascular lesions as 'atherosclerosis' is not very strongly justified in clinical or pathological terms. Nor do the two conditions always behave similarly epidemiologically: the recent vital statistics are quite different; and this small experience among doctors (Table 3) is interesting. The natural history of conditions as *group* phenomena may thus help to define syndromes. The vast unknown field of chronic chest disease – middle-aged men with respiratory symptoms – today offers particular opportunities for this application of the epidemiological method.

(The reverse is also true – that the epidemiological method may help to show or to confirm that apparently disparate phenomena are connected, by drawing attention to their related behaviour in the population – for example, malformation and rubella,[12] rheumatic fever and streptococcal infection, zoster and chicken-pox. However, I cannot think of any satisfactory illustrations from the non-infectious diseases.)

Table 3 Coronary and cerebrovascular disease among medical practitioners: number of 'first attacks', 1947–1950 (men aged 40–64)

	General practitioners	Other doctors
Coronary heart disease	82	33
Cerebrovascular disease	14	13
Man-years of observation	10 800	8620

Clues to causes

The main function of epidemiology is to discover groups in the population with high rates of disease, and with low, so that causes of disease and of freedom from disease can be postulated. The most obvious and direct examples are the original observations on the nutritional deficiencies (scurvy, beriberi, pellagra, goitre); the geographical study of cancer (especially of the skin and liver); the industrial cancers (bladder, for instance); and industrial accidents (of coal-miners or railway workers). The biggest promise of this method lies in relating diseases to the *ways of living* of different groups, and by doing so to unravel 'causes' of disease about which it is possible to do something.

'Ways of living' can usually be described only in simple terms, and the kinds of causes of health and disease postulated in them tend therefore to be in rather simple terms, not of intimate biological mechanisms, but of social factors in the satisfaction of elementary human needs, of large-scale environmental features, of major aspects of behaviour. They are thus often 'general' rather than specific factors of health, causes of *disease*, or diseases, rather than of a particular disease: as in the relations of water supply to bowel infections (not merely the cholera), living space and respiratory infections (as a class), income levels, nutrition and growth. We are only just beginning to identify such factors in ways of life, mass habits and social customs which may be related to many of the important problems of our own highly advanced society. For example, *over-nutrition* (obesity; and atherosclerosis, thrombosis, dental caries, diabetes, toxaemia of pregnancy?); *physical* inactivity ('coronary thrombosis' and how much else?); *atmospheric pollution* (lung cancer; chronic chest disease of many kinds, and acute, and other, non-respiratory conditions?); *cultural factors* (genital cancer in Jews and non-Jews); *eating customs* (alimentary cancer?); *social isolation* (schizophrenia, senile psychosis, suicide?). And, of course, there is still an overabundant heritage of nineteenth century (and earlier) *poverty* and *crowding, insanitation* and *bad habits* that contribute over-fully to modern ill-health.

Figure 7 illustrates from some recent studies, and includes a wide range of data, from the first turning of the ground to highly advanced observations. I have included (b) the famous analysis from the Metropolitan Life on the dangers of 'overweight'; an elaboration of Doll and Bradford Hill's classic data on cigarette-smoking and cancer of the lung (e); some figures (unique so far as I know) from France on consanguineous marriages in relation to stillbirth and early neonatal mortality (g); an example (h) of the recent pioneering by the General Register Officer in psychosis, the darkest area of all;

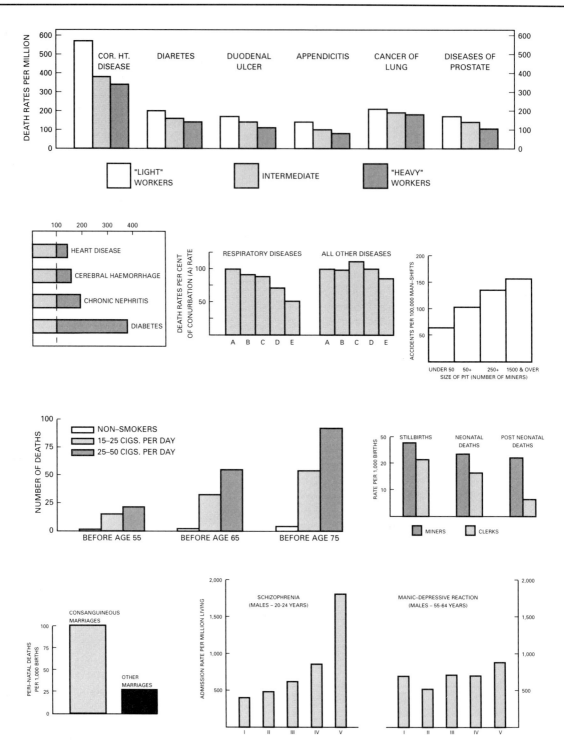

figures from Revans on the size of industrial units in relation to the frequency of accidents (d), which raise large questions of morale and the human environment, of *group* functioning as such, rather than the properties of the *individuals* who aggregate the group (compare immunity, and endemicity of infections). The distributions shown (a) on physical activity (they are different for *gastric* ulcer, incidentally, and for diabetes in *younger* persons, and do not show with other diseases), and on the disadvantages of town dwellers in respect of respiratory disease (c), merely set a stage for further inquiry; the natural experiment, or 'experiment of opportunity' provided by miners and clerks (f), provides, at least, contrast groups in which it may be profitable to seek factors that are significant in modern infant mortality.

The great advantage of this kind of approach to prevention is that it may be applicable in the early stages of our knowledge of disease, to disrupt the pattern of causation before the intimate nature of diseases is understood. Sufficient facts may be established for this by epidemiological methods alone, or in combination with others. The opportunity may thus offer to deal with one 'cause', or with various combinations of causes. Moreover, the possibility of two types of control may be opened up – environmental (as in the fluoridation of water) and personal (through alteration of diet and hygiene).

Conclusion

Epidemiology is today the Cinderella of the medical sciences. The proposition might, however, be advanced that public health needs more epidemiology, and so does medicine as a whole, and, it may be said, society at large. *Public health* needs more epidemiology – this is the most obvious intellectual basis for its further advance. Epidemiology, moreover, as a tried instrument of research – with its modern developments in sampling and surveys, small-number statistics, the follow-up of cohorts, international comparisons, field experiment and family study;

and with its extensions to problems of genetics as well as environment, to physiological norms as well as disease, the psychological as well as the physical, morbidity as well as mortality – epidemiology now offers the possibility of a new era of collaboration between public health workers and clinical medicine. Such a collaboration could be on equal terms, each making their particular contribution to the joint solving of problems. There is abundant evidence today that clinicians would very much welcome such a development.

Medicine as a whole needs more epidemiology, for without it cardinal areas have to be excluded from the consideration of human health and sickness. Epidemiology, moreover, is rich with suggestions for clinical and laboratory study, and it offers many possibilities for testing hypotheses emerging from these. One of the most urgent *social* needs of the day is to identify rules of healthy living that might do for us what Snow and others did for the Victorians, and help to reduce the burden of illness in middle and old age which is so characteristic a feature of our society. There is no indication whatever that the experimental sciences alone will be able to produce the necessary guidance. Collaboration between clinician, laboratory scientist and epidemiologist might be more successful. The possibilities are at present unlimited, if often neglected.

Summary

We may summarize what has been said in terms of some of the relations between epidemiology, and the epidemiological method, and clinical medicine.

Epidemiology studies populations, and all cases that can be defined in them. It is concerned not only with those whose troubles immediately present to particular clinical attention but with the subclinical, the undiagnosed, the cases treated elsewhere. It thus *helps to complete the clinical picture* and natural history of disease.

Epidemiology *supplements the clinical picture* by

Fig. 7 Seeking clues to causes. a, Mortality in relation to physical activity of work, men aged 45–64 in social class III (skilled workers), England and Wales, 1930–1932. b, Experiences of overweight men in comparison with standard policy holders, Metropolitan Life Assurance Company, actual number of deaths per 100 expected, ages attained 25–74. c, Mortality of town and country dwellers from bronchitis, pneumonia, respiratory tuberculosis and lung cancer, and from all other diseases (males), aged 45–64, England and Wales, 1950–1952 (A, conurbations; B, C, D, large, medium and small urban areas; E, rural areas – the trend for females is very similar). d, Frequency of accidents to miners and size of pits. e, Smoking and lung cancer: number of men per 1000 aged 25 expected to die from cancer of lung before ages shown. f, Infant mortality in the families of miners and clerks, England and Wales, 1949–1950. g, Stillbirths and deaths in the first four weeks of life, infants of consanguineous and other marriages, two French *départements*. h, Social class and admissions to mental hospitals, England and Wales, 1949.

asking questions that cannot be asked in clinical study – about the health of the community and of sections of it, present and past; by setting clinical problems in community perspective, describing their behaviour as group, not individual, phenomena, indicating their dimensions and distributions, and how much, and where, action is needed; by revealing problems and indicating where among the population these might best be studied.

Finally, epidemiology, by identifying harmful ways of living, and by pointing the road to healthier ways, *helps to abolish the clinical picture*. This is its chief function and the one in greatest need of development today.

Bibliography

1 Acton Society Trust, *Size and Morale,* 1953, London.
2 Backett, E.M., Heady, J.A. and Evans, J.C.G., *British Medical Journal,* 1954, 1, 109.
3 Baird D. and Illsley, R., *Proc. Roy. Soc. Med.,* 1953, 46, 53.
4 Baird, D. and Scott, E.M. *Eugen. Rev.,* 1955, 45, 139.
5 Baird D., Biles, E.M., Illsley R., Scott, E.M., and Thomson, A.M., personal communication, 1955.
6 Cochrane, A.L., Fletcher, C.M., Gilson, J.C. and Hugh-Jones, P., *Brit. J. Industr. Med.,* 1951, 8, 53.
7 Doll, R., Jones, F. Avery and Buckatzsch, M.M., *Spec. Rep. Ser. Med. Res. Coun. (Lond.),* No. 276, 1951.
8 Doll, R. and Hill, A. Bradford, *British Medical Journal,* 1952, 2, 1271.
9 Dublin, L.I. and Marks H., *Trans. Ass. Life Insur. Med. Dir. Amer.,* 1951, 35, 235.
10 Glover, J.A., *Monthly Bull. Minist. Hlth (Lond.),* 1950, 9, 62.
11 Heady J.A. and Barley R.G., *British Medical Journal,* 1953, 1, 1105.
12 Hill, A. Bradford, *New Engl. J. Med.,* 1953, 248, 995.
13 Kellgren, J.H., Lawrence, J.S. and Aitken-Swan, J., *Ann. Rheum. Dis.,* 1953, London.
14 Ministry of Education, *Health of the School Child,* 1946 and 1947, 1952 and 1953, London.
15 Ministry of Pensions and National Insurance, *Digest of Statistics Analysing Certificates of Incapacity,* 1951 and 1952, London.
16 Ministry of Transport, *Return of Road Accidents for 1949.*
17 Morris, J.N. *Lancet,* 1951, 1, 69.
18 Morris, J.N. and Heady, J.A., *Brit. J. Industr. Med.,* 1953, 10, 245.
19 Morris, J.N. and Heady, J.A., *Lancet,* 1955, 1, 343, 554.
20 Morris, J.N., Heady, J.A. and Barley, R.G., *British Medical Journal,* 1952, 1, 503.
21 Registrar-General (various years), *Statistical Review of England and Wales.* Tables, Part I, Medical; Text Medical Civil. London.
22 Registrar-General, *Decennial Supplement, England and Wales, 1921.* Part II, Occupational Mortality. London, 1927.
23 Registrar-General, *Decennial Supplement, England and Wales, 1931.* Part IIa, Occupational Mortality. London. 1938.
24 Registrar-General, *Supplement on General Morbidity, Cancer, and Mental Health.* 1949. London, 1953.
25 Registrar-General, *Decennial Supplement, England and Wales, 1951.* Part I. Occupational Mortality. London, 1954.
26 Rowntree, G., *Scot. J. Polit. Econ.,* 1954, 1, 201.
27 Schilling, R.S.F., quoted by author.
28 Social Medicine Research Unit and Collaborators. Unpublished.
29 Social Medicine Research Unit, with R.G. Barley. Unpublished.
30 Sutter, J. and Tabah, L., *Population,* 1953, 8, 511.
31 Thompson, E.D.B., *Med. Offr,* 1954, 91, 235.

Acknowledgement

Morris, J.N. (1955) Uses of Epidemiology. *British Medical Journal,* 13 August, 395–401.

THE ICEBERG: 'COMPLETING THE CLINICAL PICTURE' IN GENERAL PRACTICE

There is much interest in the role of the general practitioner in early detection of chronic disease and in its prevention. In this paper I have used epidemiological methods to show the nature and size of some of the problems in England and Wales, by adjusting the relevant data to a hypothetical 'average general practice'.

The practice has been given a list of 2250 (the nearest round number to the average list of general practices in England and Wales in 1960[23]), and the age and sex distribution of England and Wales in 1960[30] (Table 1). I have estimated the number of patients in this practice who would be 'known' to have certain diseases according to morbidity statistics.[3,4,6,8,12–14,17,18,21,27,30,41,42]

Table 1 Population distribution in the average general practice

	Age-group (years)				Total
	0–14	*15–44*	*45–64*	*65+*	
Male	264	441	276	104	1085
Female	251	446	304	164	1165
Total	515	887	580	268	2250

Table 2 Experience of 1 year in the average general practice (Both sexes, all ages, unless specified)

Disease recognised by the practitioner		*Total present in the practice, including undetected and potential disease*	
Pulmonary tuberculosis [18] [24] [30]		Radiological evidence of pulmonary tuberculosis [8]	12–14
Cases	6–7	Previously unsuspected pulmonary tuberculosis, patients aged 15 and over, would be detected at	
New notifications per annum	1		
Deaths per annum (1 in 7 years)	0.12	mass radiography	2–3
Cancer [22]		Suspect, probably inactive pulmonary tuberculosis	3–4
New cases per annum	7	Cancer [8] [18]	
lung	1	Cases	11–12
breast (3 in 4 years)	0.75	Lung cancer, males aged 55+, would be first	
stomach (3 in 4 years)	0.74	detected at mass radiography (1 in 2 years)	0.5
prostate and rectum (1 in 2 years)	0.52	Precancerous lesions [42]	
		Carcinoma-in-situ	2–3
cervix (1 in 4–5 years)	0.22	Haemoglobin concentration [14]	
Anaemia (all forms) [18]		Males, below 12.5 g. per 100 ml. aged 15–44	10
Males 15–44	1	45–64	23
45–64	1	65+	23
65+	1	Females, below 12 g. per 100 ml. aged 15–44	114
Females 15–44	12	45–64	37
45–64	7	65+	35
65+	5	Glycosuria and 'diabetic' blood-sugar curve	29
Diabetes mellitus [4]	14	Undetected cases	15
Aged 45+	12	aged 45+	14
Urinary infections [18]		Significant bacteriuria [12]	
Females, aged 15+	20	Females, aged 15+	40
Staphylococcal diseases [18]		Nasal carriers of *Staph. aureus* [27]	500–1500
Overt skin infection	110	penicillin-resistant	100–300
Glaucoma [18]		Early chronic glaucoma [6]	
Aged 45+	3	Aged 45+	17
Hypertension and hypertensive heart disease [18]		Casual diastolic blood-pressure 100 mm. Hg. and over [21]	
Males aged 45+	8	Males aged 45+	30
Females aged 45+	24	Females aged 45+	131
Bronchitis [18]		Symptoms and signs of bronchitis [3]	
Males aged 45–64	24	Males aged 45–64	47
Females aged 45–64	19	Females aged 45–64	24
Rheumatoid arthritis [18]		'Definite' and 'probable' rheumatoid arthritis [17]	
Aged 15+	11	Aged 15+	25
Epilepsy [18]	7–8	Epilepsy [29]	13–14
Psychiatric disorders [18]		'Conspicuous psychiatric morbidity' [13]	
Males 15+	27	Males 15+	58
Females 15+	62	Females 15+	102

By the methods described by Morris,[25] I have tried to 'complete the clinical picture' by estimating the numbers of people with undetected or potential disease who might be found on search. These numbers are mostly based on surveys of whole communities for a particular condition, and I have assumed that the hypothetical average general practice will contain the same proportion of people with these conditions. Table 2 shows the experience of a year in the practice, with disease known to the general practitioner on the left, and the undetected cases on the right. The annual number of new cases and the age-groups of all patients, with data on precursors and associated signs for some diseases, are given.

Official sources have been used to compile the 'vital statistics' given in Table 3 and for the estimate of certain other events in the practice.

Comment on tables

Subclinical disease

Community surveys have shown that epilepsy,[29] psycho-neurotic illness,[13] chronic bronchitis[3] and rheumatoid arthritis,[17] are more prevalent than is suggested by the morbidity statistics of 106 general practices in England in 1955–6.[18] No doubt there are undiscovered cases of

Table 3 Some annual events in the average general practice

Vital statistics [30]

Births		39
Illegitimate births	2	
Marriages		17
Divorces	1	
Deaths		26
Diseases of circulatory system	10	
Malignant neoplasms	5	
Vascular lesions of nervous system	4	
Bronchitis	1	
Violence	1	

Contact with other parts of NHS [18 23 31 32]

Hospital		
All admissions		208
No. of patients		96
Peptic ulcer	3–4	
Acute appendicitis	3–4	
Abdominal hernia	5	
Uterovaginal prolapse	2	
Arthritis	1–2	
Tonsillectomy	9–10	
Injuries	14	
Head injuries	2–3	
Fractured femur	1	
New outpatients		641
Casualty		277
Other departments		364
Traumatic and orthopaedic	51	
General surgery	46	
ENT	32	
Ophthalmic	31	
General medical	31	
Mental Hospital:		
All admissions	5	
First admissions	2–3	
New outpatients	8	
Diagnostic Services:		
Referred to hospital pathological		
laboratory	59	
X-ray department	99	
mass radiography by practitioner	10	
Annual number examined by mass		
radiography	177	
Domiciliary visits by consultants	16	
Domiciliary Services:		
Health visitor	600 visits	
Home nurse	1134 visits to 45 patients	
Home help	16 patients	
Maternal and Child Welfare		
Patients attending antenatal clinic	17	
postnatal clinic	2	
Domiciliary confinements:		
Attended by midwife	14	
Doctor booked	12	
Attended by doctor	2	
First attendance infant welfare clinic	31	
Seen by school medical service	107	

Miscellaneous [1 23 33]

Receiving National Assistance	100
Supplied for first time with full dentures	
(all teeth just extracted)	17
Casualties on the roads	17
Receiving war pensions	25
Registered blind	5

these diseases in most general practices. Some of these potential patients may be people living with a disability which has been recognized, and for which they have not sought treatment in the year of the inquiry. But this can hardly be true of diabetics and the tuberculous, where the figures support the dictum that for every known case there is another undiscovered.

Detection of *diabetes* has been made easier by the use of glucose-oxidase paper strips, a simple and reliable method of urine-testing. Community studies[4,41] show that middle-aged and elderly patients are most likely to have unrecognised diabetes, and the general practitioner has many opportunities to test their urine. Those with symptoms can be helped, and some complications perhaps reduced.

The figures for *tuberculosis*[8,24,30] prove that this disease is still a clinical and public-health problem. The highest rates of infection are among elderly men and delinquent and psychopathic members of the community,[8] some of whom are likely to be found in the average general practice.

It is hardly surprising that half the cases of *urinary infection* in women remain undetected. If the suggestion is correct, that bacteriuria may precede chronic pyelonephritis and hypertension,[12] the general practitioner may help to prevent these serious conditions by detecting and treating patients with 'symptomless' bacteriuria. Simple methods of detection have been described[36] though there is not yet agreement about their value.[37]

The significance of the figure for glaucoma, based on several American surveys,[6] may be debatable. Undetected cases of early chronic glaucoma will occur in the average general practice, if the incidence of the disease is comparable with American experience. These cases could be detected by a combination of techniques – measurement of visual acuity, perimetry, fundoscopy, and measurement of ocular tension – all within the competence of the well-trained and well-equipped general practitioner. The incentive is the prevention of blindness; the average general practice at present has five blind patients and at least one of these has glaucoma.

The problem of the *Staphylococcus* is demonstrated by this method of presentation; while there are about 110 cases annually of (presumably) staphylococcal skin infection in the average general practice (boils, carbuncles, impetigo, styes and so on), there may be between 500 and 1500 nasal carriers of *Staph. aureus* – perhaps a fifth of them penicillin-resistant.[27]

Anaemia

If recent community surveys[14] record the true prevalence

of anaemia, the average general practitioner deals with only about one patient in seven of those who are anaemic. In the course of a year many of the 200 with anaemia in the practice will consult their doctor for incidental disease, if not because they have symptoms due to the anaemia itself; and many are probably working below full efficiency. A small minority, especially of the elderly, have grave disease of which anaemia is an early sign.[35] Clinical examination alone will detect with certainty only those with severe anaemia, below 60 per cent Hb (9 g per 100 ml)[19]; only laboratory tests will detect all who need treatment. The average general practitioner requests only 59 examinations annually, or just over one a week. (The figure includes all pathological investigations, blood, urine and faeces tests, and many must be for antenatal cases.) Without adding an insuperable burden to the hospital laboratory service, more haemoglobin estimations for women of childbearing age, the group most likely to be anaemic, could be asked for. Better still, could not the general practitioner undertake such simple tests as estimation for haemoglobin? This can be done with reasonable accuracy using simple equipment, such as grey-wedge haemoglobinometer, though there is argument about the reliability of observations on capillary blood. Changes in the method of payment for medical services might encourage this work.

Cancer

There will be some seven new cases of cancer each year in the average general practice.[22] The commoner forms are listed in Table 2.

The presence of two or three cases of carcinoma-in-situ of the uterine *cervix*[42] is a strong argument for better facilities for exfoliative cytology. The most vulnerable women (middle-aged multiparae, particularly in the lower social classes) are more likely to attend their family doctor with complaints that justify pelvic examination and offer an opportunity to take a cervical smear, than they are to visit clinics set up for the purpose. The general practitioner is also in a good position to encourage people to attend special cancer-detection clinics, where these exist. The efficacy of the technique of cervical cytology in reducing the incidence of invasive cancer of the cervix is being convincingly demonstrated.[2]

About three new cases of cancer of the *breast* will occur every four years in the average general practice. Many of the vulnerable women are likely to attend their general practitioner under circumstances that from time to time offer an opportunity to examine their breasts, thus reinforcing whatever measures some women may take for themselves; and if this opportunity were taken, some

cancers might be detected earlier than otherwise. The incidence of the disease makes clear the need for education of patients in the technique of self-examination.

Opportunities for rectal examinations are less common, but the knowledge that there will be one new case of cancer of either the *rectum* or the *prostate* every two years (as well as an unknown number of cases of benign hypertrophy of the prostate) may be an incentive to make this examination more often.

At present there is one new case of *lung* cancer every year in the average general practice in England and Wales – and one death. The probability that this case need not have occurred if all men in the practice were non-smokers, and the lower incidence of the disease among ex-smokers than among those still smoking,[34] should encourage health counselling. It should also encourage the doctor to set the patients a good example. Of the cases that occur, perhaps one in alternate years might first be detected at mass miniature radiography if all men in the practice over the age of 55 were radiologically examined,[8] though it may be hard to decide how often such an examination would be justifiable, and whether it should be confined to vulnerable groups, such as heavy smokers.

Too little is known about the causes of cancer for much of it to be considered preventable; but by always remembering the possibility, and by using ordinary clinical skills of history-taking and physical examination, with diagnostic aids such as cervical cytology and radiology when appropriate, the general practitioner can engage in 'secondary prevention' – the earlier detection which will more surely lead to successful treatment.

The iceberg phenomenon

Disease known to the general practitioner represents only the tip of the iceberg; Morris[25] has shown that differences below the surface may be qualitative as well as quantitative. A good example of this is coronary artery disease in middle-aged men (Table 4).

The numbers are mostly approximate, and there is considerable overlap in data about the submerged parts of the iceberg. The prognostic significance of several of the factors included in the table has been clearly demonstrated,[7] and several lines of action are implied – namely, search for vulnerable individuals; health counselling, where appropriate; and epidemiological research.

Although mass serum-cholesterol estimations are hardly justifiable until we have a cheap micromethod, ordinary clinical examination could detect more men

Table 4 Coronary-artery disease in men aged 45–64

Visible

1	Death [30]
5	Cases [18]

Submerged

11	ECG evidence of left ventricular hypertrophy [11]
15	Casual diastolic blood-pressure 100 mm Hg or over [21]
24	Serum-cholesterol 300 mg per 100 ml or over [38]
28	Healed infarcts [26]
52	Smoking more than 20 cigarettes per day [34]
55	Obese, more than 10% over ideal weight [20]
140	Moderate to severe atheroma of coronary arteries [9]
???	Insufficient exercise
	Worried by responsibility
	Other emotional stress
276	At risk

with high blood pressure, some of whom might need treatment. Cheap, and easily portable, transistorised electrocardiographs could be used by general practitioners to 'screen' vulnerable groups in their practice – for example, men who are overweight, who lack opportunity or incentive to take exercise or who smoke too much. These should benefit from the good counsels of their family doctor. The question marks in the table indicate suitable subjects for research in general practice; no one has any clear idea about the leisure activities of middle-aged men, or about the relation, if any, between these and health. Is the vicarious stress of watching competitive sports related to the incidence of stress disease, such as hypertension?

Patients who commit suicide are at the tip of another iceberg. In the average general practice there will be one suicide[30] in four years, and, when it was still an indictable offence, one attempted suicide came before the courts[5] in the same period. But each year at least two more people will have made suicidal attempts.[16] A still larger number have depressive illness severe enough to make them wish to end their lives. These people do not always get appropriate medical treatment; many with milder depression are even less likely to do so.

Other events

Social pathology

The figures for illegitimate births and for divorce are given in Table 3. Others can be derived from various sources. Each year one adult criminal will be sent to prison, and five or six children under the age of 17 will be charged with offences.[5] About 100 people in the practice will

receive National Assistance.[1] Twenty five to fifty people over retiring age will live alone[40] and about 40 children under the age of 15 come from broken homes.[10] There will probably be between five and ten problem families;[28] and there will be four chronic alcoholics with mental and physical complications, and about another dozen who are addicted to alcohol.[15] Each year ten abortions will escape the notice of the medical profession, compared with the three or four who receive proper medical care.[39] Many of these numbers are only crude estimates, and regional and social variations could cause wide deviations from the average.

Uncommon events

In the same way figures can be adjusted to show how seldom some conditions will turn up in the average general practice. Diseases which were common a generation ago are now rare; the average general practitioner might wait eight years to see a case of rheumatic fever in a child under the age of 15; 60 years to see a case of typhoid or paratyphoid fever, and as long as 400 years to see a case of diphtheria.[24] A patient with schizophrenia will probably be seen once in two years,[31] a patient with leukaemia or other malignant disease of the lymphatic and haemopoietic system once in four years, and a patient with a cerebral tumour once in eight to ten years.[30]

The diversity of activities in the average general practice, and the range of tasks expected of the average family doctor, have been shown. Changing conditions of practice in recent years should not allow their clinical skills to atrophy.

Communication

If the general practitioner is to draw together the various parts of the National Health Service, much will depend on the efficiency of his lines of communication. The number of contacts with the hospital services (Table 3) are probably inflated because some patients will attend more than one hospital and some will be admitted to the same hospital more than once a year. The contrast between the figure of 208 derived from the report on the health and welfare services[23] and of 96 from the morbidity statistics from general practice[18] makes this clear. Even so, nearly 1000 contacts between the practice and the hospital services each year must represent a formidable number of letters and/or telephone calls. Considering the quantity of communications, it is hardly surprising that their quality is sometimes defective.

The discrepancies in the figures for domiciliary obstetrics cannot only be due to the division of the obstetric services into three parts. Whatever else may be said about this, it is clear that if in the average general practice a doctor is present at only two out of the fourteen home confinements that take place each year, opportunities are being lost to cement a firm doctor–patient relationship. Postnatal care may be no more satisfactory, but here the data are incomplete.

Summary

A model has been used to show a year's experience in an average general practice, particularly of the chronic diseases.

A considerable amount of undetected disease, some of which is serious and some controllable, might be found fairly easily without adding greatly to the burden of the day's work.

Ordinary clinical skills and new diagnostic aids may be used to detect cases of actual and potential disease in general practice.

The detection and control of diabetes, some forms of hypertension and their sequelae, glaucoma, anaemia, some kinds of cancer, and coronary-artery disease have been discussed.

References

1 Annual Abstract of Statistics (1961) No. 98. HM Stationery Office.

2 Boyes, D.A., Fidler, H.K. and Lock, D.R. (1962) *Brit. Med. J.*, i, 203.

3 College of General Practitioners. (1961) *ibid.*, ii, 973.

4 College of General Practitioners. (1962) *ibid.* i, 1497.

5 Criminal Statistics 1960 (1961) HM Stationery Office.

6 David, W.D. (1959) *US publ. Hlth Serv. Publ.* no. 666. Washington, DC.

7 Dawber, T.R. (1962) *Proc. R. Soc. Med.*, 55, 265.

8 Heasman, M.A. (1961) *Stud. Med. Popul. Subj.*, no. 17.

9 Hill, K.R., Camps, F.E., Rigg, K. and McKinney, B.E.G. (1961) *Brit. Med, J.*, i, 1190.

10 Illsley, R. and Thompson, B. (1961) *Social Review*, 9, 27.

11 Kagan, A., Dawber, T.R., Kannel, W.B. and Revotskie, N. (1962) *Fed. Proc.*, 21, Suppl. ll, 52.

12 Kass, E.H. (1962) *Ann. Intern. Med.*, 56, 46.

13 Kessel, W.I.N. (1960) *Brit. J. Prev. Soc. Med.* 14, 16.

14 Kilpatrick, G.S. (1961) *Brit. Med. J.*, ii, 1736.

15 *Lancet* (1962) i, 1169.

16 *ibid.*, p. 1171.

17 Lawrence, J.S., Laine, V.A.I. and de Graaff, R. (1961) *Proc. Roy. Soc. Med.* 54, 454.

18 Logan, W.P.D. and Cushion, A.A. (1958) *Clin. Sci.*, 17, 409.

19 McAlpine, S.G., Douglas, A.S. and Robb, R.A. (1957) *Brit. Med. J.*, ii, 983.

20 Metropolitan Life Insurance Company (1960) Statistical Bulletin, January, p. 4.

21 Miall, W.E. and Oldham, P.D. (1958) *Clin. Sci.*, 17, 409.

22 Ministry of Health (1960) On the State of Public Health. HM Stationery Office.

23 Ministry of Health (1961a) The Health and Welfare Services. HM Stationery Office.

24 Ministry of Health (1961b) On the State of Public Health. HM Stationery Office.

25 Morris, J.N. (1957) Uses of Epidemiology. Edinburgh.

26 Morris, J.N. and Crawford, M.D. (1958) *Brit. Med. J.*, ii, 1485.

27 Munch-Petersen, E. (1961) *Bull. World Hlth Org.*, 24, 761.

28 Philp, A.F. and Timms, N. (1957) Problem of the Problem Family. London.

29 Pond, D.A., Bidwell, B.H. and Stein, L. (1968) *Psychiat. Nuerol. Nuerochir.*, 63, 217.

30 Registrar General (1961a) Statistical Review of England and Wales, 1960, part I, tables, medical. HM Stationery Office.

31 Registrar General (1961b) Supplement on Mental Health, 1960. HM Stationery Office.

32 Registrar General (1961) Report on the Hospital Inpatient Inquiry, 1956–57. HM Stationery Office.

33 Road Research, 1960 (1961) HM Stationery Office.

34 Royal College of Physicians (1962) Smoking and Health. London.

35 Semmence, A. (1959) *Brit. Med. J.*, ii, 1153.

36 Simmons, N.A. and Williams, J.D. (1962) *Lancet*, i, 1377.

37 Smith, L.G. and Schmidt, J. (1962) *J. Amer. Med. Ass.*, 181, 431.

38 Social Medicine Research Unit (MRC) Unpublished data.

39 Tietze, C. (1948) *Amer. J. Obstet. Gynec.*, 56, 1160.

40 Townsend, P. (1959) *Bull. World Hlth Org.*, 21, 583.

41 Walker, J.B. and Kerridge, D. (1961) Diabetes in an English Community. Leicester.

42 Wilson, J.M.G. (1961) *Monthly Bull. Min. Hlth PHLS*, 20, 214.

Acknowledgement

Last, J.M. (1963) The iceberg: 'Completing the clinical picture' in general practice. *The Lancet*. 6 July, 28–31.

7 *Professor Stephen Leeder*

McAlister Gregg, N. (1941) Congenital cataract following German measles in the mother. *Transactions of the Ophthalmological Society of Australia*, 3, 35–46.

Colley, J.R.T., Holland, W.W., Leeder, S.R. and Corkhill, R.T. (1976) Respiratory function of infants in relation to subsequent respiratory disease: an epidemiological study. *Bulletin Européen de Physiopathologie Respiratoire*, 12, 651–7.

INTRODUCTION

The paper by Norman McAlister Gregg is a fine example of epidemiological observation based on clinical practice. It demonstrates the importance of intuition and insight in the definition of epidemiological research questions, however refined the subsequent methodology is that is required to address those research questions.

His initial paper in 1941 was important for several other reasons. It showed that rubella, previously regarded as a mild infectious disease, could have disastrous consequences in susceptible pregnant women. This stimulated the eventual laboratory isolation of rubella two decades later and subsequently the development of a vaccine.

His study also gave a major impetus to the development of teratology – the study of birth defects and their causes – because it showed that infections, and possibly other environmental factors, could cause birth defects.

The paper on passive smoking consolidated the observations first noted in an earlier paper by John Colley concerning the influence of parental smoking on the health of children. It took into account, in its methods, the independent effect of parental cough and sputum, which might have been a source of cross infection, and established a dose–response relationship between parental smoking and subsequent respiratory illness incidence in children in the first year of life.

CONGENITAL CATARACT FOLLOWING GERMAN MEASLES IN THE MOTHER

In the first half of the year 1941, an unusual number of cases of congenital cataract made their appearance in Sydney. Cases of similar type, which appeared during the same period, have since been reported from widely separated parts of Australia. Their frequency, unusual characteristics and wide distribution warranted closer investigation, and this report is an attempt to bring to notice some of the more important features of what might almost be regarded as a mild epidemic.

I am indebted to many of my colleagues in New South Wales, Victoria and Queensland for particulars of very many of the cases reviewed. These, for the most part, conform very closely to the general features noted in my own series of cases on which the following description is based. The total number of cases included in this review is 78. My own cases total 13, and in addition I have seen seven others included in my colleagues' lists.

General description and special features

The first striking factor is that the cataracts, usually bilateral, were obvious from birth as dense white opacities completely occupying the pupillary area. Most of the babies were of small size, ill nourished and difficult to feed, with the result that many of them came under the care of the paediatrician before being seen by the ophthalmic surgeon. Many of them were found to be suffering from a congenital defect of the heart – a fact which, as will be explained later, has adversely affected full investigation of the condition of the lens and in some cases the treatment. The pupillary reaction to light was weak and sluggish; in some cases the irides had a somewhat atrophic appearance. This was more noticeable after mydriasis when the pupillary border appeared as a flat dark band seemingly devoid of any iris stroma.

Full mydriasis was difficult to obtain; in my experience it varied from one-half to three-quarters of the normal; moreover, an unusual number of the patients showed intolerance to atropine. In a large proportion of the cases one was forced to rely upon repeated instillations of homatropine to maintain the mydriasis.

Cataract

In the undiluted condition of the pupil the opacities filled the entire area. After dilatation the opacities appeared densely white – sometimes quite pearly – in the central area with a small, apparently clear, zone between this and the pupillary border of the iris. Closer examination revealed in this zone a less dense opacity of smoky appearance, and outside this only a narrow ring through which a red reflex could be obtained.

The cataractous process seemed to have involved all but the outermost layers of the lens, and was considered to have begun early in the life of the embryo. Generally the cataract was symmetrically situated, but in a few cases it was somewhat eccentric – in these there was some sparing of more of the fibres in the lower portion of the peripheral zone. Although the general appearance was much the same in all cases, two main types were noticed in the character of the cataract. In one the contrast between the larger dense white central area and the smaller cloudy more peripheral zone was very marked. In the other density of the cataract was more uniform throughout and occupied an intermediate stage between that of the two portions of the other type. This distinction has been confirmed by the immediate results of operation. When needling was undertaken in cases of the first group, the dense white central portion was difficult to divide and sometimes separated off as a firm white disk. In others the whole lens seemed to be pushed away by the needle. Subsequent absorption in this group was delayed.

In the second type discission was easier to perform and absorption regular and uniformly progressive. In one case under my care both these types were present, the first type in the right eye and the second type in the left eye. In my opinion these variations and those described by other observers are not essentially different from each other, and the apparent differences are due merely to a variation in intensity and duration of action of the same noxious factor.

The appearance of the cataract does not, in my opinion, exactly correspond to any of the large number of morphological types of congenital and developmental lenticular opacities that have been described. I do not wish to add to what Duke Elder[1] has described as 'the confusion which has arisen from the enthusiasm of various observers in the multiplication of types which differ but little in their essential pathology and vary only in their shape and position'. I shall, therefore, merely describe the cataract as subtotal. Other descriptions by my colleagues in notes on their cases have been: central nuclear, complete discoid, nuclear plus, anterior polar, dense central with riders, complete pearly, mature and total lamellar. In 16 cases of the whole series reviewed the cataract was unilateral.

Vision

In all cases the response to light was good: the babies appeared to follow readily any movement of the light stimulus.

Nystagmus

In the very young patients nystagmus was not noted, but in older babies or in cases in which treatment had to be delayed it was present. The movements were of a coarse, jerky, purposeless nature rather than a true nystagmus. It was a searching movement of the eyeballs and indicated the absence of any development of fixation. In my own cases it was always present if treatment had been delayed beyond the age of three months. In one case, in which the parents deferred operation in order to try some other form of treatment of which they had been informed, it developed before they consented to operation. In another case it developed after operation during the process of absorption. This development during the waiting period before operation has been noticed by other observers.

Variations

One case in my series was particularly interesting. The baby was referred to me at the age of three weeks with a diagnosis of bilateral keratitis. The corneae were quite white at birth and both parents had been subjected to a Wassermann test with negative results. At examination I noted a peculiar corneal haze, denser in the centre than in the periphery. The iris was just visible through this haze in the peripheral zone. The tension was normal and there was no inflammation. I advised re-examination under anaesthesia. This was done two weeks later. By this time the cornea had cleared and the typical white cataracts were seen in the pupillary areas. This baby subsequently became very ill and it was only a few weeks ago that I was able to operate. At operation mydriasis was fuller than usual in these cases and the cataracts were the largest observed in this series.

Two other cases with similar corneal involvement have been noted – namely, by A. Odillo Maher and H. E. Robinson. Involvement was unilateral in Maher's and bilateral in Robinson's case. In these cases there had apparently been some temporary interference with the nutrition of the cornea. Maher's case is also interesting in that the mother developed cataract during pregnancy at the age of 27. This is the only instance throughout the series of any familial history of cataract.

In another case, reported by S. R. Gerstman, there was 'bilateral subluxation of the lenses, mature cataracts, accompanied by arachnodactyly and large fontanelle. Hip regions appeared normal.'

Other complications reported have been cleft palate, one; congenital stenosis of naso-lachrymal duct, three; *calcaneus varus*, one; although it is not certain these are above the average incidence in any group of infants of similar numbers.

Monocular cases

The monocular cases merit special consideration. Sixteen of these have been reported, and in ten of them definite microphthalmia has been described.

In one of my cases – there were three in all – the cataract was noted by the mother only when the child was seven weeks old, though she stated that it may have been present before that date. The affected eye was definitely microphthalmic and examination of the other eye under mydriasis revealed a large pale area with some scattered pigmentation in the lower half of the fundus suggestive of a coloboma.

In another case the mother gave a history that both eyes were said to have had conjunctivitis at birth. This inflammation, she stated, cleared up under treatment in three weeks, and then two weeks later she noticed a white mass in the left pupil. Conceding the accuracy of these histories, I have no doubt that the cataracts were present at birth in the central portion of the lens and that it was the final opacification of the more peripheral fibres which made them apparent. In all other cases the cataracts have been apparent from birth.

Reporting her case of left-sided monocular cataract, Dr Aileen Mitchell wrote:

No difference was noticed in the size of the eyes when the child was seven weeks old: when the child was aged four months there was microphthalmia of the left eye. The mother said the eye had got small. Diameter of the right cornea was about 11 millimetres, of the left cornea, 8.5 millimetres. Nystagmus, which was not present at the first examination had developed and was coarse in nature with roving movements of the eyeballs. The fundus of the right eye appeared pale, and some scattered irregular shaped spots of pigment were observed.

L. Stanton Cook described one case, monocular central opacity of the lens, and writes: 'It would appear that this cataract is a developmental defect rather than a toxic type.' As the baby also had the typical congenital defect of the heart, I feel that this is open to question.

The accompanying microphthalmia, definitely noted in 66 per cent of cases, suggests an inhibitory effect on the development of the eye generally. In an autopsy performed in a monocular case at the Royal Alexandra Hospital for Children the following measurements were recorded. Left eye (affected), antero-posterior diameter, 1.6 centimetres; transverse diameter, 1.5 centimetres. Right eye (unaffected), these measurements were respectively 1.8 centimetres and 1.9 centimetres. It was also noted that the left cornea was smaller than the right in proportion to the general variation in size of the eyes.

Microphthalmia

Microphthalmia is present so frequently (66 per cent) in the cases of monocular cataract that closer attention to the size of the eyes in the binocular cases is advisable. Is it not possible that both eyes may be smaller than normal, and that this feature may be unnoticed because it is bilateral? Further information on this aspect can be obtained from measurements at autopsies and by observation of the subsequent growth of the eyes in the living infants.

Heart

As previously mentioned, an extremely high percentage of these babies had a congenital defect of the heart. I am indebted to Dr Margaret Harper for the following description of eight cases seen by her.

All these babies were seen because of difficulty in feeding and failure to thrive. They all had symptoms suggesting a cardiac defect such as difficulty in taking the breast; they had to be fed in their cots by bottle and some by gavage. They were all in the acyanotic or potentially cyanotic groups of cardiac defects. None was cyanotic. There was a harsh systolic murmur over the base of the heart and down the sternum in all. Some had a thrill. All had signs suggesting the continuance of a foetal condition or of a malformation of the heart.

In my own series this condition was present in all but one case. In the whole series it has been present in 44 cases: in eleven cases there is no record of the cardiac condition; in ten cases it has been recorded as normal or apparently normal; in four cases in which the condition was not reported upon, the babies died and death was sudden: in another the baby was 'ill-nourished'; and in three cases the report was 'no defect noted'.

Autopsy in three cases at the Royal Alexandra Hospital for Children revealed a wide patency of the *ductus arteriosus*, and I understand that in autopsies performed elsewhere a similar condition has been found.

Additional findings

In one case at the Royal Alexandra Hospital for Children there were several additional findings worth record here.

Both lungs had a considerable degree of hypostatic congestion at the bases. Throughout the remainder of the lungs there were a very large number of haemorrhagic spots, some of which were confluent and covered considerable areas. Haemorrhagic spots were detected on the inner surface of the pericardium and on the surface of the myocardium. In addition, the visceral pericardium over the upper anterior aspect of the left ventricle bore a 'milk spot'. The right kidney was situated in such a position that the ureter entered the pelvis on the lateral side of the kidney after coursing across its anterior surface. The right kidney consisted of two distinct lobes, the upper one about twice as large as the lower. Each lobe had its own separate pelvis, and the ureter divided outside the kidney into two branches, one to each lobe. Both ovaries were cystic. The uterus was bicornuate in type.

Another complication noted in a few cases was the development of a dry scaly eczematous condition, involving the face, scalp and limbs, which was very resistant to treatment.

Sex

Thirty-three of the patients were males, 35 were females. In the remaining ten cases the reports did not specify the sex of the child.

Deaths

In this series of cases 15 deaths have been recorded. Details are not available in all cases of the mode or cause of death, but broncho-pneumonia has been noted in several. In three cases within my own knowledge there has been a sudden rise of temperature up to 105° F or even 106° F, accompanied by extreme distress, and death has followed within 24 hours.

Intolerance to atropine

Intolerance to atropine has been a noticeable feature of the cases in my own series and in no single instance has it been possible to continue its administration throughout the treatment. In most cases, even after one or two instillations, the baby has exhibited considerable constitutional disturbance with pyrexia, restlessness and irritability, and the difficulty of feeding has been intensified. In one case in which two instillations were made over a period of 24 hours, the temperature rose to 105° F. Homatropine, 2 per cent, was substituted and the temperature returned to normal, and was not subsequently elevated. Other observers have noted the same intolerance to atropine.

Aetiology

Although one was struck with the unusual appearance of the cataracts in the first few cases, it was only when other similar cases continued to appear that serious thought was given to their causation.

The remarkable similarity of the opacities in the lens, the frequency of an accompanying affection of the heart and the widespread geographical incidence of the cases suggested that there was some common factor in the production of the diseased condition, and suggested it was the result of some constitutional condition of toxic or infective nature rather than of a purely development defect.

The question arose whether this factor could have been some disease or infection occurring in the mother during pregnancy which had then interfered with the developing cells of the lens. By a calculation from the date of the birth of the baby it was estimated that the early period of pregnancy corresponded with the period of maximum intensity of the very widespread and severe epidemic in 1940 of the so-called German measles.

Special attention was accordingly paid to the history of the health of the mothers during pregnancy, and in each new case it was found that the mother had suffered from that disease early in her pregnancy, most frequently in the first or second month. In some cases she had not at that time yet realized that she was pregnant.

The investigation was then repeated in the early cases in which such a history had not been sought, and again the history of early 'German measles' infection was definite. Moreover, in all these cases the health of the mother during the remainder of the pregnancy was described as good.

As the constant involvement of the central nuclear fibres in the cataractous process suggested an early incidence of the noxious factor, it was considered that a possible solution of the problem had been obtained. Confirmation for this theory was therefore sought from any of my colleagues who had lesions of this type, and they kindly agreed to assist me by inquiry into the health of the mothers during pregnancy. The result of their inquiries confirmed the amazing frequency of the 'German measles' infection.

'Congenital cataract may be due to a maldevelopment, physical or chemical element acting on the developing lens, or inflammation during the embryonic or foetal period'.[2]

Duke Elder[3] stated: 'The aetiology of these opacities depends upon some disturbances of the development of the lens, but what the actual disturbance may be, or the precise method of its action, is a matter of considerable doubt in most cases.'

From his anatomical studies Jaensch[4] concluded that an intra-uterine inflammation was a frequent cause of a total opacity of the lens. Toxic influences also may play a part in the production of opacities, and it is inconceivable, writes Duke Elder,[5] that toxic or infective processes in the mother may cause a derangement in the lens of the foetus, or that similar causes, error of feeding and nutrition or acute exanthemata in the infant, may have a similar effect.

Ida Mann[6] has stated that exanthemata, measles, mumps, smallpox, chickenpox, scarlet fever etc. are all known to be transmissible transplacentally.

Whatever the disturbing factor may be, it is fair to assume that the earlier it acts, the more will the central portion of the lens be likely to suffer.

In the developing lens, in the 26-millimetre stage of the embryo, the original central primitive fibres, elongations of the cells of the posterior wall, have completed their growth. Then begins the development of the secondary lens fibres from the cells in the equatorial region. All subsequent growth in the lens is from these equatorial cells, which give rise to successive layers of new lens fibres, these fibres enveloping and compressing the central fibres. With the development of these fibres comes the appearance of the suturing which eventually takes on the typical 'Y' pattern of the foetal nucleus.

In the cases under review the cataractous process has involved these early fibres. Can we not fairly assume that the morbid influence began early? As successive layers of fibres were also affected, until the greater part of the lens became involved, this noxious factor must also have persisted in diminishing strength until finally with its disappearance some normal fibres were formed.

Just how and where this disturbance took place I cannot say. Much more histological evidence than is at present available will have to be obtained before any suggestions can be made. However, if we allow the possibility that the lens may be affected by infective processes in the mother, and if we find the same infection occurring at approximately the same early period in the pregnancy in almost all the cases, and if we then find that the babies of these mothers have cataracts of a more or less uniform type which involves the fibres formed at that period, then I think it is reasonable to assume that the occurrence cannot be a mere coincidence, but that there must be some definite connection between that infection and the morbid condition of the lens.

Although it is rare, cases of the exanthemata have been seen in the newborn baby. Ballantyne[7] noted 20 recorded examples of foetal measles up to 1893; while up to 1902 not more than 20 well authenticated cases of scarlet fever in the foetus had been recorded, varicella *in utero* was not unknown.

The remarkable frequency of the accompanying congenital defect of the heart and the apparent constancy in type of this defect seem to me to indicate a common causative factor. Could this not be some toxic or infective process resulting in a partial arrest of development?

Incidence of German measles in this series

In all but ten cases in this series the history of 'German measles' infection is present. In two of these ten cases the report is negative for measles; in one there was 'history of kidney trouble'; in two others the report is definitely 'history not asked for'; in the remaining five cases the report is 'no history of measles' or 'not known'. It is interesting to note that the majority of these were cases occurring in 1940 or early in 1941 before the theory of a possible association between 'German measles' and the congenital cataracts was promulgated.

Among the cases that have come under my own notice in only one is the history negative. In this case the mother stated that she was kept so busy looking after her ten children that she could not recollect any details of her own health beyond the fact that she was ill at about the sixth week of pregnancy when one of the other children died suddenly from whooping-cough. Even though she was ill, she was unable to go to bed during the last month before the baby was born one month before full term. In the vast majority of the cases infection occurred either in the first or second month of pregnancy. In a few cases it was during the third month, and in one it is reported as a severe attack occurring three months before pregnancy.

This maternal infection occurred in July or August 1940 in the majority of cases; in the minority of cases outside this period the date of infection ranged from December 1939 to January 1941.

Out of 35 cases in which the record is available, the affected baby was the first child in 26 instances; in three others it was a second child; while in the six remaining cases the baby was the third, fourth, fifth, seventh, eighth and tenth child respectively. I believe that these figures, with the noticeably high incidence in the children of *primiparae*, afford confirmatory evidence of the close association between congenital cataract in the baby and the maternal infection. For it was this young adult group, to which these *primiparae* belong, which was particularly affected by this epidemic of 'German measles'.

Geographical distribution

Although the majority of the cases reported came from the suburban districts of Sydney and Melbourne, others were from widely separated country towns in New South Wales and Victoria, and eight were from Queensland, distributed between Brisbane, Rockhampton and Ipswich.

Nature of epidemic

Within my own experience I have not previously seen German measles of such severity and accompanied by such severe complications as occurred during this epidemic in 1940. The swelling of the glands of the neck, the sore throat, the involvement of the wrist and ankle joints and the general constitutional disturbance were all very pronounced. The average stay in hospital of patients treated at the Prince Henry Hospital was eight days as against four days in previous years.

The peak period of the epidemic from returns at this hospital was from mid-June to early August.

Running concurrently with this epidemic were the epidemics of sore throat known as the Ingleburn throat or Puckapunyal throat etc., deriving its name from the military camp with which it was associated. These epidemics started in the camps and spread to the civilian population. Could they not have been streptococcal in origin and is it not possible that the rash diagnosed as 'German measles' may have been, in some cases, a toxic erythema accompanying a streptococcal infection?

In this respect it is interesting to note that the rash occurring in this so-called 'German measles' epidemic has been described to me by physicians as macular, morbilliform, scarlatiniform and toxic erythematous; in other words, it was pleomorphic. I have also been informed by two physicians that they have at present an unusual number of young patients suffering from arthritis and other rheumatic conditions, and these patients all have a history of 'German measles' last year. Because 'German measles' is not a notifiable disease it is impossible to obtain any details of the epidemic from the health authorities, but from my own observations and inquiries I have formed the opinion that the 1940 'German measles' epidemic differed greatly from the ordinary virus infection bearing that name.

Management

From the purely ocular standpoint the essential consideration is the same as in cases of the ordinary lamellar type of cataract – to permit sufficient light stimulus to reach the retina so that fixation may be developed. In this respect the time factor is of the utmost importance. If the stimulus is insufficient or delayed, nystagmus will result.

The special considerations in this series are: (a) the marked density and large size of the opacity; (b) the difficulty in obtaining mydriasis, so that the transparent area for entrance of light is minimal; (c) the high frequency of intolerance to atropine.

These factors compel us to operate at the earliest possible moment. In my opinion the only contraindication to early interference is the general state of health of the baby. In many cases this has been so bad that physicians have refused to give an anaesthetic until some improvement has been obtained in the general condition. So frequently has nystagmus been observed to develop during this waiting period that I am convinced that some risk is justified in order to operate at the earliest possible moment, particularly as later experience has shown that the babies take the short anaesthetic required more easily than had been anticipated.

When operation has to be deferred it is essential to maintain the fullest possible degree of mydriasis, by atropine if tolerated. If atropine cannot be employed, then repeated instillation of homatropine must be substituted for it.

The value of early operation is well illustrated by one case reported by E. Temple Smith in which he performed discission on a baby aged three weeks. Clear pupils resulted and there has been no sign of nystagmus developing.

Operation

Discission has frequently proved more difficult than usual. The anterior chamber is particularly shallow, and in many cases the very dense central portion of the lens has proved very resistant to the needle. Sometimes it has separated off as a firm disk, in others the whole lens has tended to move away from the point of the needle, and one has obtained the impression that it would have been possible to perform an ordinary extraction. In other cases, on the other hand, discission has been straightforward and easy.

Results of operation

Absorption has been slower than that of the ordinary lamellar cataracts. I have not yet had an opportunity to examine the fundi of any patient after absorption of the lens matter, but I propose to do so in as many cases as possible under general anaesthesia. Careful search will be made for any other defects. The unhealthy appearance of the iris in some cases suggests that there may be possibly some changes in the choroid, particularly since the patients in the monocular cases are so frequently microphthalmic.

Prognosis

It is difficult to forecast the future for these unfortunate babies. We cannot at this stage be sure that there are not other defects present which are not evident now but which may show up as development proceeds. The cardiac condition also tends to make the prognosis doubtful. One baby which survived two operations some months ago, suddenly died quite recently at the age of seven months. The possibility of the appearance of neurotropic manifestations at a later date will be kept in mind. The prognosis for vision depends on the presence or absence of nystagmus and, of course, on the condition of the retina and choroid.

I look forward to further improvements in contact glass development, for herein lies the greatest possibility for help in the future.

If we agree that these cases are the result of infection of the mother by 'German measles', what can we do to prevent a repetition of the tragedy in any future epidemic? Is the mass of modern research into the causation of senile cataract going to be helpful by the discovery of some remedy which could be given to the mother to inhibit the formation of opacity in the developing lens of the embryo?

In the present state of our knowledge the only sure treatment available is that of prophylaxis. We must recognize and teach the potential dangers of such an epidemic or, I think, any other exanthem, and do all in our power to prevent its spread and particularly to guard the young married woman from the risk of infection.

As to confirmation of the theory of causation put forward in this paper, I suggest that the following line of investigation may be helpful. In all prenatal clinics and maternity hospitals very careful histories should be taken and recorded of exposure of the mother to infection of any kind during the entire period of pregnancy.

References

1 W. Stewart Duke Elder: *Text Book of Ophthalmology*, Volume II, page 1364.
2 Daniel B. Kirby: *The Eye and Its Diseases*, edited by C. Berens, 1936, page 557.
3 W. Stewart Duke Elder: *Loco citato*, page 1365.
4 P.A. Jaensch: Anatomische Untersuchungen eines angeborenen Totalstarts. *Archiv fur Ophthalmologie*, Volume cxv, 1924, page 1366.
5 W. Stewart Duke Elder: *Loco citato*, page 1366.
6 Ida Mann: *Developmental Abnormalities of the Eye*, 1937, page 18.
7 J. W. Ballantyne: *Manual of Antenatal Pathology and Hygiene*, 1902, Part I, page 196.

Acknowledgement

McAlister Gregg, N. (1941) Congenital cataract following German measles in the mother. *Transactions of the Ophthalmological Society of Australia*, 3, 35–46.

RESPIRATORY FUNCTION OF INFANTS IN RELATION TO SUBSEQUENT RESPIRATORY DISEASE: AN EPIDEMIOLOGICAL STUDY

Introduction

Children who have made a clinical recovery from lower respiratory tract illness have been found to have lower ventilatory function than those children who have escaped such illnesses (Wahdan, 1963; Lunn *et al.*, 1967; Holland *et al.*, 1969; Colley and Reid, 1970). This lower ventilatory function may be a direct result of a respiratory illness, and thus would indicate a degree of permanent lung damage. Alternatively, children who suffer attacks of lower respiratory illness may start life with low ventilatory function. This paper reports the findings of a study in which these alternatives have been investigated.

Method

A cohort of children born in the years 1963–5 in Harrow, a suburb in north-west London, was followed over the first five years of life, together with other members of their families. The methods used in the study have been described in detail previously (Colley and Holland, 1967; Holland *et al.*, 1969; Colley *et al.*, 1974). In brief, all families living in six wards of the borough of Harrow who had a newborn infant born on 1 July 1963 to 30 June 1965 were included in the study, the only exclusions being families of infants who died within seven days of birth. A total of 2365 families had a newborn infant during this period. However, 160 families out of this total could not be visited or declined to participate in the study, leaving 2205 (93 per cent) of the original population for investigation.

Health visitors, who had been specially trained to act as observers, visited infant and mother at home within 14 days of the infant's birth, administered a questionary and measured crown–rump length and chest circumference. The questionary sought, among other items, birth weight of the infant and details of health since birth. A one in three systematic sample of these families were subsequently visited by a field team, the questionary was re-applied and the body measurements were repeated. In addition, ventilatory function of the infant was measured using a portable pneumotachograph (Colley, 1964, 1969). This instrument measures air flow during crying.

From these flows peak inspiratory and expiratory air flow rates in 1 minute and, by integration inspiratory and expiratory volumes in millilitres were obtained. These measurements, and in particular inspiratory volumes, have been shown in earlier studies to be valid indices of ventilatory function in children of up to 18 months old (Colley, 1969). Recordings of crying air flow were made with the infant lying supine on the mother's lap. A rubber face mask with pneumotachograph attached was placed on the infant's face and recording made of the air flow during three crying complexes. Apart from placing the mask on the face, no other stimulus was used to make the infant cry.

For each child the three crying complexes with the largest peak flow rates were measured, as were the volumes. The mean of these flows and volumes have been used in the analysis.

These infants were subsequently visited annually by members of the field team. At the first follow-up, when the infant had just passed the first birthday, crying air flows were again recorded. Various items of medical history were collected at each annual follow-up visit using a questionary. The parents were asked if the child had suffered a lower respiratory tract illness, such as pneumonia or bronchitis, since the last visit by the team. The parents' account of such illnesses were checked, in a sample, by examination of their general practitioners' case notes, and the level of agreement of these two sources was adequate.

The recording pneumotachography was not available at the start of the study and 98 children did not have initial measurements of ventilatory function. These omissions are unlikely to be important as there are no differences in the crown–rump length, chest circumference and age between this group and those who had crying air flow measurements.

Measurements of crying air flow were made between November 1963 and September 1965 on the one in three sample. A total of 623 infants were eligible for these measurements. In 80 infants the record could not be used due to recorder malfunction (46), the infant did not cry (29) or parents refused the test (5), leaving 543 (87.2 per cent) in whom satisfactory recordings of crying air flow were made. Out of these, 56 did not have annual follow-ups to age five, leaving 487 infants with complete information. The main cause of failure to obtain a measurement was recorder malfunction. This appeared to be a random occurrence. Most of the infants who did not cry had been fed just prior to the team's visit and were sleepy. It seems unlikely that the absence of recordings for these groups of infants would lead to any serious bias in the comparisons reported in the paper.

133

Table 1 Crying ventilatory function at birth by history of pneumonia or bronchitis in the first years of life

Crying ventilatory function[a]	Attack of pneumonia or bronchitis in first five years of life				t	P
	None (n = 358)		One or more (n = 129			
	Mean	SEM	Mean	SEM		
Peak inspiratory flow rate (1/min)	25.7	0.3	25.2	0.5	0.86	0.3<P<0.4
Peak expiratory flow rate (1/min)	21.6	0.4	20.4	0.7	1.51	0.1<P<0.2
Inspiratory volume (ml)	91.6	1.4	89.2	2.3	0.89	0.3<P<0.4
Expiratory volume (ml)	87.2	1.4	85.4	2.3	0.66	0.5<P<0.6

[a] Adjusted for birthweight and age.

At the first follow-up visit, when the infants had just passed their first birthday, the whole one in three sample was eligible for measurement of crying ventilatory function. A total of 550 had satisfactory measurements at this age (i.e. 76 per cent of the initial one in three sample of 721 infants).

Results

Crying measurements of ventilatory function for the 487 infants with satisfactory records have been classified by their history of bronchitis or pneumonia. Differences were found between these groups of infants in their birth weight and in the age at which crying ventilatory function was measured. The crying ventilatory function measurements have therefore been adjusted for difference in these two factors. These adjusted measurements are set out in Table 1. Inspection of these measurements do not suggest any large or consistent difference in initial crying ventilatory function between infants who suffered, and who escaped attacks of pneumonia or bronchitis over the subsequent five years of life. No difference reaches statistical significance.

At the age of approximately one year crying ventilatory function measurements were made on those infants in the original one in three sample who still resided in the area, a total of 550 infants. These included some of those who were not measured on the first occasion after birth. These measurements have, as with the initial measurements, been adjusted for difference in age at which the crying measurements were made and birth weight. Adjusted measurements for those infants who suffered an attack of pneumonia or bronchitis in the first year of life, and those who escaped these illnesses, are presented in Table 2. At this age, apart from crying peak expiratory flow rates, no statistically significant differences were observed between the measurements in those infants who suffered an attack of pneumonia or bronchitis in the first year of life and those who did not.

Discussion

No large or consistent difference has been found in this study between the crying ventilatory function of children who subsequently suffer attacks of pneumonia or bronchitis and those who escaped such illnesses. These findings therefore provide no evidence to support the hypothesis that children who subsequently develop pneumonia or bronchitis start life with low ventilatory function.

At the age of one year infants who had made a clinical recovery from an attack of pneumonia or bronchitis had a rather inconsistent pattern of crying ventilatory function in relation to infants who did not have such attacks. While crying peak expiratory flow rates in the two groups differed significantly ($t = 2.84$, $0.005 < P < 0.01$), no such differences were found with the other crying measurements. Measurements of peak expiratory flow rate using the Wright Peak Flow Meter were made in these same children at the age of five years. These measurements demonstrated deficits in those with a documented history of pneumonia and bronchitis in the previous five years compared with those without such illnesses (Leeder et al., 1976).

It is, as expected, more difficult to obtain wholly satisfactory records of crying ventilatory function in infants than it is to obtain measurements of lung function, such as peak flow rate, in older children. Although rigorous standardization of the technique was achieved in the field study, the variation in infants' crying performance under field conditions of measurement may still be substantial. This variation could obscure small differences in crying ventilatory function between infants with differing respiratory experience. The technique used to

Table 2 Crying ventilatory function at one year of age by history of pneumonia or bronchitis in the first year of life

Crying ventilatory function[a]	Attack of pneumonia or bronchitis in first year of life				t	P
	None (n = 480)		One or more (n = 70			
	Mean	SEM	Mean	SEM		
Peak inspiratory flow rate (1/min)	49.2	0.5	47.3	1.4	1.28	0.2<P<0.3
Peak expiratory flow rate (1/min)	38.5	0.7	33.1	1.8	2.84	0.005<P<0.01
Inspiratory volume (ml)	263.8	3.6	274.7	9.5	1.07	0.2<P<0.3
Expiratory volume (ml)	274.5	4.1	269.2	10.7	0.47	0.6<P<0.7

[a] Adjusted for birthweight and age.

measure crying ventilatory function does, however, have adequate validity for detecting reductions in ventilatory function in infants with severe acute lower respiratory tract illnesses studied while in hospital (Colley, 1969). Major deficits in crying inspiratory flow rates and inspiratory and expiratory volumes were found in such infants in comparison with measurements made on recovery. These differences were considered to be the result of acute disease in the lungs and airways rather than reduced ventilatory effort when crying at the time the infants were ill.

In calculating the optimum size of sample required to be sure of detecting a true difference between groups of infants, we are handicapped by having no knowledge of the likely size of the difference we are looking for. Although the test of ventilatory function may have adequate sensitivity, the sample studied could have been too small for real differences in crying ventilatory function to be detected, if these differences are, in fact, very small. In a study of older children, differences in peak expiratory flow rate, measured using the Wright Peak Flow Meter, of up to 5 per cent have been found between groups of children with and without a past history of lower respiratory illness (Colley and Reid, 1970).

In the present study, differences in peak expiratory flow rate of 7.5 per cent were found at the age of five years between children with and without a history of previous lower respiratory illness (Leeder et al., 1976). Crying peak flow rates cannot be directly equated with peak expiratory flow rates measured using the Wright Peak Flow Meter. However, if we assume that in infants and young children the difference in lung function between groups with and without a past history of lower respiratory tract illness is relatively the same for these two measurements, we can use this estimate to calculate the optimal sample size for this study.

With this in mind, the initial sample size needed in this study has been calculated assuming that the variance in

measurements of lung function is roughly the same in children irrespective of whether they have a respiratory illness or not, and also that the incidence of bronchitis or pneumonia in children during the first five years of life has been accurately estimated at 26 per cent. With these assumptions a minimum of 234 infants would be required to detect a 7.5 per cent difference in initial crying inspiratory flow rate with a power of 95 per cent and a difference to be significant at the 5 per cent level, using a two-tailed test. The corresponding sample size for crying peak expiratory flow rate is 568, inspiratory volume 334 and expiratory volume 393.

Clearly, on this basis the sample eventually examined was adequate to have reliably detected differences of 7.5 per cent for all but the measurement of crying peak expiratory flow rate. On a one-tailed test, the sample size was more than adequate to detect differences of this size in all four measurements.

Assuming, therefore, that the sample size is adequate to detect a significant difference in ventilatory function between those children who suffered from a respiratory illness, and those who do not, then we must either look to the sensitivity of the test of ventilatory function to explain why we found no difference between these children, or accept the fact that no such difference really exists at this age. Doubts must remain about the sensitivity of the test, but it is possible that the effects of such illnesses do not become apparent until their influence upon rate of lung growth, or the combined effect of environmental factors on a damaged lung, become detectable.

As this is the first occasion in which an attempt has been made to measure the ventilatory function of children in a large epidemiological field survey during their first year of life, it may be no surprise that the study has raised more questions than it has answered. The acceptability and ease with which this technique can be employed is such that measurements could easily be made on the large majority of infants in a field study, and should encourage others, better placed than ourselves, to evaluate and develop the method further. One aspect of further evaluation would be to determine if changes in ventilatory function could be detected using other, possibly more sensitive, respiratory function tests in one year old children with a history of respiratory illness; a group in whom we found no changes. Such an investigation might resolve the present uncertainty on the sensitivity of the crying ventilatory function test.

References

Colley, J.R.T. (1964) A method for measuring lung function in babies suitable for the epidemiologist. *J. Physiol., Lond.,* 177, 40–1.

Colley, J.R.T. (1969) The evaluation of a test of infant lung function for use in epidemiological field studies. Thesis for MD degree, University of London.

Colley, J.R.T. and Holland, W.W. (1967) Social and environmental factors in respiratory disease: a preliminary report. *Arch. environm. Hlth,* 14, 157–61.

Colley, J.R.T., Holland, W.W. and Corkhill, R.T. (1974) Influence of passive smoking and parental phlegm on pneumonia and bronchitis in early childhood. *Lancet* ii, 1031–4.

Colley, J.R.T. and Reid, D.D. (1970) Urban and social origins of childhood bronchitis in England and Wales. *Brit. Med. J.* ii, 213–17.

Holland, W.W., Halil, T., Bennett, A.E. and Elliott, A. (1969) Factors influencing the onset of chronic respiratory disease. *Brit. Med. J.* ii, 205–8.

Holland, W.W., Kasap, H.S., Colley, J.R.T. and Cormack, W. (1969) Respiratory symptoms and ventilatory function: a family study. *Brit. J. prev. soc. Med.,* 23, 77–84.

Leeder, S.R., Colley, J.R.T., Corkhill, R.T., Wysocki, M. and Holland, W.W. (1976) The influence of personal and family factors on ventilatory function in children. *Brit. J. prev. soc. Med.* 30, 219–22.

Lunn, J.E., Knowelden, J. and Handyside, A.J. (1967) Patterns of respiratory illness in Sheffield infant school children. *Brit. J. prev. soc. Med.* 21, 7–16.

Wahdan, M. (1963) Atmosphere pollution and other environmental factors in respiratory disease of children. Thesis for PhD degree, University of London.

Acknowledgement

Colley, J.R.T., Holland, W.W., Leeder, S.R. and Corkhill, R.T. (1976) Respiratory function of infants in relation to subsequent respiratory disease: an epidemiological study. *Bulletin Européen de Physiopathologie Respiratoire*, 12, 651–7.

8 *Professor Klim McPherson*

McPherson, K., Wennberg, J.E., Hovind, O.B. and Clifford, P. (1982) Small-area variations in the use of common surgical procedures: an international comparison of New England, England and Norway. *New England Journal of Medicine*. 307, 1310–14.

Cochrane, A.L., St Leger, A.S. and Moore, F. (1978) Health service 'input' and mortality 'output' in developed countries. Journal of Epidemiology and Community Health, 32, 200–5.

INTRODUCTION

Epidemiology is the study of the distribution and causes of disease. Two major problems which bedevil studies require enormous amounts of detailed attention to minimize their insidious effect. The first is measurement error of both the fact of disease itself and the exposures which may or may not be implicated in its causes. The second is the confounding of any exposure being investigated with a risk factor, particularly one that is as yet unknown and poorly understood.

It is sometimes incumbent on the epidemiologist to study surrogate measures of disease. Those which receive a great deal of attention are hospital admissions and cause-specific mortality rates, because they are easily measured. The first might be an early event in the process of having a disease, while the latter clearly may be a late outcome.

The first paper is an epidemiological investigation into the causes of hospital admission and the second seeks to test the hypothesis that mortality rates are negatively correlated with the supply of health services. The first is concentrating in part on the extent of possible measurement error associated with using hospital admission for surgery as an index of disease incidence. The expectation would have been that the complexities of the historical, social and economic processes which determine admission to hospital would mean that admission rates would have hardly any relationship with relevant disease incidence, which cannot usually be measured.

This study shows that by comparing the variation, at two levels of population aggregation, in admission rates several useful insights into the process can be gained that are not available from the rates alone. In particular, hospital admission rates vary differently for different kinds of admission and the amount of relative variation is surprisingly similar among dissimilar health systems. Most importantly, to regard hospital admission as largely a biological phenomenon is likely to be most misleading, and hence useless as a surrogate measure of disease.

The second paper is a wonderful example of confounding in epidemiological investigations of mortality, when the expectation would naturally have been that health care provision would be negatively associated with all-cause mortality. This study calculates the correlation of mortality at different ages with the most obvious and measurable aggregated indices of health care and consumption inputs. Surprisingly, among the highest positive correlations found were those between doctors per thousand population and mortality at young ages. Even the association of cigarette consumption and mortality at ages 55–64 was not as strong as the correlation between numbers of doctors and perinatal mortality – usually thought to be a sensitive index of appropriate health care provision.

These papers, while not answering many questions, give rise to uncertainties which may not have been acknowledged. Thus epidemiology is as useful in illuminating complicated casual pathways in medicine as it is in raising questions whose importance may not otherwise have been appreciated.

SMALL-AREA VARIATIONS IN THE USE OF COMMON SURGICAL PROCEDURES: AN INTERNATIONAL COMPARISON OF NEW ENGLAND, ENGLAND, AND NORWAY

Systematic and persistent differences have been documented in the standardized rates for use for common surgical procedures in the United States and the United Kingdom,[1] as well as among the political subdivisions within these countries, such as states, health regions and counties.[2-4] Generally, both rates of surgery and resources invested in surgery are lower in the United Kingdom than in the United States. In the New England states the use of surgery varies considerably among hospital service areas.[5,6] Because these areas, which are defined according to the pattern of use among local hospitals, usually contain only one or two hospitals, most of the procedures of a given kind are performed by a small number of local surgeons. Hospital service areas are thus well suited to an investigation of the influence of physicians' decision making on surgical rates.

This article compares variations in surgical rates among the resident populations of hospital service areas in three countries. We wanted to know whether services were provided more homogeneously in areas served by the nationally organized health systems of Norway and the United Kingdom than in areas served by the decentralized American system. We were particularly interested in the distribution of procedures such as tonsillectomy, hysterectomy and prostatectomy, for which rates of use are highly variable in the United States. In England and Norway, where the rates of use for these procedures are considerably lower, are the relative variations lower, suggesting less discretion in professional decision making when supply is smaller or differently organized? Alternatively, are the variations the same or greater, suggesting a similar latitude in clinical decision making, despite differences in the supply and organization of health care and in average rates of use?

Methods

Data sources

In England most of the 14 regional health authorities record all inpatient episodes in the Hospital Activity Analysis. We obtained these data for 1976 to 1978 in the 21 health districts of the West Midlands Regional Health Authority. The rates exclude private and day cases. Omission of day-care surgery had a small effect on the recorded rates of hernia repair and a moderate effect on the rates of haemorrhoidectomy. Omission of private cases did not have a marked effect on any of the rates for the period of study. Estimates of the national incidence of private surgery[3] indicate that approximately 4 per cent of these operations are excluded from the National Health Service statistics. In the West Midlands the proportion is unlikely to be very different from the national average. The effect of these omissions on the estimation of variance between adjacent areas would be expected to be even smaller. Our data consist of all admissions to National Health Service hospitals that resulted in a cholecystectomy, appendectomy, hysterectomy or prostatectomy. Data on the same procedures are available for Maine, Rhode Island and Vermont from 1974 to 1976, and for seven counties in southern Norway for 1977. The data for New England are from regional data systems: the Co-operative Health Statistics Centre of Vermont, the Maine Data Service and Rhode Island Health Services Research. The Norwegian data were collected by the national government. In all cases the rates refer to operations performed on residents of a hospital service area, including the small numbers of operations performed outside the area of residence.

Study populations

The study populations were selected to correspond as closely as possible to hospital service areas. The population of Maine, Rhode Island and Vermont was subdivided into 81 areas, according to frequency of use of hospitals. Only the 18 areas with populations greater than 50 000 in 1975 (range 50 000 to 180 000) were used in the study, because they correspond most closely with European hospital areas in terms of size and medical-care complexity. Estimates of populations for April 1975 were provided by state agencies. In England the boundaries of the health districts correspond closely to hospital service areas. The 21 districts had populations that ranged from 90 000 to 500 000. Estimates of district population were supplied by the Office of Population Censuses and Surveys. In Norway hospital services are organized by county, and these geopolitical boundaries correspond to seven hospital areas in our study. Population estimates, provided by the national government, ranged from 100 000 to 300 000.

Standardization of rates

Using age-specific and sex-specific rates of surgery for England and Wales in 1975, we indirectly standardized all crude rates for each country in terms of age and sex.

Table 1 Age- and sex-standardized surgical rates per 100 000 population in three New England states, southern Norway and the West Midlands Regional Health Authority

Surgical procedure	New England	Norway	West Midlands
Hernia repair	276	186	137
Appendectomy	128	150	177
Cholecystectomy	238	86	89
Prostatectomy[a]	264	236	132
Hysterectomy[a]	540	118	220
Haemorrhoidectomy	76	45	28
Tonsillectomy	289	64	172

[a] Rates for hysterectomy and prostatectomy are for women and men, respectively.

For estimating variation within each country, rates were internally standardized according to the age-specific and sex-specific rates for that country.

Measuring variation

Two statistics commonly used to measure variation in a sample are variance and standard deviation. Both measure absolute variation; that is, they are influenced by the scale of measurement. If the average rate of surgery in a particular region is high, we can expect the absolute variation within the region to be correspondingly large. Comparisons of the uses of surgery – between countries and between types of surgery – involve not only the average rates of surgery but also the internal variability of these rates. Our concern in this study was to supplement existing knowledge of the disparity between average rates with information on internal variation. For this purpose we attempted to devise a measure of variation that was not merely a reflection of differing average rates.

The obvious candidate for such a measure is the coefficient of variation, which is the standard deviation of the sample divided by the mean. However, if sampling error is the dominant source of variation – i.e. if the surgical rate is low or the population is small – then the calculated coefficient of variation will tend to be large, whereas the sample variance and other measures of absolute variation will tend to be small. Furthermore, since the sizes of the populations in the areas selected for study are themselves variable, the random component is not a constant proportion of the total variation in rates.

To overcome these difficulties, we developed a measure of variation that takes account of scale sensibly and permits comparisons between units of different sizes and procedures with different prevailing rates. Details are

given in the Appendix. Briefly, the statistic is based on a model of variation adapted from the proportional hazards model. It estimates the relative systematic component of variation between areas by subtracting the random component of variance from the estimate of total variance. This measure permits comparisons of the variability of surgical rates among countries but makes few assumptions about the nature of the variation and allows for appropriate amounts of sampling variation in the data. Differences in intrinsic variability among the surgical procedures were tested by examining the ratios of the variance estimates and comparing them to standard tables of the F distribution.

Results

Table 1 gives the surgical rates, standardized for age and sex, in the three New England states, the southern Norwegian counties and the West Midlands Health Authority. The British and Norwegian rates were lower than the New England rates for all procedures except appendectomy, which appeared to be performed at a similar rate in all three countries. Women and children residing in the states of Maine, Rhode Island and Vermont were four times as likely to have had a hysterectomy and a tonsillectomy, respectively, as were residents of the Norwegian counties. Similarly, men in New England were twice as likely to have had a prostatectomy as were men in the West Midlands. Indeed, for all procedures except appendectomy, international comparisons showed a twofold or greater difference between at least two of the three countries for each procedure.

Figure 1 shows the distribution (mean and range) and of standardized surgical rates among the New England hospital service areas, the health districts within the West Midlands Health Authority and the seven Norwegian counties. The incidence of surgery differed widely, depending on place of residence. For most of the procedures, the range of rates in one country overlapped the range in at least one other country. For example, although the mean tonsillectomy rate for the New England areas was 4.5 times the rate for the Norwegian counties, the rate for one hospital service area was the same as the highest rate for Norwegian counties. Also, the distribution of rates differed according to the particular procedure. For example, the range of rates within each country for hysterectomy and tonsillectomy appeared to be considerably wider than the range for appendectomy or hernia.

The relative variation in rates for individual procedures within the three New England states, the Norwegian

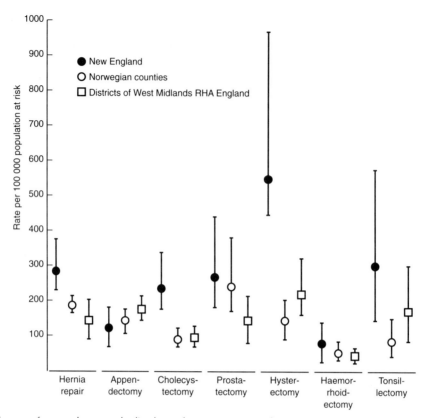

Fig. 1 Mean and range of age- and sex-standardized rates for common surgical procedures in New England, Norway and the West Midlands.

counties and the West Midlands health region is summarized in Table 2. In spite of the differences in average rates between countries, the amount of variation within one health-care system appeared to be similar for all three countries. Domestic variation followed a characteristic pattern, with tonsillectomy rates showing the most variation, followed by haemorrhoidectomy, hysterectomy and prostatectomy. To evaluate international differences in the intrinsic variability of surgical rates, we examined the ratios of the variance estimates, using an F test. On this basis, hernia repair was the only operation that showed significant heterogeneity of use; Norway was less variable ($P < 0.05$) and the West Midlands much more variable ($P < 0.005$) than the New England areas. Otherwise, Norwegian counties appeared to be significantly more variable than the West Midlands health districts ($P < 0.05$) in the use of hysterectomy, but compared with New England service areas, the difference was of borderline significance.

Discussion

Small-area analysis of hospital service areas is well suited to an investigation of differences in clinical decision making, because the rates in a given area are the direct consequence of decisions made by a small group of physicians. On the basis of their small-area studies in New England, Wennberg and his colleagues concluded that differences among physicians in either their diagnostic style or their belief in the efficacy of specific treatment contributed substantially to the observed variation in rates of use. Also, a particular procedure had a characteristic pattern of variation, which was related to the degree of professional uncertainty concerning the diagnosis or treatment of the common condition (or conditions) for which surgery was one possible treatment.[7,8] The results of our study indicate that, for most of the procedures we examined, a specific pattern of variation exists across international boundaries and is independent of the

Table 2 Indexes of variation in age- and sex-standardized surgical rates among selected hospital services in New England, Norway and the West Midlands

	Hernia repair	Appen-dectomy	Cholecys-tectomy	Prosta-tectomy	Hysterec-tomy	Haemorrhoid-ectomy	Tonsil-lectomy	All seven procedures
Coefficient of variation (%)								
New England	0.11	26	18	30	22	30	36	14
Norway	0.20	16	18	33	31	47	48	11
West Midlands	0.20	16	16	24	20	35	31	12
Range (high/low)								
New England	1.7	2.3	1.9	2.2	2.2	4.8	4.2	1.69
Norway	1.3	1.6	1.5	2.2	3.0	2.9	4.7	1.34
West Midlands	2.0	2.0	1.5	2.1	2.1	4.6	3.3	1.55
Systematic component ($\times\,100\,\sigma^2$)								
New England	0.6	1.7	1.7	5.0	4.8	12.7	12.2	2.08
Norway	0.2	2.4	1.9	9.3	10.4	14.7	27.5	1.28
West Midlands	4.4	2.9	2.1	6.2	3.7	12.2	18.5	1.33

national method of organizing or financing medical care. Furthermore, procedure-specific variation occurs in countries where prevailing rates of use are considerably lower than in the United States.

Tonsillectomy illustrates the case of a procedure with a highly variable rate of use. There is documented controversy concerning the appropriate use of tonsillectomy, including diagnosis of the condition for which it is used, as well as the value of the surgical procedure, once the diagnosis has been made.[9,10] Although mean tonsillectomy rates were lower in Norway and in the United Kingdom than in the United States, their distribution among hospital service areas was as variable in the two European countries as it was in the United States, suggesting that Norwegian and British clinicians are as uncertain as their American colleagues about recommending tonsillectomy. The similarity in pattern of variation is evidence against the notion that decision making in the low-rate countries reflects a clear threshold above which everyone receives the treatment and below which decisions are carefully balanced on the basis of competing needs and priorities for alternative uses of surgical resources.

A similar interpretation seems plausible for the other procedures with highly variable rates for use. Haemorrhoidectomy is one treatment of a condition for which reasonable alternative treatments exist.[11,12] Indeed, in common applications the procedure has been labelled 'unnecessary surgery'.[13] Disagreements among clinicians appear to influence practice patterns similarly on both

sides of the Atlantic. The use of hysterectomy for non-cancerous conditions is a continuing source of professional controversy.[14] Perhaps more surprising is the highly variable use of prostatectomy in each country, even though the prevailing rate in the West Midlands is substantially lower than the rates in the United States and in Norway. The relatively high fatality rate associated with this procedure suggests the importance of clarifying the implications of differences in rates of use.[15]

The procedures with little variation in use appear to be those for which there is a consensus among physicians concerning their appropriate application. Inguinal herniorrhaphy is undertaken for a readily apparent condition whose treatment is not controversial. Indeed, in the United States and Norway, for patients who are reasonable operative risks, there is no accepted alternative therapy.[16] This consensus contrasts with the situation in the United Kingdom, where a truss is sometimes prescribed. We believe this difference in clinical practice is reflected in the greater variation in use of inguinal herniorrhaphy in the United Kingdom.

There was little variation in the use of appendectomy in each country, and the mean rates of distribution were similar, suggesting similar incidence rates of appendicitis. Appendectomy is generally recognized as the only acceptable treatment for this acute condition. Despite evidence of differences in diagnostic acumen among physicians,[17] the pattern of variation for appendectomy described here suggests greater professional consensus in the use of this procedure than in the use of the other six procedures. The rates of use of cholecystectomy, which also varied little in each country, were higher in the United States than in the European countries, perhaps because of different attitudes towards the removal of asymptomatic gallstones,[18] as well as a lower threshold for diagnostic tests in the United States. Despite these possible differences, the measures of variation were similar for the three countries.

Appendix

Estimated rates of surgery vary from area to area because of sampling error and systematic area-dependent factors. Since all surgical rates vary with age and sex, the systematic component depends on the age and sex composition of each area. Adjustments to observed rates are commonly made by means of indirect standardization. The basic assumption underlying this method of standardization is that each age and sex grouping changes the risk of surgery by a fixed multiplicative factor.[19]

To allow for the possibility that, even after this adjustment is made, area differences remain, we introduced an additional multiplicative factor, which varies from area to area. If the factor is 1 for all areas, then obviously we are assuming that age and sex adjustments are sufficient. If the factor varies with a non-zero variance σ^2, then we conclude that there are unexplained area differences.

In each geographic region, let there be k hospital service areas. The age-specific and sex-specific rates for all the areas combined are known, and the numbers of people at risk in each age and sex group for each area are known. It is routine to note the observed number of operations in each area (O_i) for a particular period and to calculate the expected number of operations (E_i) given the regional age-specific and sex-specific rates. Let λ_1 be the multiplicative factor associated with the ith area. Since surgery is a relatively rare event, we conclude that the distribution of O_i is approximately Poisson, with mean $\lambda_i E_i$. If we now consider λ_i as a random variable with an expected value of 1 and a variance of σ^2, we have

$$\text{Variance } (O_i) = E_i^2 \sigma^2 + E_i,$$

and if we define Y_i as the logarithm of the ratio of O_i to E_i, we have

$$Y = \log\left(\frac{O_i}{E_i}\right) \simeq \frac{O_i - E_i}{E_i}$$

It follows that the expected value of Y_i is approximately zero and $E(Y_i^2)$, the expected value of Y_i^2 is approximated by

$$E(Y_i^2) = \frac{1}{E_i^2} \text{Variance } (O_i - E_i)$$

$$= \frac{1}{E_i^2} (E_i^2 \sigma^2 + E_i)$$

$$= \sigma^2 + \frac{1}{E_i}$$

so that

$$\left(\sum_{i=1}^{k} Y_i^2/k\right) = \sigma^2 + \frac{1}{k}\sum_{i=1}^{k}\left(\frac{1}{E_i}\right)$$

and therefore σ^2 can be estimated by

$$\hat{\sigma}^2 = \sum_{i=1}^{k} \frac{Y_i^2}{k} - \frac{\sum_{i=1}^{k}\left(\frac{1}{E_i}\right)}{k}$$

Thus, the area-dependent component of variance in rates standardized for age and sex can be estimated by subtracting the random component from the observed variance of the logarithm of the observed over the expected ratios. In this way we are comparing relative variation around a regional norm; therefore, the estimate should not be affected by differences in prevailing operation rates. Also, because the contribution of random variation to the total observed variation in the logarithm of observed over the expected ratios varies according to the total number of operations in each area, this method adjusts for unequal contributions to the variance estimate that are introduced by differences in prevailing rates and population denominators between areas and between regions.

Each estimate has approximately $k - 1$ degrees of freedom. A plot of the $\ln(O_i/E_i)$ in each region for each operation does not show any systematic departure from a symmetric Gaussian distribution. Therefore, a test of the null hypothesis (no difference in systematic variance for each operation across regions) can be performed using an F test for independent samples.[20] Moreover, the estimated values of σ^2 can be compared for pairs of operations in a single region.

References

1 Bunker J.P., Barnes B.A., Mosteller F., eds. *Costs, risks, and benefits of surgery.* New York: Oxford University Press, 1977.
2 American College of Surgeons and the American Surgical Association. *Surgery in the United States: a summary report of the Study on Surgical Services for the United States.* Baltimore: American College of Surgeons and the American Surgical Association, 1975.

3 McPherson K., Strong P.M., Epstein A., Jones L. Regional variations in the use of common surgical procedures: within and between England and Wales, Canada and the United States. *Soc. Sci. Med.* 1981; 15A: 273–88.

4 Lewis C.E. Variations in the incidence of surgery. *N. Engl. J. Med.* 1969; 281: 880–4.

5 Wennberg J., Gittlesohn A. Small area variations in health care delivery. *Science* 1973; 182: 1102–8.

6 Wennberg J., Gittlesohn A. Health care delivery in Maine. I. Patterns of use of common surgical procedures. *J. Maine Med. Assoc.* 1975; 66: 123–30, 149.

7 Wennberg J.E., Barnes B.A., Zubkoff M. Professional uncertainty and the problem of supplier-induced demand. *Soc. Sci. Med.* 1982; 16: 811–24.

8 Wennberg J., Gittlesohn A. Variations in medical care among small areas. *Sci. Am.* 1982; 246: 120–34.

9 American Child Health Association. *Physical defects: the pathway to correction.* New York: Research Division, American Child Health Association, 1934.

10 Bolande R.P. Ritualistic surgery – circumcision and tonsillectomy. *N. Engl. J. Med.* 1969; 280: 591.

11 Ferguson J.A., MacKeigan J.M. Hemorrhoids, fistulae, and fissures: office and hospital management – a critical review. *Adv. Surg.* 1978; 12: 111–53.

12 To tie; to stab; to stretch; perchance to freeze. *Lancet* 1975; ii: 651.

13 Outpatient treatment of haemorrhoids. *Br. Med. J.* 1975; ii: 651.

14 Dyck F., Murphy F.A., Murphy J.K. *et al.* Effect of surveillance on the number of hysterectomies in the province of Saskatchewan. *N. Engl. J. Med..* 1977; 296: 1326–8.

15 Wennberg J.E., Bunker J.P., Barnes B. The need for assessing the outcome of common medical practices. *Annu. Rev. Public Health* 1980; 1: 277–95.

16 Koontz A.R. *Hernia.* New York: Appleton-Century-Crofts, 1963.

17 deDombal F.T., Leaper D.J., Horrocks J.C., Staniland J.R., McCann A.P. Human and computer-aided diagnosis of abdominal pain: further report with emphasis on performance of clinicians. *Br. Med. J.* 1974; 1: 376–80.

18 Ingelfinger F.J. Digestive disease as a national problem. V. Gallstones. *Gastroenterology* 1968; 55: 102–4.

19 Breslow N.E., Day N.E. Indirect standardization and multiplicative models for rates, with reference to the age adjustment of cancer incidence and relative frequency data. *J. Chronic Dis.* 1975; 28: 289–303.

20 Snedecor G.W., Cochran W.G. *Statistical methods.* 6th edn. Ames, Iowa: Iowa State University Press, 1967.

Acknowledgement

McPherson, K., Wennberg, J.E., Hovind, O.B. and Clifford, P. (1982) Small-area variations in the use of common surgical procedures: an international comparison of New England, England, and Norway. *New England Journal of Medicine.* 307, 1310–14.

HEALTH SERVICE 'INPUT' AND MORTALITY 'OUTPUT' IN DEVELOPED COUNTRIES

Health services in developed countries, both state and private, are based upon many common assumptions about what constitutes adequate health care. Doctors and their paramedical colleagues in different developed countries receive similar educations to more or less the same standards, and their approaches to clinical and preventive medicine are unlikely to differ in fundamental principles. However, these countries show marked differences in their mortality rates and in health costs per head. In this paper, we seek to discover some factors to explain these differences in mortality.

Materials and methods

We employed the following criteria in selecting our countries:

1 Gross national product (GNP) exceeding $2000 per caput. We made an exception for the Republic of Ireland (GNP $1949 per caput).

2 Population of more than two million.

3 Data available for 1970, but if not, data for 1969 or 1971 accepted if available.

4 We excluded countries where genetic factors may account for a substantial proportion of the difference in mortality between them and our other countries. This excluded Japan.

The data recorded on our countries are of two types: 'input' and 'output'. The input variables were selected according to two criteria: firstly, availability; secondly, an expectation that the variables might be related to the health of the communities. There are three types: health care indices, dietary consumption, and other demographic or economic variables. The output is measured by age-specific mortality rates up to the age of 64; we excluded the older ages because these are less likely to be associated with environmental factors.

The set of input variables is far too large in relation to the number of countries, and it was necessary to reduce the numbers to produce a more manageable set of relevant variables. This was accomplished by studying scatter diagrams of the mortality rates against each of the input factors, and by examining the correlation matrix of all the variables. Regression analysis of the output variables also helped to determine which variables may

Table 1 Countries used in the study

Australia	Republic of Ireland
Austria	Italy
Belgium	Netherlands
Canada	New Zealand
Denmark	Norway
England and Wales	Scotland
Finland	Sweden
France	Switzerland
German Federal Republic	United States of America

explain differences in mortality. Our criteria for the inclusion of factors in the subsequent analysis were:

1 The intrinsic importance of the variable; that is, we included variables such as prevalence of doctors, and availability of hospital beds, which many people consider to be self-evidently related to mortality.
2 A factor had to show a large product-moment correlation with at least one mortality rate, or it had to show a consistent pattern of association with several mortality rates.
3 A factor had to contribute a large proportion to the sums of squares of regression in a consistent manner in spite of changes in the composition of the other variables in the regression.

With only 18 countries, and many possible input variables, problems arise if we seek to apply standard methods of statistical inference, such as significance testing, to the data. If no allowance is made for multiple comparisons, then a correlation coefficient must exceed ± 0.44 in order to be significantly different from zero at the 5 per cent level of significance (assuming normality, etc.). It is arguable, however, that problems of statistical inference may not be relevant to our 18 countries because these cannot be regarded as being a random sample from some large set of developed countries. We think that there are so many possible sources of error in this sort of data, and so many pitfalls in interpretation, that a slavish adherence to significance testing, if relevant, would give our results a spurious and perhaps misleading aura of precision. We have used the criteria set out above in our analysis, and we have placed particular emphasis on the criterion of consistency. We believe that the results outlined in the next section are both interesting and amusing, and we make no apology for the necessarily subjective nature of some stages in our analysis.

Results

On the basis of the criteria listed earlier, we had a set of 18 countries, which are shown in Table 1.

The input and output variables, their median values and their ranges across the 18 countries are shown in Tables 2 and 3.

The principal findings on examination of the raw correlations (Table 4) were as follows:

1 The correlation between prevalence of doctors and paediatricians and mortality is large and positive in the younger age groups, is positive in young adult life, and only becomes negative in the two oldest age groups.
2 The correlation between alcohol consumption and mortality shows a similar pattern to that for doctors, but with a particularly strong correlation between alcohol consumption and maternal mortality.
3 The prevalence of nurses shows a negative association with maternal, perinatal, infant and early childhood mortality. Their association with other mortality rates is positive or negligible.
4 The prevalence of acute hospital beds shows an erratic association with mortality rates; most of the associations are weak.
5 Cigarette consumption has a positive association with all the death rates, and this association is strongest in the two age groups 45 to 54 and 55 to 64.
6 The dietary factors, other than sugar consumption, have consistently positive associations with mortality. In particular, total calorie intake and protein consumption are strongly positively associated with all mortality rates.
7 Sugar consumption has a large negative association with maternal mortality and with mortality in the younger age groups, and the association remains negative up to 44 years of age.
8 Gross national product per head is negatively associated with mortality except in the age groups 5 to 14 and 15 to 24 years.
9 The intervention index (per cent of health care provided by public funds) has a consistently negative association with all mortality rates, and these associations are large in the age groups 15 to 24 and 25 to 34 years. There is reason to believe, however, that in the 25 to 34 age group this correlation may be spurious, because the United States of America, with a high mortality rate and a low index, stands far away from the other countries, which appear to form a random cluster. Exclusion of the USA halves the correlation coefficient.

Table 2 Input variables

	Minimum	Median	Maximum
Health service indices			
Doctors[a]	10.2	13.7	18.5
Nurses[a]	6.7	35.4	56.0
Acute hospital beds[a]	39.5	52.3	97.7
Paediatricians[b]	3.9	23.6	68.8
Obstetricians[b]	12.6	27.3	50.8
Midwives[b]	10.2	106.0	399.7
% Gross National Product spent on health	4.7	5.2	7.1
Dietary indices			
Cigarette consumption per caput per annum	630	2440	3810
Alcohol consumption in litres per caput per annum	3.7	7.2	17.5
Calories per caput per day	2805	3195	3410
Grams protein per caput per day	83.9	90.5	108.2
Grams total fat per caput per day	124.3	148.3	173.8
Grams sugar per caput per day	75.8	120.0	138.5
Economic and demographic factors			
Average population per km^2	1.6	77.2	324.2
Gross National Product per caput	1949	4236	6652
Education index	10.0	16.3	49.4
Intervention index (% of health expenditure covered by public expenditure)	40.5	80.7	94.8

[a] per 10 000 population.
[b] per 10 000 live births.

Table 3 Output variables

Mortality rates	Minimum	Median	Maximum
Maternal per 100 000 live births	8.5	21.5	54.5
Perinatal per 1000 live births	16.5	22.9	31.7
Infant per 1000 live births	11.0	18.2	29.6
1–4 years per 10 000 population	5.3	8.5	10.2
5–14 years per 10 000 population	3.2	4.1	4.7
15–24 years per 10 000 population	6.8	8.8	13.0
25–34 years per 10 000 population	8.0	10.9	15.9
35–44 years per 10 000 population	16.9	22.9	32.2
45–54 years per 10 000 population	43.6	56.2	72.8
55–64 years per 10 000 population	107.9	150.0	183.2

The correlations for smoking and for GNP per head accord with expectation, and lead us to suppose that our method of study gives sensible results. Many of the other results are confusing, and interpretation is made more difficult by the cross-correlations among the input variables.

Regression analysis is a useful aid to sorting out the relationships between sets of moderately intercorrelated variables. There are too many input variables relative to the output variables to allow one large analysis, so we performed a series of regression analyses on various overlapping subsets of the input variables in order to seek a small subset, should it exist, of variables with most explanatory power. The main findings from these analyses were:

1 None of the health service factors was consistently negatively related to mortality. Prevalence of doctors was positively associated with mortality in all age groups except 45 to 54 years, and the association was

Table 4 Correlation coefficients between the death rates and the input variables[a]

	Mortality rates			Age groups (years)							
	Maternal	Perinatal	Infant	1–4	5–14	15–24	25–34	35–44	45–54	55–64
Doctors	0.45	0.60	0.67	0.37	0.42	0.32	0.23	0.04	−0.27	−0.20
Nurses	−0.39	−0.53	−0.50	−0.28	0.37	0.12	0.06	0.19	0.27	0.11
Beds	0.04	−0.32	−0.10	0.07	0.18	0.37	0.06	−0.02	−0.14	−0.14
Paediatricians	0.40	0.47	0.51	0.23	0.31	0.35	0.37	0.15	−0.11	−0.12
Obstetricians	0.04	0.18	0.18	−0.17	0.29	0.48	0.54	0.36	0.09	0.04
Midwives	−0.10	−0.15	−0.14	−0.29	−0.33	−0.57	−0.28	0.00	0.26	0.28
% GNP on health	−0.12	0.01	−0.10	−0.23	0.27	0.39	0.30	0.00	0.23	0.36
Cigarettes	0.17	0.22	0.22	0.11	0.31	0.36	0.35	0.32	0.46	0.49
Alcohol	0.68	0.52	0.61	0.33	0.32	0.26	0.27	0.09	−0.18	−0.14
Calories	0.41	0.59	0.58	0.58	0.41	0.31	0.30	0.31	0.38	0.52
Protein	0.43	0.37	0.33	0.44	0.20	0.47	0.50	0.50	0.49	0.43
Fat	0.10	0.29	0.23	0.32	0.46	0.43	0.37	0.21	0.10	0.16
Sugar	−0.61	−0.57	−0.56	−0140	−0.31	−0.17	−0.20	−0.05	0.26	0.21
Population density	0.17	0.24	0.21	0.07	−0.03	−0.30	−0.35	−0.45	−0.30	−0.10
GNP per caput	−0.29	−0.48	−0.46	−0.41	0.18	0.25	0.17	−0.13	−0.36	−0.53
Education index	−0.13	−0.22	−0.20	0.28	−0.43	−0.79	−0.61	−0.47	−0.27	−0.21
Intervention index	−0.15	0.15	−0.02	−0.13	0.12	0.44	0.48	0.30	0.26	0.07

[a] The input variables are defined in Table 2.

particularly marked for infant mortality, being even stronger than that suggested by the raw correlations.

2 The main factors consistently negatively associated with mortality were GNP per head, population density, sugar consumption and the intervention index.

3 The principal factors, other than doctors, which were mainly positively associated with mortality were cigarette consumption and alcohol consumption.

4 Consumption of calories and protein showed very much weaker associations with mortality than their adjusted correlations suggested, particularly when the regression equations contained GNP with protein and of GNP with calorie consumption are −0.29 and −0.30 respectively. Gross national product per head appeared to have an independent association with the mortality rates over and above the association which may be attributed to its cross-correlation with the dietary variables. We therefore retained GNP per head and rejected protein and calorie consumption as contributing little additional explanatory power. Incidentially, total calorie intake and sugar consumption have a correlation coefficient of 0.02, and the correlations between sugar consumption and fat and protein consumption are −0.12 and −0.04 respectively. It therefore follows that the contribution to the regression made by sugar consumption is unlikely merely to reflect a general dietary contribution.

On the basis of these analyses, we were able to select seven variables, each of which appeared to have some independent effect upon mortality in at least one age group. The set of variables as a whole had most of the explanatory power of our input data. The resulting regression equations seemed to be reasonably stable in the sense that adding other variables singly, in turn, to the set of seven did not bring about major alterations in the first seven regression coefficients. Table 5 displays the results of regressing mortality rates on the chosen seven variables. The figures in the first seven columns are the percentage change in a given death rate (denoted by the row) for a one standard deviation increase in the input variable (denoted by the column) from its mean value, all other input variables being fixed at their mean values. This enables a comparison to be made, for example, between the effects of the prevalence of doctors, of maternal mortality and of GNP on the same mortality rate; or between the effect of prevalence of doctors on maternal mortality and that of GNP on infant mortality. The figures described above are not regression coefficients but they are derived from them. The legitimacy of the comparisons depends partly upon the stability of our regression equations over the input variables at our disposal and over others unknown to us, and partly on the fact that all the regression equations being compared have an identical set of independent (input) variables. The final column

Table 5 Regression analysis of mortality rates on the seven variables with greatest explanatory power

Mortality rate	Input variables							% Total sums of squares explained by 7 variables
	Doctors	GNP	Cigarettes	Alcohol	Population density	Intervention index	Sugar consumption	
Maternal	1	−15	25	18	−3	2	−29	72
Perinatal	8[a]	−11[a]	8[a]	0	0	−2	−8[a]	90
Infant	17[a]	−16[a]	10[a]	5[a]	−2	0	−4	97
Age groups (years)								
1–4	3	−8[a]	1	1	1	−6	−5	55
5–14	1	1	5	−1	−2	−2	−6	42
15–24	0	0	2	0	−7[a]	−16[a]	−8	79
25–34	−4	1	5	0	−7	−10[a]	−11	65
35–44	−3	−5	4	−1	−9[a]	−9	−8	57
45–54	−3	−7	7	−3	−4	−4	−3	55
55–64	−1	−9[a]	7	−3	−1	−3	−3	62

The figures in the first seven columns are the percentage changes in the death rates following a one standard deviation increase in the input variables, the other input variables remaining fixed.
[a] t value for inclusion of variable in regression exceeds 2. Note, however, that even when not formally 'significant' the values given are best estimates.

of Table 5 displays the percentage of the total (corrected) sums of squares of a given death rate explained by the set of seven variables.

The findings for infant mortality are particularly interesting. The seven variables explain 97 per cent of the variance in infant mortality rates. In fact GNP per head alone explains 21 per cent of the variance while the prevalence of doctors alone explains 45 per cent of the variance. Doctors and GNP per head together explain 82 per cent of the variance. Doctors and GNP per head are not themselves highly correlated ($r = 0.2$) in these developed countries.

Other points of interest in Table 5 are the positive association between alcohol consumption and maternal and infant mortality; the positive association between cigarette consumption and mortality, which is strongest with infant, perinatal and maternal mortality, and is also strong in the two oldest age groups; and the negative association between population density and mortality in young adults. Gross national product is negatively associated with mortality in all age groups except 5 to 34 years, where it becomes negligible. Sugar consumption is negatively associated with mortality in all age groups. The intervention index becomes prominent in the age groups 15 to 24 and 25 to 34 years, although, as noted earlier, caution is required in interpreting it in the latter age group. Caution is also advisable in interpreting the results for maternal mortality, because this is a very uncommon cause of death in our 18 developed countries.

We repeated a similar correlation and regression analysis on a smaller set of variables based upon data in 1960. Our main findings from the 1970 data concerning GNP per head, doctors and some other health care variables were replicated on the 1960 data. Our analysis of the 1960 data, although cursory, does suggest that our findings are fairly stable over time and cannot too easily be dismissed as a chance curiosity.

Discussion

In the previous sections, we have remarked on the statistical difficulties associated with this study. We must now examine the broader issue of the general validity of studies which seek to draw inferences about the relationship between diet, environment and mortality on the basis of a statistical comparison of countries.

The first objection to our study is that we have a highly selective collection of countries. This is indeed so, but this circumstance was forced upon us by the lack of developed countries for which extensive and reliable information was available. We may nevertheless claim the advantage that because our selected countries are all 'Western' or 'European' in their styles of life and outlook, they may be expected to be fairly homogeneous with respect to many variables which we have been unable to consider. A more serious methodological objection is that both the mortality rates and the input variables are averaged across each country, so that we cannot examine or allow for the undoubted heterogeneity of these factors within each country. We do not even have the comfort of knowing that their frequency distributions within each country are identical, and this throws greater doubt upon the representativeness of the simple averages. It may well be that these difficulties serve to dilute or underestimate any true associations, in which case any positive findings that we display are of enhanced interest. We cannot, however, dismiss the possibility that these problems cause entirely false associations. We do not claim that any of the associations are causal, although in one or two cases this hypothesis is attractive.

The striking relationship between the prevalence of doctors and mortality in the younger age groups deserves serious consideration. Stewart (1971), Hinds (1974) and Richardson (1976) have each commented on this association but have not found a totally convincing explanation. We have examined the possibility that this association could be explained in terms of other variables in our data see, but, as Table 5 shows, we were unable to make the doctor anomaly go away. In spite of the possibility that there is some variable unknown to us which is cross-correlated with doctor prevalence and is capable of explaining the anomaly, we shall attempt a few explanatory hypotheses.

One possibility is that each country, consciously or unconsciously, adjusted the supply of doctors to meet the demand of medical problems. We attempted to test this by seeing whether the increase in the number of doctors between 1960 and 1970 was related to infant mortality in 1960. No such relationship was found.

Another hypothesis is that increasing doctor prevalence increases 'dependency', but even Ivan Illich (1975) never suggested that the dependency was lethal. Similarly, 'iatrogenesis' might be suggested as a linking factor, but the wrong age groups are affected and the effect on mortality is too large.

Two factors suggest that the doctor and mortality relationship is not causal. Firstly, there is no evidence of a relationship between doctor prevalence and infant mortality rates when the regions of England and Wales are studied (West and Lowe, 1976). Secondly, the correlation and regression coefficients are still positive, but much weaker, if doctors are replaced by obstetricians and paediatricians, both of whom are likely to influence infant mortality more strongly than other doctors.

In general, however, we must admit defeat and leave it to others to extricate doctors from their unhappy position.

It is also difficult to explain the roles of population density and the intervention index (proportion of health service spending coming from government funds), both of which are strongly negatively associated with mortality in young adults. An interpretation of the effect of the intervention index is that the more nationalised the health services, the more effective is delivery of health care for potentially lethal illness. This may well be so, but in referring to our analysis, great caution is necessary before drawing this inference. Why should the intervention index be most strongly associated with deaths in young adults? A tentative explanation might be that deaths in young adults are primarily due to accidents, particularly road accidents, and non-fatal outcome following an accident may be dependent upon an an efficient accident service.

Private medicine would not be interested in funding an accident service which by its nature must often provide treatment before questions of fees are broached, and therefore this may be highly dependent upon public funding. If state financing of health services in developed countries is truly effective, however, then the intervention index should be strongly associated with other causes of death, particularly perinatal and infant mortality; and this we have not found. We originally thought that the population density effect could be explained by a negative association with road accidents but this is not so, and in the light of other findings we can hardly argue that nearness to medical help is important.

The results for gross national product per caput accord with expectations. Its association with mortality is strongest in the youngest and oldest age groups, and its negative sign is consistent with the idea that increasing overall wealth reduces mortality. In the intermediate age groups, its negligible association with mortality is consistent with the view that older children and young adults, having survived thus far, are little affected, with respect to mortality, by those social and environmental factors which correlate with wealth. This view is, of course, tenable only for societies in which overall wealth exceeds subsistence level, as is true of all our 18 developed countries.

It is not surprising that cigarette consumption should be associated with mortality rates in older age groups. The strong association with infant and perinatal mortality is not easy to explain, although it is perhaps now generally recognised that smoking in pregnancy has a deleterious effect on the foetus, but we cannot claim to have shown this.

Our finding that sugar consumption is not positively associated with mortality is inconsistent with the belief that unrefined sugar is generally harmful, and associated with coronary heart disease in particular (Yudkin, 1957). We would not, however, wish to place too much weight upon our own findings. In any case, severe doubts about the harmful role of sugar have been raised by other workers in studies designed to test this issue (Bennett et al., 1970; MRC Working Party, 1970).

We believe that one overall conclusion may be drawn

from this study. It is that health service factors are relatively unimportant in explaining the differences in mortality between our 18 developed countries. There is nothing new in this. The case has been argued particularly well by Fuchs (1974). As a corollary to this, it could also be argued that there is probably a considerable element of inefficiency in the way some developed countries spend so much more than others on health services. As to the overall value of the results, we consider them to be interesting and provocative, and perhaps capable of generating worthwhile new hypotheses which may be tested in appropriate studies.

References

Bennett, A.E., Doll, R. and Howell R.W. (1970) Sugar consumption and cigarette smoking. *Lancet,* i, 1011–14.

Fuchs, V.R. (1974) *Who Shall Live?* Basic Books: New York.

Hinds, M.W. (1974) Letter. *New England Journal of Medicine,* 291, 741.

Illich, I. (1975) *Medical Nemesis – the Expropriation of Health.* Calder and Boyars: London.

Medical Research Council (1970) Working Party on the relationship between dietary sugar intake and arterial disease. *Lancet,* ii, 1265–71.

Richardson, J. (1976) The dependency hypothesis – That more doctors will result in lower quality health. Research paper No. 113, School of Economics and Financial Studies. Macquarie University: Sydney.

Stewart, C.T. (1971) Allocation of resources to health. *Journal of Human Resources,* 6, 103–22.

West R.R. and Lowe, C.R. (1976) Regional variations in need for and provision and use of child health services in England and Wales. *British Medical Journal,* ii, 843–6.

Yudkin, J. (1957) Diet and coronary thrombosis. *Lancet,* ii, 155–62.

Appendix: Sources of data and indices

Mortality data and population density data: World Health Organisation (1973) *World Health Statistics Annual. Vol. 1. Vital Statistics and Causes of Death for 1970.* WHO: Geneva.

Doctors, nurses and beds per 10 000 population: World Health Organisation (1973) *World Health Statistics Annual. Vol. 3. Statistics of Health Personnel etc.* WHO: Geneva. (With help from Dr Robert Maxwell.)

Alcohol (litres per head per year): Produkschap voor Gedistilleerde Dranken 1975. *Hoeveel alcoholhoudende dranken worden er in de wereld gedronken?* Schiedam, Netherlands.

Manufactured cigarettes per adult (aged over 15) per annum: Tobacco Research Council (1972) *Tobacco Consumption in various countries.* Tobacco Research Council: London.

GNP per head (we used data for 1960 and 1970 at constant 1973 prices as we hope to study changes later): International Bank for Reconstruction and Development, Washington. (Through the kindness of Dr Schrieber, 1977.)

Per cent GNP spent on health: United Nations *Year Book of National Accounts.* Statistics for 1970. Office of Health Economics: London. Dr Robert Maxwell.

Per cent of health expenditure covered by public expenditure (intervention index): OECD Paris Working Party on Economic Policy. (Through the kindness of Dr J.P. Poullier.)

Education index, 'percentage of the cohort continuing education after age 18' (both sexes): UNESCO, Paris. (Through the kindness of Dr S. Fauchette.)

Dietary data: OECD (1975). *Food consumption statistics 1955– 1973.* OECD: Paris.

Acknowledgement

Cochrane, A.L., St Leger, A.S. and Moore, F. (1978) Health service 'input' and mortality 'output' in developed countries. *Journal of Epidemiology and Community Health,* 32, 200–5.

9 *Professor Jerry Morris*

Orr, J.B. (1936) *Food Health and Income. Report on a Survey of Adequacy of Diet in Relation to Income.* London: Macmillan.

Morris, J.N. (1992) Exercise versus heart attack: history of a hypothesis. *Coronary Heart Disease Epidemiology: from Aetiology to Public Health*, eds M. Marmot and P. Elliott. Oxford: Oxford University Press, 242–55.

INTRODUCTION

When I received the Editor's invitation my thoughts immediately turned to Boyd Orr. *Food Health and Income* was my first solid text in 'social medicine'; I was already exploring these issues and have been concerned with them ever since[1,2]. I have, however, been unable to find a published account of the book appropriate for a reader in epidemiology. So, as it has long been out of print, I compromised by piecing together extracts from it that will, it is hoped, adequately represent the book's main contents and at the same time convey its special flavour, its Victorian echoes and its inspiration.[3]

Food Health and Income pioneered a combination of social-economic analysis and survey with the newer knowledge of nutrition in the service of public health. The emphasis throughout was on *optimal* rather than politically correct, safe *minimal* standards for 'health and working capacity' (see the British Medical Association's report of 1933[4]). Boyd Orr, of course, was mainly concerned with the deficiencies and deprivation exposed among the poorer *half* of the population who spent very nearly *half* of their total income on food.

The book was weakest in its account of the physiological-clinical associations of the unequal levels of nutrition that were demonstrated. Its sequel in 1937–9[5] (though not published until 1955) took this aspect, as well as the actual dietary assessment, much further. Young Drs John Pemberton and Angus Thomson were enlisted for the medical examination of samples of children. All in all, the Boyd Orr oeuvre made a major contribution to the food and nutrition policy which was such a remarkable success during the Second World War.

This classical illustration of epidemiology as the basic science of public health will, I hope, stimulate lively discussion. Here are a few issues: the shifting paradigm of healthy diet[6–8] in our age of comparative plenty (in one of the dietary 'deficiencies', however, were the poor disadvantaged?); the short- and long-term fates of children and adults with such diverse documented life experiences; the abiding problems of method in nutritional epidemiology;[9] the political responsibilities of public health; and the grand question, What are we learning from history . . . and failing to learn?

Notes and references

1 Morris J.N. and Titmuss, R.M. (1942) Epidemiology of juvenile rheumatism. *Lancet*, ii, 59–63.
2 Morris, J.N. (1990) Inequalities in health: ten years and little further on. *Lancet*, 336, 491–3.
3 Where I have included linking sentences in my own words they have been printed in italics.
4 Report of BMA Nutrition Committee (1933) *Br. Med. J.*, 25 November, suppl., 1–16.
5 Family Diet and Health in Pre-war Britain. (1955) A Dietary and Clinical Survey. Dunfermline: Carnegie United Kingdom Trust.
6 Secretary of State for Health (1992) *The Health of the Nation: a Strategy for Health in England*. London: HMSO.
7 Gregory, J., Foster, K., Tyler H. and Wiseman, M. (1990) *The Dietary and Nutritional Survey of British Adults*. London: HMSO.

8 Department of Health (1991) *Dietary Reference Values for Food Energy and Nutrients for the United Kingdom.* Report on health and social subjects 41. London: HMSO.

9 Bingham, S. (1987) The dietary assessment of individuals. *Nutr. Abstr. Rev.*, 57, 705–42.

FOOD HEALTH AND INCOME

Foreword

The state of nutrition of the people of this country is surveyed here on a broad scale and from a new angle. Instead of discussing minimum requirements, about which there has been so much controversy, this survey considers optimum requirements. Optimum requirements are based on the physiological ideal, which we define as 'a state of well-being such that no improvement can be effected by a change in the diet'. The standard of adequacy of diet adopted is one which is designed to maintain the standard of perfect nutrition.

The average diet of each of six groups into which the population has been divided according to income are compared with these requirements for perfect nutrition. The health of the population is reviewed to see to what extent inadequacy of diet is reflected in ill-health and poor physique.

It is difficult in the present state of knowledge to lay down precise and detailed criteria of perfect nutrition. The basis of comparison taken for health is, therefore, the state of health and physique of those groups of the population who can choose their diets freely, without any economic consideration seriously affecting their choice. For the purposes of this large-scale survey individual errors of diet can be ignored. These errors are undoubtedly common. The diets, even of those who are able to purchase unlimited amounts of any foodstuff available, will improve as the knowledge of dietetics extends. Meantime, however, the state of nutrition of the higher income groups, whose diet is not limited by income, can be taken as a standard which can be attained with the present dietary habits of the people of this country.

The tentative conclusion reached is that a diet completely adequate for health, according to modern standards, is reached at an income level above that of 50 per cent of the population. This means that 50 per cent of the population are living at a level of nutrition so high that, on the average, no improvement can be effected by increased consumption.

The important aspect of the survey, however, is the inadequacy of the diets of the lower income groups, and the markedly lower standard of health of the people, and especially of the children, in these groups, compared with that of the higher income groups.

The method of grouping the population according to income is new and may be open to the criticism, among others, that it over-emphasises the importance of children as an economic factor affecting standard of living. The basis of the grouping is the total family income divided by the number of persons, including children, supported by it. Thus an average income of 30s. per head per week is reached by a man earning £550 a year, with a wife, four children and one domestic servant. It is also reached by a manual worker earning £3 a week with only a wife to support. The 'higher income' and 'lower income' groups cannot be simply identified with 'rich' and 'poor' in the generally accepted sense of these terms.

The lowest of the six income groups contains a disproportionately high number of children – rather more than a fifth of all the children in the country. This is the group whose diet falls furthest below the standard of adequacy for health. Great improvements in health have been and are being effected in these children by improved nutrition. The picture presented in the survey justifies all and more than all the efforts which have already been made, but opens up a prospect of still further improvement.

As is noted in the report, the data are too scanty to yield a picture fully accurate in detail. Moreover, both the technique of the investigation and the standard of dietary requirements adopted are new and must be regarded as still on trial. There is need for further investigation and further discussion of the whole question in all its complicated relationships, in order that the measures taken to deal with the situation may be based on generally accepted facts and well-informed public opinion.

Methods and data

To get an idea of the nature of the diet in different sections of the community, the whole population was classified in six groups according to family income, and an estimate based on family budget data was made of the consumption of the various foodstuffs in each of the groups.

The classification of the population into groups according to income was based on income tax statistics, wage statistics and data relating to unemployment, old age pensions and other forms of social income, combined with a sample investigation of the 1931 Population Census designed to yield information as to the sizes of

Table 1 Classification of the population by income groups and average food expenditure per head in each group

Group	Income per head per week	Estimated average expenditure on food	Estimated population of group	
			Numbers	Percentage
I	Up to 10s.	4s.	4 500 000	10
II	10s. to 15s.	6s.	9 000 000	20
III	15s. to 20s.	8s.	9 000 000	20
IV	20s. to 30s.	10s.	9 000 000	20
V	30s. to 45s.	12s.	9 000 000	20
VI	Over 45s.	14s.	4 500 000	10
Average	30s.	9s.	–	–

Table 2 Quantities of food consumed per head per week at different income levels in 1152 family budgets

	Group I	Group II	Group III	Group IV	Group V*	Group VI*	Weighted average of groups
Proportion of the population (%)	10	20	20	20	20	10	
Number of budgets	411	152	233	156	136	64	–
Beef and veal (oz.)	9.5	11.5	11.7	11.3	10.2	9.5	10.8
Mutton and lamb (oz.)	2.1	3.1	4.3	6.2	6.8	9.7	5.3
Bacon and ham (oz.)	2.6	4.1	4.6	5.7	5.7	6.6	4.9
Other meat[a] (oz.)	2.8	2.9	4.2	5.4	3.6	3.5	3.8
Total meat[b] (oz.)	17.0	21.6	24.8	28.6	26.3	29.3	24.8
Bread and flour (excl. biscuits and cakes)[g] (oz.)	64.5	62.0	63.3	64.7	54.6	47.7	60.1
Milk, fresh (pints)	1.1	2.1	2.6	2.9	4.5	5.4	3.1
Milk, condensed[c] (pints)	0.6	0.4	0.4	0.3	0.2	0.1	0.3
Eggs (no.)	1.9	2.8	3.7	4.8	4.7	5.2	3.9
Butter (oz.)	2.7	5.7	7.4	8.8	8.9	9.7	7.4
Cheese (oz.)	1.5	2.1	2.8	3.2	2.9	2.5	2.6
Margarine (oz.)	4.9	2.9	2.2	1.9	2.5	1.4	2.5
Tea (oz.)	2.2	2.5	2.5	2.8	2.5	2.1	2.5
Potatoes[f] (oz.)	51.2	50.8	55.5	57.4	42.8	39.4	50.4
Lard, suet and dripping (oz.)	2.5	3.4	4.5	4.7	3.5[e]	3.2[e]	3.8
Fish[d] (oz.)	2.4	2.6	3.9	5.4	5.9	8.1	4.6
Sugar purchased as such (oz.)	13.5	15.9	18.1	20.1	19.0	18.1	17.8
Jams, jellies and syrups (oz.)	4.3	5.5	5.7	5.8	6.5	5.6	5.7

[a] Sausage, corned beef and pork only. [b] The total of the four items above. [c] In terms of liquid milk equivalent. [d] Excludes fried and tinned. [e] For the two middle class groups, lard only. [f] Excludes purchased 'chipped' potatoes. [g] In terms of flour. * Group V has been calculated as a straight average of one working class group with income of 30 to 40s. per head, and two middle class groups with family incomes of £200–300 and £300–400 (30s. and 40s. per head per week respectively). Group VI has been calculated as a straight average of four middle class groups with family incomes of £400–500, £500–600, £600–700, £700–800 per annum.

families and the ratio of earners to dependants in different occupation groups.

The composition of the average diet of each group was examined, the amounts of each of the constituents present being compared with the amounts required for health.

The estimates of the distribution of the total food supply between the different groups were based on the data from family budgets. (*1152 of these budgets were assembled, from across the country but mainly from North England; these data all refer to 1933–5*).

Standards

The standard of health adopted is the physiological or ideal, viz., a state of well-being such that no improvement can be effected by a change in the diet. It is based on fundamental physiological principles, and it will not alter with any change either in dietary habits or in average health of the community. In an investigation of this nature the standard by which adequacy of diet is measured obviously determines the degree of inadequacy which will be found.

The standards of dietary requirements adopted are those of Stiebeling of the Government Bureau of Home Economics, USA. These standards have been set up to provide what was estimated to be a sufficiency of essential dietary constituents.

The national population

Table 1 shows the final approximate estimates of the distribution of the national income. The population has been classified into six groups, consisting of 10 per cent at the top and the bottom, and four intermediate groups of 20 per cent.

Here also the figure given for income per head is the income of the family divided by the number of persons supported. Thus, a man and wife with £2 10s. a week with no children or dependants would fall into group IV; with one child into group III; with two or three children into group II; and with four or more children into group I. The poorest 10 per cent of the population consist in the main of families in which there is a disproportionate number of children or other dependants per earner. It is estimated that half the persons in group I are children under 14 and that between 20 and 25 per cent of the children in the country are in the lowest income group.

Included in the table is a column showing average food expenditure per head per week. It is obvious, of course, that as income falls the percentage spent on food, which is a prime necessity of life, will increase. The average expenditure on food represents a proportion rising from below 20 per cent in group VI to nearly 50 per cent in groups I, II and III.

Dietary assessment

Table 2 gives the estimates of food consumption derived from the family budgets.

The national picture

The information derived from the family budgets was extrapolated, with much qualification, to provide national estimates of food consumption by income group. Figure 1 gives some interesting examples.

Nutrients

The next step translated these data into the main nutrients, as these were then understood. Table 3 is a fascinating picture of stability and change.

Nutrition and health

Several aspects are briefly considered. The rate of growth in children is illustrated with the marked difference in height attained by boys drawn from different social classes. The incidence (we would say prevalence) of 'deficiency disease' in children in terms of residual rickets (major manifestations having become rare through application of the new knowledge of nutrition), 'bad teeth' and nutritional anaemia, which appeared still to be widespread in lower income groups.

There is a brief reference to tuberculosis mortality by social class but surprisingly little reference to the Registrar Generals' decennial supplements, though of course that based on the 1931 census had not yet appeared.

Finally, feeding experiments on animals and children are mentioned. The Carnegie Survey followed this up with its own trial.

Summary and conclusion

The food position of the country has been investigated to show the average consumption of the main foodstuffs at different income levels. The standard of food requirements and the standard of health adopted are not the present average but the optimum, i.e. the physiological standard, which, though ideal, is attainable in practice with a national food supply sufficient to provide a diet adequate for health for any member of the community. The main findings may be summarized as follows:

1 Of an estimated national income of £3750 million, about £1075 million are spent on food. This is equivalent to 9s. per head per week.
2 The consumption of bread and potatoes is practically uniform throughout the different income level groups.

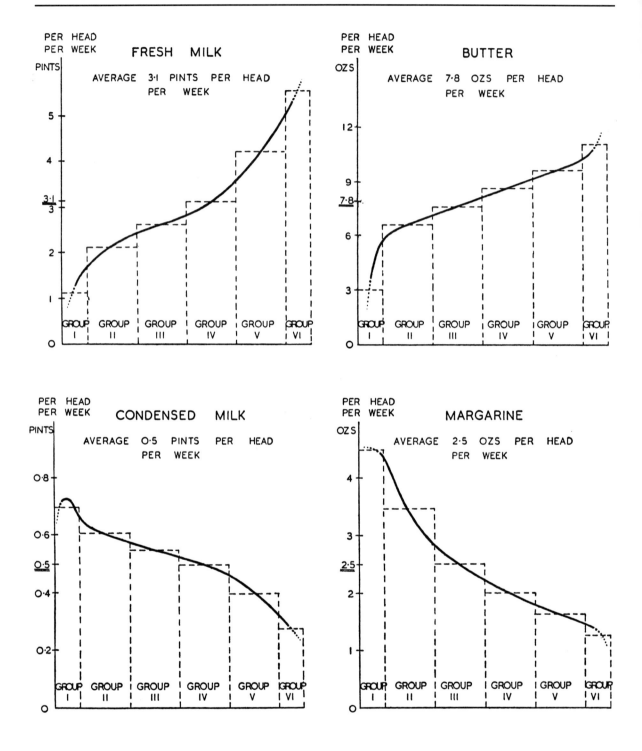

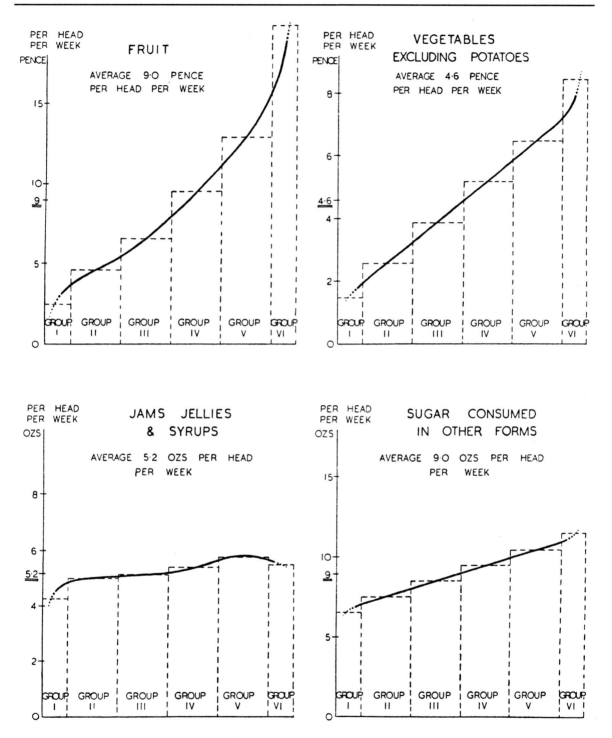

Fig. 1 Estimated consumption per head of certain foodstuffs by income groups.

Table 3 Composition of the diet (per day) by income groups of the population

	Group I		Group II		Group III		Group IV		Group V		Group VI		Standard requirements per unit of population
	grams	per cent	grams	per cent	grams	per cent	grams	per cent	grams	per cent	grams	per cent	grams
Protein													
Plant	40.9	64.5	43.5	57.2	44.0	52.6	43.8	49.0	42.8	45.3	40.5	41	–
Animal	22.5	35.5	32.5	42.8	39.6	47.4	45.6	51.0	51.6	54.7	57.8	8	–
Total	63.4	100.0	76.0	100.0	83.6	100.0	89.4	100.0	94.4	100.0	98.3	100.0	68
Fat													
Plant	20.9	29.2	17.9	18.1	14.5	13.2	13.3	11.0	12.2	9.4	11.1	7.9	–
Animal	50.7	70.8	80.9	81.9	95.1	86.8	107.3	89.0	118.3	90.6	130.4	92.1	–
Total	71.6	100.0	98.8	100.0	109.6	100.0	120.6	100.0	130.5	100.0	141.5	100.0	98
Carbohydrate	348	–	381	–	395	–	403	–	406	–	396	–	–
Minerals													
Calcium	0.37	–	0.52	–	0.61	–	0.71	–	0.83	–	0.95	–	0.6[a] 0.9[b]
Phosphorus	0.81	–	1.04	–	1.17	–	1.28	–	1.42	–	1.54	–	1.23
Iron	0.008	–	0.0099	–	0.011	–	0.012	–	0.0127	–	0.0137	–	0.0115

	Sherman units	International units	Sherman units	International units	Sherman units	International units	Sherman units	International units	Sherman units	International units	Sherman units	International units	Sherman units	International units
Vitamin A	1548	774	2500	1250	3248	1624	4030	2015	4420	2210	5750	2875	3800	1900
Vitamin C	57	838	78	1134	90	1314	108	1577	126	1832	158	2323	95	1400
Calories	2317		2768		2962		3119		3249		3326		2810	

[a] Minimum for positive balance. [b] Minimum plus 50 per cent for safety margin.

Consumption of milk, eggs, fruit, vegetables, meat and fish rises with income. Thus, in the poorest group the average consumption of milk, including tinned milk, is equivalent to 1.8 pints per head per week; in the wealthiest group 5.5 pints. The poorest group consume 1.5 eggs per head per week; the wealthiest 4.5. The poorest spend 2.4d. on fruit; the wealthiest 1s. 8d.

3 An examination of the composition of the diets of the different groups shows that the degree of adequacy for health increases as income rises. The average diet of the poorest group, comprising four and a half million people, is, by the standard adopted, deficient in every constituent examined. The second group, comprising 9 million people, is adequate in protein but deficient in all the vitamins and minerals considered. The third group, comprising another 9 million, is deficient in vitamins and minerals. Complete adequacy is almost reached in group IV, and in the still wealthier groups the diet has a surplus of all constituents considered.

4 A review of the state of health of the people of the different groups suggests that, as income increases, disease and death rate decrease, children grow more quickly, adult stature is greater and general health and physique improve.

5 The results of tests on children show that improvement of the diet in the lower groups is accompanied by improvement in health and increased rate of growth, which approximates to that of children in the higher income groups.

6 To make the diet of the poorer groups the same as that of the first group whose diet is adequate for full health, i.e. group IV, would involve increases in consumption of a number of the more expensive foodstuffs, viz., milk, eggs, butter, fruit, vegetables and meat, varying from 12 to 25 per cent, nationally.

If these findings are accepted as sufficiently accurate to form a working hypothesis, they raise important economic and political problems. Consideration of these is outwith the scope of the investigation. It may be pointed out here, however, that one of the main difficulties in dealing with these problems is that they are not within the sphere of any single Department of State. This new knowledge of nutrition, which shows that there can be an enormous improvement in the health and physique of the nation, coming at the same time as the greatly increased powers of producing food, has created an entirely new situation which demands economic statesmanship. The prominence given to this new social problem at the Assembly of the League of Nations in 1935 and 1936 shows that it is occupying the attention of all civilised countries. It is gratifying that the lead in this movement was taken by the British Empire.

Finally, a parting salvo from Boyd Orr's Foreword to the second edition of Food Health and Income.

It has been suggested that the standard adopted, viz. what is needed to enable people to attain their maximum inherited capacity for health and physical fitness, is so high that it is impracticable. One writer terms it 'utopian'. In animal husbandry, an optimum standard, far from being utopian, is regarded as good practice. Every intelligent stock farmer in rearing animals tries to get a minimum diet for maximum health and physical fitness. A suggestion that he should use a lower standard would be regarded as absurd. If children of the three lower groups were reared for profit like young farm stock, giving them a diet below the requirements for health would be financially unsound. Unfortunately, the health and physical fitness of the rising generation are not marketable commodities which can be assessed in terms of money.

From the point of view of the State, the adoption of a standard of diet lower than the optimum is uneconomic. It leads to a great amount of preventable disease and ill-health which lay a heavy financial burden on the State, and on the public-spirited citizens who support hospitals and other charitable organisations. It is probable that an inquiry would show that the cost of bringing a diet adequate for health within the purchasing power of the poorest would be less than the cost of treating the disease and ill-health which would thereby be prevented. A few years hence, when the connection between the poor feeding of mothers and children and subsequent poor physique and ill-health is as clearly recognised as the connection between a contaminated water supply and cholera, the suggestion that a diet fully adequate for health should be available for everyone will be regarded as reasonable and in accordance with common sense, as is the preservation of our domestic water supply from pollution.

Acknowledgement

Orr, J.B. (1936) *Food Health and Income. Report on a Survey of Adequacy of Diet in Relation to Income.* London: Macmillan.

EXERCISE VERSUS HEART ATTACK: HISTORY OF A HYPOTHESIS

The observation that physical activity can protect against heart attack was first made in studies of men in a variety of occupations. Conductors on London's double-decker buses (up and down stairs 11 days a fortnight, 50 weeks a year, often for decades) experienced half or less the incidence of acute myocardial infarction and 'sudden death' ascribed to coronary heart disease (CHD) in the sedentary bus drivers. Postmen (70 per cent of their shift walking, cycling and climbing stairs to deliver the mail) were similarly protected by comparison with postal clerks and miscellaneous other groups of sedentary government workers (Morris *et al.*, 1953). The self-selection issue soon presented: conductors were manifestly more lightly built than drivers. Perhaps the conductors were generally healthier than the drivers (as manifest in their leanness) and so less likely to suffer heart attack – and more likely to choose more active jobs? However, prospective analysis of rates of sudden death in relation to uniform trouser-waist (central obesity?) in the bus population found that slim, average or portly conductors suffered about half or less the incidence of the drivers (Heady *et al.*, 1961). Subsequent occupational studies in the UK and elsewhere mostly confirmed the main observation and its 'independence' from a variety of other relevant, possibly confounding factors (Paffenbarger *et al.*, 1970; Powell *et al.*, 1987; Kristensen, 1989).

By the 1960s it had already become evident that if physical activity was to contribute in the years ahead to prevention of CHD it would increasingly have to be the exercise taken off the job, in leisure time, by a population increasingly employed in physically undemanding work and otherwise physically inactive. Therefore a survey was mounted among a group of male sedentary/physically very light workers in the executive grade of the civil service to test the hypothesis drawn (not very perceptively) from these occupational studies that such men with high totals of physical activity in their leisure time would suffer less CHD than comparable men with low totals. There was no support for this in prospective study. Instead, it was found that only the men engaging in vigorous activity showed a reduced incidence of the disease (Figure 1). Vigorous activity was defined as that liable to reach peaks of energy expenditure of 7.5 kcal/min (31.5 kJ/min), over six times basal oxygen uptake, say, and a gross oxygen uptake of 1.5 l/min or about 20 ml/kg/min. Furthermore, the men reporting dynamic vigorous aerobic exercise, in sports and getting about, showed much stronger and more consistent protection than those reporting heavy recreational 'work', the other form of vigorous activity (Morris *et al.*, 1973, 1980).

Again, the benefits of such vigorous aerobic exercise were statistically independent of the other factors that were studied. For example, Table 1 shows the age-standardized percentage CHD incidence rates for men

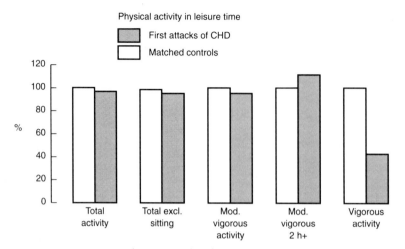

Fig. 1 Prospective survey (1968/1970–1978) of 16 882 British male executive grade civil servants, aged 40–64 at entry. The first 214 fatal and non-fatal clinical attacks of coronary heart disease and 428 controls. Activity was logged, 5 min × 5 min, on sample Friday and Saturday.

classified according to cigarette smoking and vigorous exercise at 8.5 years follow-up. The reductions were substantially greater in men aged 50–64 than in the younger entrants.

Variations of CHD

The advantage of men engaging in vigorous aerobic exercise was evident in the incidence of acute myocardial infarction (non-fatal and fatal), sudden death, angina pectoris and coronary insufficiency.

In a cross-sectional approach a sample of 509 men was drawn from the cohort. Of these, 74 reported vigorous aerobic exercise. Their resting electrocardiograms (ECGs) were compared using the Minnesota Code (Rose and Blackburn, 1968) with those of the 384 men reporting no vigorous exercise: 2.9 per cent of the former (age-standardized) showed definite or possible ischaemia against 10.4 per cent of the latter. Less expected were the differences in the frequency of ectopic beats (Ebs). These were 2.9 per cent in the 74 men reporting exercise versus 7.1 per cent in the 384 others: 0 versus 10 instances of supraventricular EBs, 2 versus 17 instances of ventricular EBs, and 0 versus 14 instances of EBs comprising 10 per cent or more of recorded cycles. Electrical instability?

Exclusion of men with evidence of clinical or subclinical cardiovascular disease did not affect this contrast. The 51 men reporting heavy recreational work showed no such immunity (Epstein *et al.*, 1976).

Table 1 CHD incidence (per cent)

	VE	No VE
Non-smokers		
Non-fatal first clinical attack	1.3	3.2
Fatal first clinical attack	0.85	1.7
Smokers		
Non-fatal	1.6	4.4
Fatal	3.3	5.2

VE, vigorous aerobic exercise.

Next steps

The indication that a threshold of intensity of exercise has to be reached for protection against CHD, and the further suggestion that vigorous *aerobic* exercise is distinctively effectual, raised questions for theory (Fentem *et al.*, 1988; Pollock and Wilmore, 1990) and for public health. Thus we could be identifying a level of activity in this homogeneous population of middle-aged middle-class office workers whose health was average or above, sufficiently intense on average, i.e. entailing over 50–60 per cent of individual maximal aerobic power, and of sufficient quantity to produce 'overload' and a 'training' stimulus. And this could be improving cardiorespiratory fitness to moderately high levels. Plainly, health education messages would be affected if such a proposition superseded that of the benefits of high total physical activity levels

Table 2 Vigorous aerobic exercise, other CHD factors, and the attack rate of CHD (1976–1986) in male executive grade civil servants aged 55–64 at entry (rates per 1000 man-years)

	Group 1 (frequent vigorous aerobic exercise)	Group 2 (next lesser degree of this)	Group 3 (residual vigorous aerobic exercise)	Group 4 (no vigorous aerobic exercise)	P^a
Vigorous aerobic exercise	2.3	3.3	4.5	5.9	< 0.001
Standardized for other factors[b]	2.4	3.6	4.8	5.6	< 0.005

Non-fatal first events, 55–59 years; fatal, 55–73 years.
[a] Tests for trend; tested for heterogeneity, the results are similar.
[b] Other factors, from data reported at entry, were premature parental mortality from CVD, stature, cigarette smoking, body mass index, history of high blood pressure, history of diabetes, positive/negative on LSHTM angina questionnaire (Rose and Blackburn, 1968).

(Morris, 1975). Therefore a further survey was mounted in 1976 to test the new hypothesis directly.

Fresh hypothesis

The prospective survey of 1976–86, again in men of the executive grade in the civil service, was designed to test the following propositions.

1 Vigorous habitual frequent aerobic exercise in sports and in getting about would offer substantial protection against CHD.
2 More tentatively, heavy (vigorous) recreational work in jobs and hobbies in and about the house and garden and on the car (the other main form of physical activity in leisure time), which had shown an inconsistent and weaker association with incidence of CHD in the previous survey, would also confer some protection.
3 Other physical activity would not be protective.
4 High totals of energy expenditure *per se* would not be protective (Morris *et al.*, 1990).

Exercise and incidence

Table 2 orders the data of this second survey in terms of the principal proposition 1. The total cohort consisted of 9375 men having no history or record of CHD. There were 474 first clinical events in a 9.3 year follow-up and 87 563 man-years' observation. Table 2 shows the data for men aged 55–64 at entry which relate to proposition 1.

Group 1 consists of the men (9 per cent of the cohort) reporting vigorous sports (swimming, jogging, hill-climbing, rowing, soccer and hockey (mostly refereeing), racket games, etc., at least twice a week), and/or rating the usual pace of their regular walking to and from work and in their leisure time as 'fast' (over 4 m.p.h. or

6.4 k.m.p.h.), and/or recording considerable cycling. Group 2 comprises the next highest degree of such vigorous aerobic exercise, i.e. vigorous sports at least once but less than twice a week, and/or 'fairly brisk' walking for over 30 minutes per day, and/or other cycling. Group 3 includes the residual vigorous aerobic exercise, i.e. very little, occasional sports and/or shorter 'fairly brisk' walks. Group 4, the largest, comprising just over half the men, is made up of those who reported no vigorous aerobic exercise. This category includes the very popular non-vigorous sports and games, the commoner regular walking at 'normal' pace or 'strolling', and a huge volume of recreational work in gardening and do-it-yourself, whether vigorous, moderate or light.

Group 1 of the cohort had low CHD attack rates compared with the rest of the men ($P < 0.001$). This was evident in both non-fatal and fatal first clinical events. For younger men, aged 45–54, there were no differences in attack rates among groups 2–4. However, the attack rate in entrants aged 55–64 was significantly lower in group 2 than in groups 3 and 4 ($P \simeq 0.01$). Moreover, keep-fit exercises five or more times a week, and climbing 500 plus stairs each day – dynamic aerobic activities, plausibly vigorous items from the previous survey – which were not associated with incidence in the younger entrants did show significantly lower CHD rates in these older men. Therefore they have been included in group 2. This makes sense in terms of both the probable greater variability in intensity of these two activities on the one hand, and the reduction with age of the oxygen utilization capacity of muscles on the other, so that less exercise is required for overload and a training stimulus (though of course it still has to be more intense than customary). The net result is that 30 per cent of the older entrants showed such exercise-related reduction of heart disease.

In group 3 there is a non-significant continuation of the favourable trend in the older men. Thus there was some

Table 3 Miscellaneous activities in leisure time and mortality from CHD in male executive grade civil servants (1976–1986) aged 60–73 (rates per 1000 man-years)

Episodes in previous 4 weeks[a]	Ballroom dancing	Golf	Long walks[b]	Do-it-yourself		
				Heavy	Moderate	Light
0	4.2	4.2	4.4	4.3	4.2	4.0
1–3	4.3	4.0	3.8	3.9	3.9	3.6
4–7	5.5	5.1	4.1	4.7	5.4	5.1
≥ 8	(3.1)	6.2	4.2	6.5	3.4	4.6

Regular walking to and from work, and elsewhere, regardless of pace, per day: 0, 3.9 per 1000 man-years; ≤ 30 min, 4.2 per 1000 man-years; > 30 min, 3.7 per 1000 man-years. (The 0 is an overstatement since episodes of activity < 5 were disregarded throughout.)
[a] Reported at entry in 1976 (Rates for less than five cases in parentheses.)
[b] Walks of at least an hour, additional to 'regular' walking.

indication of dose–response of CHD with frequency/intensity in vigorous aerobic exercise. A threshold effect of such exercise alone is seen in younger men, at the highest level of intensity that was identified (group 1). High coronary incidence at all ages was recorded in group 4.

Table 3 further illustrates the failure of popular non-vigorous sports and games (dancing was reported by 14 per cent of the men and golf by 10 per cent) to affect CHD rates. The outcome is similar with the quantity of regular walking if pace is disregarded. The negative findings with the detailed and more representative record in this survey of 'recreational work' are clear; the results are the same for gardening. The situation chosen in Table 3 is that most likely to elicit association with coronary disease: first clinical events in men over 60 and the harder mortality data. At ages under 60 the results are the same for both non-fatal and fatal events. Because of the popularity and appeal of the non-vigorous sports and games, they were subjected to an intensive study, searching, for example, for possible associations with CHD in vulnerable groups such as cigarette smokers, the overweight, those with subclinical CVD and so on, which might be expected to show a response to such exercise of lower intensity. Again, none was found.

Multivariate analysis

The lower line of Table 2 controls for possible confounding by some CHD risk factors. The familiar dilemmas and limitations of such adjustment arise (Davey Smith and Phillips, 1990), including circularity and double-counting of such factors as body mass and subclinical cardiovascular disease (and blood cholesterol levels). These factors themselves are likely to be lowered by exercise, and may indeed be mechanisms of the effect of exercise on CHD.

Therefore their introduction into the multivariate analysis may misleadingly reduce the value of the exercise factor itself in the outcome. This can be illustrated by data on 'personal control'.

In these men, there is a significant association between confidence in the possibility of personal control of future health and future coronary incidence. When the psychological variable is 'adjusted' for vigorous aerobic exercise, the association is considerably weakened, and if cigarette smoking is then introduced it disappears altogether. It is possible that this belief/attitude/knowledge is effectual through or mediated by these (and other health-directed) behaviours. This is attractive, but for understanding of aetiology – and for public health and its need to understand motives – how much is being lost by such computation and the summary dismissal of antecedent by later stages in the long natural history of CHD? (The difference in the precision of classification of exercise and smoking compared with that of the attitude, and how far this is responsible for the result, need not detain us now.)

Be all this as it may, the striking feature of Table 2 is the similarity of before and after profiles, again pointing to 'statistical independence' of the exercise factor and some freedom from its confounding by the other factors studied. Of course, multivariate analyses are now ritual in epidemiological research, and in the relation between physical activity and CHD they have included all the standard risk factors and show the same general picture (Powell et al., 1987).

Overview

A few points can be made about some recent reports. First, a remarkable variety of populations have shown lower CHD rates with high physical activity. Thus the two most detailed studies are of elite affluent Harvard alumni (Paffenbarger *et al.*, 1978) and our own British civil servants (social class II in the national scale), on modest incomes and generally without tertiary educational qualifications. The Finnish general population sample is from an area with a notably high prevalence of CHD (Salonen *et al.*, 1988). The Honolulu Study follows a cohort of men of Japanese ancestry (Donahue *et al.*, 1988). The Multiple Risk Factor Intervention Trial (MRFIT) is an experiment on American men selected for high risk of CHD by elevated lipid and blood pressure levels (Leon *et al.*, 1987).

There are difficulties in interpreting discrepancies between the findings of these studies. Thus, in contrast with our findings, Paffenbarger *et al.*, (1978) report substantial benefit from more than 2000 kcal per week of leisure time activity, however this is accomplished. On analysis, two-thirds of the men with such high totals engaged in vigorous sports, but those reporting other non-vigorous aerobic exercise also show some, albeit less, advantage. Could it be that the American cohort is basically less active and less fit than the British and thus capable of benefiting from less intense exercise? (The same point has previously been made on age.) Other obvious differences in the populations are that the British are subject to governmental medical recruitment and retirement policies and that they are men actually in post and hence are a 'healthy worker' cohort. Comparative physiological studies on American and British men could be rewarding.

Another question arises with regard to the methods of assessment of physical activity that are being used and, in particular, on their probability of identifying training or conditioning exercise. Because of the frequency of do-it-yourself and gardening in our British study (90 per cent of the men gardened and 80 per cent reported other moderate or heavy 'work'), overall assessment of activity by totals of energy expenditure blur the picture: neither of these two classes of activity contain much of the sustained rhythmic contraction/relaxation of large muscle groups that is required for cardiorespiratory training. Again, as previously found, total physical activity estimates do not identify groups with different CHD risk in this population. Thus, in group 4, who reported no vigorous aerobic exercise, incidence rates per 1000 man-years by total physical activity in leisure time per week, summing all the forms previously considered, were as follows: < 2000 kcal, 5.9; 2000–2999 kcal, 6.5; > 3000 kcal, 7.0.

The other studies mentioned above are uniform and total in their assessments and do not seek to report predominantly aerobic exercise, vigorous or not, so that rival hypotheses can be tested. The fact that these studies produce positive results could mean that it is not training

and fitness that matter but high total energy expenditure, thus refuting the British findings, or perhaps indicating that they apply only to a relative healthy population. Alternatively, the overall profiles among those scoring high totals in these other studies may include enough vigorous aerobic exercise for benefit in their populations. It should be possible to disaggregate the data and extract such information. Highlighted by this discussion is the lack, exposed by the needs of epidemiological research, of physiological information on real-life everyday physical activities in leisure time (in people of disparate occupation): on caloric expenditures, dynamic/static components, vascular reactions, metabolic responses, and short-, medium- and long-term risk factor relationships. (The contrast with the richness of data on athletes and athleticism (Reilly *et al.*, 1990) is striking.) Clinical and psychological data are frequently equally sparse.

Mechanisms of protection

With little qualification it can be said that exercise improves all physiological function, and of course there are also psychological and social benefits. In that sense exercise is a 'general cause' of good health (Morris, 1975). Therefore, not surprisingly, major risk factors for CHD are liable to be diminished: lipid profiles, blood pressure, insulin sensitivity, glucose levels and body mass (Powell *et al.*, 1987; Fentem *et al.*, 1988). At the same time, exercise both counteracts these risk factors and is some defence against them, as seen in the data previously given on smoking. Thus it might be expected that coronary atherosclerosis will be retarded or reduced, but so far the evidence in man is not impressive.

The more interesting suggestion in our study is that in such a different body of data it confirms and amplifies the observation by Paffenbarger *et al.*, (1978) that, for benefit, the exercise has to be current. A history of exercise in the past, which has been abandoned, confers no protection. For example, Table 4 reports the experience among men who reported no vigorous sports in the 1976 survey. By the same token, men who reported taking part in vigorous sports in 1976 had the same low incidence over the period 1976–86 whether or not they had been 'athletic' when young (as attested by a record of the most vigorous sports, such as squash, rugby, athletics and wrestling). The future rates in men reporting vigorous sports at least once a week in 1976 were 3.2 and 3.0 per 1000 man-years respectively in those with and without such a record.

These observations point to the acute phase of the heart disease rather than the slow build-up of chronic coronary

Table 4 Men with no vigorous sport activity in 1976

	Cases 1976–86	Rate per 1000 man-years
Played no vigorous sports previously	128	5.7
Played up to 25 years of age	27	4.1
Played up to 30 years of age	54	6.4
Played up to 40 years of age	92	5.7
Played past 40 years of age	112	6.2

atherosclerosis as the main locus of protection by exercise: to acute ischaemia, thrombosis, occlusion, dysrhythmia and electrical instability. Evidence that exercise is related to improved haemostatic profile in particular is increasing (Davey Smith *et al.*, 1989; Meade, 1991). This is a field ripe for systematic study.

An alternative or complementary interpretation of the necessity for the exercise to be maintained is that the protection is related not so much to the exercise itself, for example the dynamic exercise that raises the level of high density lipoprotein cholesterol, as to the cardiorespiratory fitness and improved cardiac performance that is induced. It is well known that fitness cannot be stored; it depends on the maintenance of adequate aerobic exercise (Saltin *et al.*, 1968). Studies of CHD incidence in relation to fitness are accumulating, mostly with positive results (Gyntelberg *et al.*, 1980; Blair *et al.*, 1989). A difficulty here is that endurance capacity or stamina, the manifestation of cardiorespiratory fitness likely to be most responsive to the exercise under consideration, cannot yet be readily measured in the field, and estimates of maximum aerobic power (VO_2 max) are not satisfactory substitutes. Interestingly, the association of cardiorespiratory fitness with CHD risk factors, as distinct from CHD incidence, is more controversial (Sedgwick *et al.*, 1989, 1990; Bouchard *et al.*, 1990a).

Restatement of hypothesis

The initial hypothesis has undergone several transformations in the course of its 40 years. It can now be stated as follows.

Adequate aerobic exercise in leisure time, which is habitual and ongoing, and the training and improved cardiorespiratory fitness and performance this produces, confer substantial protection against the occurrence of CHD in middle-aged and elderly men. The total death rate is also lowered. This is the case whatever the risk status of the men with respect to other factors. Protection

by exercise is effectual mainly in the acute phases of the disease, in particular against thrombosis, though there is also some benefit from reducing and counteracting standard risk factors and the build-up of chronic coronary atherosclerosis.

In this statement 'adequate' refers to both vigour (intensity) and quantity (frequency/duration) of exercise. The hypothesis refers to ordinary relatively healthy men engaged in sedentary and physically light occupations, and not to athletes.

From aetiology to public health

There is now good reason to believe that the decline of physical activity in work, recreation, transport and daily living is an integral part of the modern epidemic of CHD in developed industrial societies. This decline may well have been greatest in adequate aerobic exercise, and hence in cardiorespiratory fitness. Moreover, the increase in CHD has entailed an increase in coronary thrombosis – perhaps the main pathological change (Morris, 1951) – and again a link with physical activity/inactivity can be postulated.

The UK is underachieving in several aspects of health, particularly in its persistent high rates of CHD, and the need to address major possible causes is now, at last, widely recognized. Exercise is today's best buy in public health, not only because of the need and potential, but because it is positive and acceptable, has insignificant side-effects and can be inexpensive. Also, the opposition to be overcome is feeble in comparison with the tobacco barons and the Common Agricultural Policy, for instance.

In seminal papers, Rose (1981, 1985) has interpreted modern aetiological research for public health practice in the prevention of CHD. He describes two strategies: the individual high-risk strategy involving case-finding and personal care, and the population strategy which, by attacking the causes of incidence, seeks to reduce the mean level of risk factors and 'to shift the whole distribution of exposure in a favourable direction'. Each has its advantages and its drawbacks, though there is no question about the importance of the population strategy for this mass scourge.

However, two points can be made in applying Rose's thesis to our present concern with exercise. Only a minority of the population takes anything worthy of the name of exercise, and only a small minority of the lower social classes that are most vulnerable to heart attack (*General Household Survey*, 1989). Thus the majority, or the great majority, of the population is probably at high risk in these terms, and the approach to them and to the population at large must be much the same. Moreover, the 'prevention paradox' of the population strategy, that participating individuals will themselves derive little benefit from their contribution to the common good (for example by lowering their blood pressure), may not apply in the case of exercise. Altruistic participating individuals can be assured that by taking exercise, as encouraged, they will rapidly feel and function better as a result of the manifold benefits that exercise confers.

The evidence on CHD can be matched by that on the general benefits of exercise to physical capacity and mobility, mental and social function, and well-being, all perhaps most notably in the elderly; to the prevention of obesity, maturity onset diabetes, osteoporosis and so on; and to the relief of anxiety and depression. Equally, benefits in the rehabilitation of chronic disease and in the life of people with disabilities could be included (Bouchard et al., 1990b). In this paper we have dealt with only one aspect.

Practical application

There are several practical messages for public health practice from the kind of positive and encouraging observations reported in this paper. The commitment to exercise manifestly has to be continuing and serious (Department of Health and Human Services, 1980; American College of Sports Medicine, 1986). Examples given here are vigorous aerobic exercise at least twice a week and the expenditure of more than 2000 kcal per week in leisure time activities. Therefore such a commitment has to be emphasized in health education. However, aetiological studies are urgently required in other social and occupational samples, particularly among the lower socio-economic groups, to aid the formulation of population strategy.

Congruent with the philosophy that, with adequate exercise, training is possible at all ages, there is encouragement for middle-aged men to start exercising and for the elderly to continue. Direct evidence on the former will soon be available (Paffenbarger 1991), and there is already some evidence of protection against CHD in the elderly (Donahue et al., 1988) and our own data for individuals up to 73 years of age.

Individual and family, society and culture

The appeal must be seen to apply to the whole population. At the same time exercise typifies the individual–social, personal–environmental, and private–public interactions and partnerships that health promotion and prevention of disease require today (Morris, 1975). The

individual takes exercise and can continue to do so. The individual alone can tell when he or she is taking enough exercise for 'overload' or too much for safety. We are slowly learning about individual and family motivations. However, culture and society have to reinforce motivation, help with education and research, and, above all, provide support facilities. Among the civil servants in our study, swimming is the most popular and beneficial exercise: the provision of pools to generate and meet growing demand is under perennial threat from local government financial constraints. Similarly, both walking and cycling entail the partnership of individual and government; the latest British national plan to spend more than £12 billion on roads considers neither walking nor cycling.

The return of physical activity as the norm in everyone's everyday life – the 'restoration of biological normality' in Rose's words – will require cultural change on a scale similar to that which has occurred with smoking. Meanwhile, there is little advance among those who need it most. Hopefully, the findings of the National Fitness Survey (1990–1) may provide the impetus. The challenges to epidemiology are great: in a wide range of research; in information of the public, health service and government; in teaching; in the example we set; and, as part of the wider public health movement, in our collective political message.

References

American College of Sports Medicine (1986) *Guidelines for exercise testing and prescription* (3rd edn), Lea & Febiger, Philadelphia.

Blair, S.N., Kohl, H.W. III, Paffenbarger, R.S. Jr, Clark, D.G., Cooper, K. H. and Gibbons, L.W. (1989) Physical fitness and all-cause mortality: a prospective study of healthy men and women. *J. Am. Med. Assoc.*, 262, 2395–401.

Bouchard, C., Leon, A.S., Rao, D. C., Skinner, J.S. and Wilmore J.H. (1990a) Cross-sectional and longitudinal relationships between physical fitness and risk factors for coronary heart disease in men and women: 'The Adelaide 1000'. *J. Clin. Epidemiol.*, 43, 1005–7.

Bouchard, C., Shephard, R.J. Stephens, T., Sutton, J.R. and McPherson, B.M. (eds) (1990b) *Exercise, fitness and health: a consensus of current knowledge,* Human Kinetics, Champaign, IL.

Connelly, J.B., Cooper, J.A. and Meade, T.W. (1992) Strenuous exercise, plasma fibrinogen and factor VII activity. *Br. Heart J.,* 67, 351–4.

Davey Smith, G. and Phillips, A. (1990) Declaring independence: why we should be cautious. *J. Epidemiol. Community Health,* 44, 257–8.

Davey Smith, G., Marmot, M.G., Etherington, M. and O'Brien, J. (1989) A work stress-fibrinogen pathway as a potential mechanism for employment grade differences in coronary heart disease rates. Abstracts, 2nd Int. Conf. on Preventive Cardiology, Washington, DC.

Department of Health and Human Services (1980) *Promoting health/preventing disease: objectives for the nation,* US Government Printing Office, Washington, DC.

Donahue, R.P., Abbott, R.D., Reed, D.M. and Yano, K.C. (1988) Physical activity and coronary heart disease in middle-aged and elderly men. *Am. J. Public Health,* 78, 683–5.

Epstein, L., Miller, G.J., Stitt, F.W. and Morris, J.N. (1976) Vigorous exercise in leisure-time, coronary risk factors, and resting electrocardiogram in middle-aged male civil servants. *Br. Heart J.,* 38, 403–9.

Fentem, P.H., Bassey, E.J. and Turnbull, N.B. (1988) *The new case for exercise,* Health Education Authority and Sports Council, London.

General Household Survey (1989) HMSO, London.

Gyntelberg, F., Lauridsen, L. and Schubell, K. (1980) *Scand. J. Work and Environ. Health,* 6, 170–8.

Heady, J.A., Morris, J.N., Kagan, A. and Raffle, P.A.B. (1961) Coronary heart disease in London busmen: a progress report with particular reference to physique. *Br. J. Prev. Social Med.,* 15, 143–53.

Kristensen, T.S. (1989) Cardiovascular diseases and the work environment. *Scand. J. Work and Environ. Health,* 15, 165–79.

Leon, A.S., Connett, J., Jacobs, D.R. Jr and Rauramaa, R. (1987) Leisure-time physical activity levels and risk of coronary heart disease and death. *J. Am. Med. Assoc.,* 258, 2388–95.

Morris, J.N. (1951) Recent history of coronary disease. *Lancet,* i, 1–7, 69–73.

Morris, J.N. (1975) *Uses of epidemiology* (3rd edn), Churchill Livingstone, London (reprinted 1983).

Morris, J.N., Heady, J.A., Raffle, P.A.B. and Parks, J.W. (1953) Coronary heart disease and physical activity of work. *Lancet,* ii, 1053–7, 1111–20.

Morris, J.N., Chave, S.P.W., Adam, C., Sirey, C. and Epstein, L. (1973) Vigorous exercise in leisure-time and the incidence of coronary heart disease. *Lancet,* i, 333–9.

Morris, J.N., Everitt, M.G., Pollard, R., Chave, S.P.W. and Semmence, A.M. (1980) Vigorous exercise in leisure-time: protection against coronary heart disease. *Lancet,* ii, 1207–10.

Morris, J.N., Clayton, D.G., Everitt, M.G., Semmence, A.M. and Burgess, E.H. (1990) Exercise in leisure-time: coronary attack and death rate. *Br. Heart J.,* 63, 325–34.

Paffenbarger, R.S. Jr, Hyde, R.T., Wing, A.L., Lee, I.M., Jung, D.L. and Karnpert, J.B. (1993) The association of changes in physical activity levels and other lifestyle characteristics with mortality among men. *N. Engl. J. Med.* 328, 538–45.

Paffenbarger, R.S. Jr, Laughlin, M.E., Gima, A.S. and Black, R.A. (1970) Work activity of longshoremen as related to death from coronary heart disease and stroke. *New Engl. J. Med.,* 282, 1109–13.

Paffenbarger, R.S. Jr, Wing, A.L. and Hyde, R.T. (1978) Physical activity as an index of heart attack risk in college alumni. *Am. J. Epidemiol.,* 108, 161–75.

Pollock, M. and Wilmore, J.H. (1990) *Exercise in health and disease* (2nd edn), W.B. Saunders, Philadelphia.

Powell, K.E., Thompson, P.D., Caspersen, C.J. and Kendrick, J.S. (1987) Physical activity and the incidence of coronary heart disease. *Ann. Rev. Publ. Health.,* 8, 251–87.

Reilly, T., Secher, N., Snell, P. and Williams, C. (eds) (1990) *Physiology of sports,* Spon, London.

Rose, G. and Blackburn, H. (1968) *Cardiovascular survey methods,* World Health Organization, Geneva.

Rose, G. (1981) Strategy of prevention: lessons from cardio-vascular disease. *Br. Med. J.,* 282, 1847–51.

Rose, G. (1985) Sick individuals and sick populations. *Int. J. Epidemiol.,* 14, 32–8.

Salonen, J.T., Slater, J.S., Tuomilehto, J. and Rauramaa, R. (1988) Leisure-time and occupational physical activity: risk of death from ischaemic heart disease. *Am. J. Epidemiol.,* 127, 87–94.

Saltin, B., Blomquist, G., Mitchell, J. H., Johnson, R.L., Wildenthal, K. and Chapman, C.B. (1968) Response to exercise after bed rest and after training. *Circulation,* 38 (Suppl. VII), 1–77.

Sedgwick, A. W., Thomas, D.W., Davies, M., Baghurst, K. and Rouse, I. (1989) Cross-sectional and longitudinal relationships between physical fitness and risk factors for coronary heart disease in men and women: 'The Adelaide 1000'. *J. Clin. Epidemiol.,* 42, 189–200.

Sedgwick, A. W., Thomas, D.W., Davies, M., Baghurst, K. and Rouse, I. (1990) Cross-sectional and longitudinal relationships between physical fitness and risk factors for coronary heart disease in men and women: 'The Adelaide 1000'. *J. Clin. Epidemiol.,* 43, 1007–12.

Acknowledgement

Morris, J.N. (1992) Exercise versus heart attack: history of a hypothesis. *Coronary Heart Disease Epidemiology: from Aetiology to Public Health,* eds M. Marmot and P. Elliott. Oxford: Oxford University Press, 242–55.

Reprinted by permission of Oxford University Press.

10 *Professor Peter Pharoah*

Farr, W. (1885) Infant and child mortality. From *Vital Statistics: a Memorial Volume of Selections from the Reports and Writings of William Farr, MD, DCL, CB, FRS*. London: Offices of the Sanitary Institute, 188–209.

Pharoah, P.O.D. and Hornabrook, R.W. (1974) Endemic cretinism of recent onset in New Guinea. *Lancet*, ii, 1038–40.

INTRODUCTION

The contributions of William Farr using vital statistics for epidemiological analysis are legion. The originality of his observations were so far ahead of the time that many are being rediscovered. While the range of topics he covered was all-embracing, his analysis of mortality rates in infancy was outstanding. He drew attention to the importance of social conditions; for example, he associated the high infant mortality rates in the textile manufacturing towns with the high proportion of women employed away from home and contrasted them with the lower rates in hardware manufacturing towns with fewer women employed in factories. Farr also examined the causes of high death rates in infants in large towns, with lung and tubercular diseases, convulsions, atrophy and diarrhoea heading the list, and attributed them to bad sanitary arrangements, improper food and neglect. These observations predated, by a century, those of McKeown, which were influential in focusing attention on infant mortality rates and what they signified.

The subdivision of the period of infancy was recommended by Farr because 'the mortality diminishes so rapidly after the date of birth and at such various rates under different conditions, that it is necessary to subdivide the first year into months and even days to get conditions that are exactly comparable', and he noted that 'so unfavourable to infant life are the unsanitary conditions of large towns that not only is the mortality at some months of age twice as high as it is in some districts, but at seven months of age and upwards it is three times as high.' Yet it was not until 1971 that the World Health Organization started to publish post-neonatal mortality statistics in their own right.

For anyone approaching afresh the analysis of infant mortality statistics, a perusal of the writings of William Farr will prove a profitable investment.

My own study reproduced here came at a time when I was being pulled away from the field of clinical medicine and being pushed unwillingly into public health. It started with an amateurish dabbling in epidemiology and gradually brought awareness of the enormous contribution epidemiology could make. The relationship between incidence and prevalence became manifest. Here was a local well-recognized condition, endemic cretinism, which had risen sharply in prevalence within less than a decade. The local community were convinced that the disease post-dated first contact with the white man, but my arrogant assumption was that the rise in prevalence was owing to better survival and not a change in incidence. Subsequent investigations proved the local community right, and the lessons of humility and of listening to the patient, be they individual or community, had to be learnt.

Awareness of the importance of social change and its impact on health also grew. Merely changing, quite inadvertently and for entirely logical reasons, from one brand of salt (iodine rich) to another (iodine deplete), precipitated an epidemic of children who were mentally handicapped, with cerebral palsy, and deaf-mute, a result having enormous social consequences to that community.

There was pleasure in the study of carrying out 'shoe leather' epidemiology, of putting on a rucksack and walking a beautiful valley on paths through jungle and grasslands and of sharing a very different culture. There was a sense of achievement in getting to the remote salt pools where the traditional salt had been made and being told that I was the first white man to visit the pools; of having legislation enacted that ensured that all salt imported into the country would be iodinated; and of seeing an international programme develop to prevent iodine deficiency disorders. Inevitably, this is tinged with a little sadness that barriers are still being erected in some countries to the implementation of the programme.

INFANT AND CHILD MORTALITY

Mortality of children

It must be borne in mind that the proportions of the deaths of children, though showing a high mortality in some places as compared with that of others, must not be regarded as true criterions of the comparative mortality, unless the proportions of living children to living adults were in those different places the same. Neither must it be supposed that the proportion of children dying out of 1000 deaths at all ages, whether given for the whole or any part of England and Wales, will afford the means of expressing correctly the proportion of such deaths to the living population. This would not be the case unless the population were stationary, the deaths being equal to the births; but in England and Wales the number of births greatly exceeds that of the deaths, as will appear from the following abstracts. Even though the registration of births is still deficient (and there is reason to believe that the number registered in every one of the 25 divisions falls short of the actual number), yet, even with this admitted probable deficiency, the number of births, if applied as an element of calculation, will show a mortality much less than it appears in the Comparative Table of Deaths. Neither of these, however, can be accepted as correct; and even the proportion of deaths under one year to 1000 registered births is a little higher than the truth (2nd Annual Report, p. 16).

Mortality of infants

As there are difficulties in determining the ages of the oldest people in the population, so there are great difficulties in determining the rate of mortality among infants, from the want of exactly observed facts. The infants in the first year of life are to some extent mixed up with infants in the second year of age; and their numbers fluctuate from year to year, owing to fluctuations in the births, and the mortality from zymotic and other diseases, so that the years of infant life cannot be accurately deduced from decennial enumerations of the infants living at the date of the Census. Again, the mortality diminishes so rapidly after the date of birth, and at such various rates under different conditions, that it is necessary to subdivide the first year into months, and even days, to get results exactly comparable. The still-born children in England are not registered; and a certain number of infants that breathe for a short time are, it is believed, to save the burial fees, interred as the still-born are buried, and so escape registration. Upon the other hand, the deaths of premature children born alive are registered; and they amounted to 45 814 out of 626 340 deaths of infants under one year of age in the six years (1858–63) that they have been distinguished from infants dying of debility. The recognised proportion is 7.315 per cent, so that to obtain the rate of mortality among children *born at the full term of nine months*, the premature children, if we had the means, should be struck out of the account of both the living and dying. This is impossible in the present state of statistical observation. But it happens that these deaths of premature children serve as probably more than a sufficient set-off against the infants of full term dying soon and escaping registration.

The age of man is reckoned from the date of birth; but before that date the foetus has lived its intra-uterine life, and the instant in which the sperm-cell and germ-cell intermingle is the true time of the embryo's origin. Respecting the rate of embryonic mortality there is little definite information; but it is probable that as the mortality in the first year of breathing life rapidly increases as we proceed backwards from the twelfth to the third, second and first month, the same law prevails during embryonic life, until we arrive at the destruction of an immense proportion of the spermatozoa and ova which are provided to secure the continuation of the species. This question well deserves the attention of the Obstetric Society, and is intimately connected with abortions, miscarriages and still-births.

Table 1, from the English Life Table, shows the estimated numbers of males and females surviving each month, and the annual rates of mortality in each month. It will be observed that the rate of mortality rapidly declines month by month; and that the mortality of boys in every month exceeds that of girls, so that at the end of the first

Table 1 English Life Table for each month of the first year of age, and annual rate of mortality of children in each month under one year of age

Age $\frac{x}{12}$ (months)	Living at 0 and at the end of each month of age $\frac{l_x}{12}$			Deaths in each month of age $\frac{d_x}{12}$			Annual rate of mortality (per cent) in each month under 1 year of age $\frac{m_x}{12}$			Age $\frac{x}{12}$ (months)
	Both sexes	Boys	Girls	Both sexes	Boys	Girls	Both sexes	Boys	Girls	
0	1 000 000	511 745	488 255	46 503	26 787	19 716	57.132	64.501	49.455	0–
1	953 497	484 958	468 539	17 195	9640	7555	21.837	24.093	19.507	1–
2	936 302	475 318	460 984	12 178	6758	5420	15.710	17.184	14.192	2–
3	924 124	468 560	455 564	10 100	5598	4502	13.187	14.423	11.918	3–
4	914 024	462 962	451 062	9550	5320	4230	12.604	13.869	11.306	4–
5	904 474	457 642	446 832	9033	5044	3989	12.050	13.299	10.761	5–
6	895 441	452 598	442 843	8547	4771	3776	11.509	12.717	10.276	6–
7	886 894	447 827	439 067	8087	4498	3589	10.992	12.114	9.849	7–
8	878 807	413 329	435 478	7657	4229	3428	10.501	11.502	9.484	8–
9	871 150	439 100	432 050	7253	3959	3294	10.033	10.868	9.184	9–
10	863 897	435 141	428 756	6872	3691	3181	9.584	10.222	8.936	10–
11	857 025	431 450	425 575	6518	3424	3094	9.161	9.561	8.756	11–12
12	850 507	428 026	422 481	–	–	–	–	–	–	–

This table was calculated from the corrected births and from the deaths registered in the 17 years 1838–1854 under 3 months, at 3 and under 6 months, and at 6 months and under 1 year. Of 1 000 000 persons born, 953 497 were living at the end of the first month of age, 46 503 having died in the interval, of whom 26 787 were males and 19 716 were females; 936 302 were living at the end of the second month, and the deaths in that month were 17 195, of whom 9640 were males and 7555 were females. The *annual* rate of mortality of infants under 1 month was 57.132, males 64.501, females 49.455, and so on for other ages.

year the number of boys does not greatly exceed the number of girls.

The mortality of infants in France was such in the first year as to reduce 1 000 000 to 820 065, according to the experience acquired by following the births in 1856–60 for the twelve months following. The deaths were 179 935, and the probability of dying 0.179 935.

The French returns show the deaths in the first week of life; and by the returns of 1856 the mortality was at the rate of 154 per cent per annum in the first seven days, 120 in the second seven days, and 54 in the 16 days following. The mean births were 927 226; the deaths in the three periods were 27 002, 20 517, and 20 618, making 68 137 deaths in the first month of life. So out of 1 000 000 births 29 121 die in the first week, 22 128 in the second week and 22 236 in the 16 days following.

In England and Wales the deaths of 2 374 379 infants in the first year of age were registered in the 26 years 1838–63; and of the number 1 329 287 were boys and 1 045 092 were girls. The deaths at the same age registered in the ten years 1851–60 were 996 630; of boys 557 213, and of girls 439 417. Nearly 100 000 infants

died annually; in the proportion of about 56 boys to 44 girls (Supplement to 25th Annual Report, pp. v–vi).

Mortality of infants under one year, and its causes

The high rate of infant mortality continues to occupy the earnest attention of medical statists. The death-rate of infants in England and Wales, in 1875, was 158 per 1000, or four per 1000 above the average rate in the ten years 1861–70. This implies that the mortality among infants is increasing.

Table 2 shows the death-rate of infants from all causes in eighteen large towns. The highest rates in 1875 prevailed in Leicester, at 245 per 1000, Liverpool 210, Norwich 210, Bradford 200, Nottingham 199, Leeds 197, Birmingham 196 and Hull 191. Portsmouth had the lowest rate, 133 per 1000.

What are the causes of such high death-rates of infants in large towns? This is a question of vital importance, and to assist in giving a satisfactory answer, the average annual death-rates of infants from each of 11 cases, in the

Table 2 Mortality of children under one year of age from all causes in 18 large towns, 1870–1875

Boroughs, etc.	Proportional number of deaths under one year to every 1000 births registered in 52 or 53 weeks in each year						
	1870	1871	1872	1873	1874	Average number in the 5 years 1870–4	1875
Portsmouth	160	144	146	139	151	148	133
London	163	171	159	159	155	161	162
Bristol	196	165	151	157	153	164	166
Wolverhampton	163	185	176	175	169	174	161
Sunderland	150	222	177	163	166	176	169
Oldham	–	188	178	169	190	181	177
Birmingham	181	190	166	180	180	179	196
Hull	176	177	204	174	172	181	191
Sheffield	180	208	185	180	188	188	176
Nottingham	186	187	207	172	195	189	199
Salford	191	221	173	185	189	192	178
Norwich	221	200	210	159	177	193	210
Newcastle-on-Tyne	183	223	177	186	198	193	187
Bradford	208	209	197	206	189	202	200
Manchester	203	221	191	198	197	202	184
Leeds	217	205	212	192	200	205	197
Leicester	235	241	228	213	215	226	245
Liverpool	259	269	222	213	233	239	210

three years 1873–5, have been calculated for 15 large towns. The results are shown in Table 3.

Table 3 deserves careful study, for the agencies which destroy infant life are many, and they vary in different localities. Some of the principal causes are improper and insufficient food, bad management, use of opiates, neglect, early marriages and debility of mothers; but whatever may be the special agencies at work which are so prejudicial to infant life, it must be borne in mind that a high death-rate is in a great measure also due to bad sanitary arrangements.

In towns such as Sunderland, Wolverhampton and Newcastle-upon-Tyne, where the iron and coal mining industries prosper, and where the marriages of minors are in excess, mismanagement through ignorance is probably one of the causes of a high infant death-rate, while in towns such as Oldham, Norwich, Salford, Nottingham, Leeds, Leicester and Manchester, where the women are more or less employed away from home in the manufacture of textile fabrics, it is probable that one of the causes of the high rates of infant mortality is maternal neglect. In the hardware manufacturing towns, such as Sheffield and Birmingham, comparatively few women are employed in the factories.

As regards illegitimate infants, the chief causes of the high mortality are no doubt improper food and neglect; but the death-rate of children born out of wedlock will be discussed further on.

The causes of death which are more directly the result of neglect and mismanagement are convulsions, diarrhoea and atrophy.

In Scotland, infant mortality is not so high as it is in England. In the ten years 1861–70, the average death-rate was 154 per 1000 in England and 121 in Scotland, and it is remarkable that the excess in the number of deaths from convulsions, diarrhoea, atrophy and premature birth accounts for nearly the whole of the difference in the high rate of infant mortality in England, compared with that of Scotland. The number of deaths of infants in England, in the ten years 1861–70, from convulsions, was 208 320, and from diarrhoea, 119 430. In Scotland the respective numbers were 5801 and 6156. The births registered during the same period in England were 7 500 096, and in Scotland 1 120 791. Thus the average annual death-rate of infants in 1861–70, in England, from convulsions, was 27.8, and from diarrhoea 15.9 per 1000, whereas in Scotland the respective death-rates were only 5.2 and 5.5 per 1000. In Table 3, average annual rates of infant mortality in England and Scotland are shown from each of 11 causes of death.

Table 3 Mortality of children under one year of age from different causes in England, in Scotland and in 15 large towns, 1873–1875

Boroughs, etc.	Annual number of deaths of children under one year of age in the three years 1873–5, to every 1000 births												
	All causes	The 11 causes	Measles	Scarlet fever	Whooping-cough	Teething	Diarrhoea	Con-vulsions	Lung diseases	Tubercular diseases	Atrophy	Premature birth	Suffo-cation
England[a]	152.7	131.6	2.2	1.4	5.9	2.9	17.1	25.1	26.3	9.8	26.7	12.8	1.4
Scotland[b]	125.7	94.3	2.2	1.9	6.4	3.4	7.0	5.5	25.2	11.1	30.7		.9
Portsmouth	145.9	130.9	2.8	.3	5.3	3.0	32.2	21.5	24.2	11.7	22.7	6.1	1.1
London	159.1	135.6	3.1	1.1	8.3	3.6	20.4	18.5	31.9	13.8	20.5	10.4	4.0
Wolverhampton	166.0	140.9	2.4	1.5	5.9	1.1	22.0	30.4	31.2	9.4	26.4	10.2	.4
Sunderland	167.6	147.5	1.5	.6	7.3	3.2	21.3	28.2	25.4	6.4	39.4	13.6	.6
Oldham	180.1	150.9	3.0	1.6	7.5	4.8	16.4	26.0	36.2	11.8	27.3	16.3	–
Norwich	183.4	161.8	.6	–	9.8	2.0	27.2	22.9	20.8	6.9	63.0	8.6	–
Salford	183.9	151.7	7.0	1.7	4.2	2.2	31.5	25.0	27.7	9.1	32.4	10.3	.6
Sheffield	186.1	148.8	1.6	3.2	6.5	5.2	31.0	33.0	36.9	8.0	10.4	12.5	.5
Birmingham	187.0	160.0	2.0	2.4	7.5	1.6	33.9	13.4	28.3	7.1	39.7	14.1	10.0
Newcastle-upon-Tyne	190.6	164.5	2.0	2.7	5.2	2.6	24.4	37.7	24.5	13.9	37.9	12.0	1.6
Manchester	192.9	157.4	3.1	2.1	6.5	2.9	28.7	28.1	31.3	9.0	33.9	11.1	.7
Nottingham	199.5	184.8	3.9	1.9	5.3	2.7	33.7	32.1	25.4	15.4	47.0	16.8	.6
Leeds	201.1	162.7	2.0	2.6	5.5	3.5	30.9	26.2	32.4	9.8	32.2	16.6	1.0
Leicester	217.3	203.1	2.8	1.1	6.0	4.1	54.5	31.6	23.1	11.8	50.7	16.6	.8
Liverpool	218.9	191.2	6.1	4.9	9.0	2.2	31.9	28.6	39.4	12.6	37.7	10.6	8.2
Mean	185.3	159.5	2.9	1.8	6.7	3.0	29.3	26.9	29.3	10.4	34.8	12.4	2.0

The results for the fifteen large towns are deduced from returns supplied by the Medical Officers of Health. As far as practicable differences in nomenclature have been adjusted.

[a] In England, in the three years 1873–5, the causes of death of 5354 infants (1.4 per cent) were not stated.

[b] The results for Scotland are for the three years 1870–2. The causes of death of 2894 infants (6.6 per cent) were not stated in those three years. Dr Robertson, the Superintendent of the Statistical Department of the General Register Office, Edinburgh, states that it cannot be assumed that the popular but utterly unscientific term 'bowel hives' is now used by informants in any large proportion of these 2894 cases; the term being rarely observed in the certificates of death.

The cause of this high mortality of infants from convulsions and diarrhoea in England, compared with Scotland, is supposed to be due to bad feeding.

In Table 4 (columns 6, 7 and 8) the death-rates from each of the 11 causes in seven textile manufacturing towns (Leeds, Leicester, Manchester, Norwich, Nottingham, Oldham, Salford) in the aggregate are compared with those in London, and the results indicate in a striking manner that – over and above a certain proportion of the mortality which may be attributable to indifferent sanitary arrangements – the causes most fatal to infant life in factory towns, and which are inseparable from bad nursing and feeding, are diarrhoea, convulsions and atrophy. The mortality from premature birth was also in excess. Thus the respective death-rates of infants in London, and in the seven factory towns, were, from diarrhoea 20.4 and 31.9, from convulsions 18.5 and 27.4, from atrophy 20.5 and 40.9, from premature birth 10.4 and 13.8 per 1000.

The death-rates in the seven factory towns from whooping-cough, teething, lung-diseases, tubercular diseases and suffocation were lower than those in London.

Mortality of illegitimate infants

As the law of bastardy was essentially altered by the new poor law, has been again amended in one of its most important principles, and has latterly attracted a good deal of public attention, I have thought it right to submit to you a general abstract of the number of illegitimate children registered in England, and to point out some of the particulars to be attended to in drawing inferences from results collected under a great variety of circumstances. But the most important matter, in a political point of view, is the condition of the illegitimate children themselves. If the mortality were not greater among them than among legitimate children, every fifteenth person in England must be of illegitimate extraction. But the mortality of illegitimate children is, as in other countries, no doubt greatly above the average; for, without any

Table 4 Causes of infant mortality in towns in the three years 1873–1875

Causes of death	Mean death-rate per 1000 in 15 towns	Portsmouth		Liverpool		London	The seven textile manufacturing towns	
		Death-rate per 1000	In defect or excess of the mean	Death-rate per 1000	In excess or defect of the mean	Death-rate per 1000	Death rate per 1000	In excess or defect of London
	1	2	3	4	5	6	7	8
All causes	185.3	145.9	−39.4	218.9	+33.6	159.1	194.0	+34.9
The 11 subjoined causes	159.5	130.9	−28.6	191.2	+31.7	135.6	167.5	+31.9
Measles	2.9	2.8	−0.1	6.1	+3.2	3.1	3.2	+0.1
Scarlet fever	1.8	0.3	−1.5	4.9	+3.1	1.1	1.6	+0.5
Whooping-cough	6.7	5.3	+1.4	9.0	+2.3	8.3	6.4	−1.9
Teething	3.0	3.0	0.0	2.2	−0.8	3.6	3.2	−0.4
Diarrhoea	29.3	32.2	+2.9	31.9	+2.6	20.4	31.9	+11.5
Convulsions	26.9	21.5	−5.4	28.6	+1.7	18.5	27.4	+8.9
Lung diseases	29.3	24.2	−5.1	39.4	+10.1	31.9	28.1	−3.8
Tubercular diseases	10.4	11.7	+1.3	12.6	+2.2	13.8	10.5	−3.3
Atrophy and debility	34.8	22.7	−12.1	37.7	+2.9	20.5	40.9	+20.4
Premature birth	12.4	6.1	−6.3	10.6	−1.8	10.4	13.8	+3.4
Suffocation	2.0	1.1	−0.9	8.2	+6.2	4.0	0.5	−3.5

crime whatever of his own, the illegitimate child is often exposed to dangers, hardships and ignominy from his infancy; the law pronounces him *filius nullius*; he, nevertheless, escapes in England the tender mercies of the foreign foundling hospital, and in our great towns and colonies has probably a better chance of attaining the station to which his personal conduct may entitle him than in any other country in Europe.

To make the statistical information respecting illegitimate children as complete as it might be, the age and occupation of the mothers should be ascertained, as well as the proportion of children who are formally recognised by the fathers. I conclude my remarks upon this subject with the judicious observations of one of the ablest statistical writers of the present day.

The proportion of illegitimate children cannot serve as a standard of morality; nevertheless a remarkable frequency of such children is without doubt in many respects a great evil. The invariable fact that the mortality among the illegitimate is far greater than among the legitimate, and that many more of them are still-born, shows clearly enough how much more unfavourable their position is from the first. Who can doubt that their bringing up is much harder and more difficult; that the existence of a class of men, bound

to society by few or no family ties, is not a matter of indifference to the State? The great majority of foundlings are illegitimate, which of itself shows how little, as a general rule, the mothers can or will care for these children. It is beyond doubt that fewer illegitimate children grow up to maturity; that they get through the world with more trouble than children born in wedlock; that more of them are poor; and that therefore more of them become criminals. Illegitimacy is in itself an evil to a man; and the State should seek to diminish the number of these births, and carefully inquire to what circumstances any increase is to be ascribed.

(6th Annual Report, pp. xxxvii–viii)

In the five years 1871–5, infant mortality was excessively high in the districts of Leicester, Liverpool and Preston, where the respective rates were 229, 223 and 222 per 1000, and as the death-rate among illegitimate infants is known to be higher than it is among legitimate infants, it was believed that the rate of illegitimacy in 1871–5 (the number of children born out of wedlock to every 1000 births) would bear some relation to infant mortality, but such is not the case, the rate of illegitimacy in Leicester and in Liverpool being 44 per 1000, while in Preston it was 71 per 1000.

Table 5 Death-rates of legitimate and of illegitimate infants; percentage of marriages of minors to total marriages, and illegitimate births to 1000 births, in 24 districts, in five years 1871–1875

Name of district	Deaths of				Percentage of marriages of minors to total marriages 1871–5		Children born out of wedlock to every 1000 births 1871–5
	Legitimate and illegitimate infants to 1000 births in 1871–5	Legitimate and illegitimate infants to 1000 births in 1875	Legitimate infants to 1000 legitimate births in 1875	Illegitimate infants to 1000 illegimate births in 1875	Men	Women	
Twelve districts with high rates of infant mortality							
Leicester	229	245	239	386	16.2	29.3	44
Liverpool	223	214	205	418	6.8	24.3	44
Preston	222	230	214	418	13.5	22.0	71
Radford	196	204	187	547	17.3	31.2	54
Nottingham	193	202	191	365	12.1	24.8	65
Goole	175	196	192	257	8.3	30.2	58
Keighley	175	181	175	325	9.8	20.2	51
Guisborough	174	206	202	292	8.5	34.2	44
Mansfield	174	189	180	324	17.3	34.3	80
Haslingden	174	189	181	355	13.8	24.1	44
Driffield	172	206	168	596	6.5	26.9	116
Basford	170	179	169	341	20.1	38.4	64
Mean	190	203	192	388	12.5	28.3	61
Twelve districts with low rates of infant mortality							
Ledbury	96	102	94	222	4.9	17.5	74
Reeth	100	107	106	118	2.4	25.9	89
Kendal	103	105	91	329	6.3	20.7	67
Stratford-on-Avon	106	83	69	293	5.1	16.6	55
Leominster	108	104	95	240	2.6	12.5	72
Easingwold	109	97	84	227	5.6	21.2	95
Wetherby	112	104	99	182	4.8	15.8	66
Shipston-on-Stour	113	120	112	237	6.9	18.5	73
Helmsley	114	87	75	184	7.5	23.9	133
Richmond	117	122	114	231	3.8	19.4	75
Hereford	119	128	114	313	3.4	13.9	75
Market Harborough	120	121	116	286	5.8	13.9	50
Mean	110	107	97	239	4.9	18.3	77

The results in Table 5 show that the rate of illegitimacy bears no relation to the death-rate of infants, and it is remarkable that the districts with a high rate of infant mortality are generally those with a comparatively low rate of illegitimacy, and vice versa. Thus in the 12 urban districts with a high mean death-rate among infants, in 1871–5, of 190 per 1000, the rate of illegitimacy was 61 per 1000, while in the 12 rural districts with a comparatively low mean death-rate among infants of 110 per 1000, the rate of illegitimacy was 77 per 1000.

It is not improbable that a certain number of illegitimate children are registered as legitimate in towns, while in the country they are correctly registered as illegitimate, the circumstances connected with their birth being too well-known to allow of any false representation being made: some illegitimate births have no doubt escaped registration altogether.

It will be observed in Table 5 that in the districts where there was an excess of early marriages, the mortality of infants born in wedlock was comparatively high. Thus the

Table 6 Life Table and annual death-rate for each month of the first year of age, in the healthy districts of England and Wales; in England and Wales generally; and in the district of Liverpool

Age $\frac{x}{12}$ (months)	Living at 0 and at the end of each month of age $\frac{l_x}{12}$			Deaths in each month of age $\frac{d_x}{12}$			Annual rate of mortality at each month of age (per cent) $\frac{m_x}{12}$		
	In healthy districts	By English Life Table	In Liverpool district	In healthy districts	By English Life Table	In Liverpool district	In healthy districts	By English Life Table	In Liverpool district
0	100 000	100 000	100 000	3661	4650	5449	44.751	57.132	67.219
1	96 339	95 350	94 551	1161	1720	2463	14.549	21.837	31.672
2	95 178	93 630	92 088	806	1218	1724	10.205	15.710	22.678
3	94 372	92 412	90 364	683	1010	1563	8.716	13.187	20.937
4	93 689	91 402	88 801	631	955	1506	8.109	12.604	20.525
5	93 058	90 447	87 295	584	903	1469	7.554	12.050	20.365
6	92 474	89 544	85 826	542	855	1453	7.054	11.509	20.489
7	91 932	88 689	84 373	504	808	1458	6.597	10.992	20.917
8	91 428	87 881	82 915	470	766	1482	6.185	10.501	21.642
9	90 958	87 115	81 433	441	725	1528	5.832	10.033	22.730
10	90 517	86 390	79 905	416	687	1594	5.528	9.584	24.180
11	90 101	85 703	78 311	396	652	1680	5.286	9.161	26.023
12	89 705	85 051	76 631	–	–	–	–	–	–

By moving the decimal one place to the right in each of the last three columns, the results will represent the annual rate of mortality per 1000.

mean infant mortality in the 12 urban districts, in the year 1875, was 192 per 1000, and the mean proportion of girls who married under age to 100 marriages in these districts was 28, whereas in the 12 rural districts, where the mean infant mortality was 97 per 1000, the proportion was only 18.

Since it has been ascertained that the mortality among illegitimate infants is about double that among the legitimate, then from the mean proportions observed in the 12 urban and in the 12 rural districts, it follows that the lives of 7020 illegitimate infants were sacrificed through neglect and improper food in the year 1875. This is on the assumption that the death-rate among illegitimate infants should be the same as that which prevailed among legitimate infants, viz., 148 per 1000.

But the general death-rate of infants, instead of being 158 per 1000, should at least be as low as that in some of the healthiest parts of England. By the healthy district life table, it was only 111 per 1000. If 111 per 1000 be taken as a standard rate, for the present, which is 47 per 1000 less than the rate for all England, then no less than 40 197 deaths of infants occurred in 1875, in excess of the number that would have been registered at the rate that prevailed in the healthy districts.

Mortality of infants at each month of the first year of age: England, healthy districts and Liverpool

According to the life table (Table 6) of 100 000 children born in the healthy districts of England, 96 339 are alive at the end of the first month, 3661 having died in the interval. Of the same number born in Liverpool, only 94 551 are alive at the end of the first month, 5449 having died in the interval.

At the end of the second month, 95 178 are alive in the healthy districts, 1161 having died in that month; in Liverpool, only 92 088 are living, 2463 having died in the month; and so on until at the age of seven months the numbers living are reduced to 91 932 in the healthy districts, and to 84 373 in Liverpool.

In the healthy districts, the mortality rapidly decreases, month by month. Thus, the rate was 448 per 1000 living under one month of age, 145 at one month of age, 102 at two months, 76 at five months, 71 at six months and 53 at eleven months of age.

In Liverpool the mortality was 672 per 1000 under one month of age, 317 at one month, 227 at two months and 204 at five months, after which age, the mortality, instead

Table 7 Number and proportion of deaths at different months of age to 1000 births in the healthy districts and in Liverpool in the eight years 1839–1846

Months	Deaths		Proportion of deaths at each month of age to 1000 births		Excess in Liverpool
	In 63 healthy districts	In Liverpool	In 63 healthy districts	In Liverpool	
Total under 1 year	52 833	16 133	110.5	228.9	118.4
0	18 790	3762	39.3	53.4	14.1
1	5956	1700	12.5	24.1	11.6
2	4135	1190	8.6	16.9	8.3
3	3505	1079	7.3	15.3	8.0
4	3239	1040	6.8	14.7	7.9
5	2997	1014	6.3	14.4	8.1
6	2781	1003	5.8	14.2	8.4
7	2586	1007	5.4	14.3	8.9
8	2411	1023	5.0	14.5	9.5
9	2264	1055	4.7	15.0	10.3
10	2136	1100	4.5	15.6	11.1
11	2033	1160	4.3	16.5	12.2

The total births in the eight years 1839–46 were 478 048 in the Healthy Districts, and 70 491 in Liverpool.

of decreasing, as in the healthy districts, increases to 205 at six months, 216 at eight months, 242 at ten months and 260 at eleven months of age.

So unfavourable to infant life are the unsanitary conditions of large towns – especially Liverpool – that not only is the mortality at some months of age twice as high as it is in the healthy districts, but at seven months of age and upwards it is three times as high. The mortality of infants by lung diseases is higher in Liverpool than in any other large town.

The mortality of children under one year of age is 111 per 1000 in the healthy districts of England, and 229 in Liverpool, but the rate at each month of age differs considerably, decreasing rapidly from birth, as will be seen by reference to Table 6.

Table 7 shows in a striking manner how much depends, at the starting point of life, whether infants breathe the poisoned air of large towns or the fresh pure atmosphere of healthy districts.

Thus in Liverpool the mortality of children under one year of age was at the rate of 229 deaths per 1000, 53 of which deaths were of infants under one month of age, 24 of one month of age, and so on for each month of age in Table 7.

In the healthy districts the mortality of children under one year of age was at the rate of 111 deaths per 1000, 39 of which deaths were of infants under one month of age, and 13 of one month of age.

The difference, therefore, in the rate of mortality of children under one year of age in Liverpool, and in the healthy districts, was 118, of which 14 were by deaths under one month of age, eight by deaths at two months of age and so on.

There is no doubt great negligence on the part of the parents, great ignorance of the conditions on which health depends and great privation among the masses of the poor, but there is no reason to suspect that any great number of the infants in these districts fall victims to deliberate crime; yet the children of the idolatrous tribe who passed them through the fire to Moloch scarcely incurred more danger than is incurred by the children born in several districts of our large cities.

A strict investigation of all the circumstances of these children's lives might lead to important discoveries, and may suggest remedies for evils of which it is difficult to exaggerate the magnitude.

The weaklier lives, it is said, are, under this state of things, cut off; but it must also be borne in mind that many of the strongest children are wounded and are left weakly for life.

Mortality of children (0–5), 1861–70

The first thing to observe is that the fatality children encounter is primarily due to the changes in themselves. Thus 1 000 000 children just born are alive, but some of them have been born prematurely; they are feeble; they are unfinished; the molecules and fibres of brain, muscle and bone are loosely strung together; the heart and the blood, on which life depends, have undergone a complete revolution; the lungs are only just called into play. The baby is helpless; for his food and all his wants he depends on others. It is not surprising then that a certain number of infants should die; but in England the actual deaths in the first year of age are 149 493, including premature births, deaths by debility and atrophy, diseases of the nervous system are 30 637, and of the respiratory organs 21 995. To convulsions, diarrhoea, pneumonia, bronchitis, their deaths are chiefly ascribed; little is positively known; and this implies little more than that the brain and spinal marrow, nerves, muscles, lungs and bowels fail to execute their functions with the exact rhythm of life. The first two are said by pathologists to be often rather symptoms of diseases unknown than diseases in themselves. The total dying by miasmatic diseases is 31 266; but it is quite possible that several of the children dying of convulsions die in the early stages of some unrevealed zymotic disease whose symptoms have not had time for development. Convulsion is a frequent precursor in children of measles, whooping-cough, scarlet-fever, fever: indeed, Dr C. B. Radcliffe well remarks, 'in the fevers of infancy and early childhood, especially in the exanthematous forms of these disorders, convulsions not unfrequently takes the place occupied by rigor in the fevers of youth and riper years.' Many of the cases of pneumonia may also in like manner be whooping-coughs and other latent zymotic diseases. In the second year of life pneumonia, bronchitis and convulsions are still the prevalent, and most fatal, diseases; many also die then of measles, whooping-cough, scarlatina and diarrhoea. Scarlet fever asserts its supremacy in the second, third, fourth and fifth years of age. Whooping-cough is at its maximum in the first year, measles in the second, scarlatina in the third and fourth years. Thus these diseases take up their attacks on life in succession and follow it onwards.

The deaths from all causes under the age of five years are 263 182. The number ascribed to infanticide is very few; but the deaths by suffocation (overlaying) etc. are more numerous; and so the deaths directly referred to the 'want of breast-milk'. The total deaths by burns, injuries, drowning and all other kinds of violence are 5175.

By a physiological law 511 745 boys are born in England to 488 255 girls; and by another law 141 387 boys and 121 795 girls die in the first five years of life; so that at the end of five years the original disparity in the numbers of the two sexes is so much reduced that at the age of five the boys only slightly exceed the girls in number. The greater mortality of boys is due to difference of organisation, for the external conditions are substantially the same in which boys and girls are placed.

Great as is the influence of organisation itself, the difference of external circumstances and sanitary condition exercise a very real influence on life, disease and death in childhood.

Thus, even in the healthy districts of the country, out of 1 000 000 born, 175 410 children die in the first five years of life; but in Liverpool District, which serves to represent the most unfavourable sanitary conditions, out of the same number born, 460 370, nearly half the number born, die in the five years following their birth. This is 284 960 in excess of the deaths in the healthy districts.

Table 8 shows how many children die from the several groups of causes (1) in the healthy districts, (2) in all England and (3) in the Liverpool District. There is a greater increase in Liverpool from small-pox and measles than from scarlet-fever; and diphtheria was more fatal in the healthy districts than in all England. Diarrhoea and cholera were greatly aggravated in the other districts of England; so were whooping-cough and fever, under which were registered typhus, typhoid, infantile remittent and relapsing fever. The diseases of the lungs are more fatal to children in Liverpool than diseases of the brain.

The children of Norway fare better than the children of sunny Italy; to which it may well be still an *officina gentium*. Out of 100 children born alive the deaths in the first five years of life are in Norway 17, Denmark 20, Sweden 20, England 26, Belgium 27, France 28, Prussia 32, Holland 33, Austria 36, Spain 36, Russia 38, Italy 39. Russia is almost as fatal to her children as Italy.

The mortality of infants evidently depends, to some extent, on the midwifery of a country; on the way the children are fed by the mothers; on the water; and on the cleanliness observed, as well as the other sanitary conditions.

Mortality of children in European states

In the first place, let us ask how many children out of 1 000 000 born alive see their fifth birthday – live five years?

In the north, there is the fine free population of Norway, scattered over the habitable parts of a large well-watered territory, in some parts fruitful or covered with pine forests, in other parts sterile: in addition to fish in their waters and agricultural produce, they derive profits from timber, mines and ships. The climate is severe, but on the western Atlantic slope the severity is softened by the Gulf Stream. In some of its features we are reminded of Scotland.

Table 8 Of 1 000 000 children born alive in the healthy districts in all England, and in the district of Liverpool, the numbers dying under five years of age from 19 groups of causes

	Healthy districts	England	Liverpool district
Deaths from all causes	175 410	263 182	460 370
Total zymotic diseases	49 761	87 099	171 009
Small-pox	602	3331	5175
Measles	5257	11 507	25 514
Scarlatina	11 373	17 959	26 818
Diphtheria	4184	2425	3395
Whooping-cough	9650	14 424	32 551
Fever (typhus, enteric and simple)	2807	5401	9297
Diarrhoea and dysentery	9354	20 344	51 911
Cholera	399	1129	4255
Other zymotic diseases	6135	10 579	12 093
Cancer	110	71	62
Scrofula and tabes mesenterica	5335	8115	11 694
Phthisis	2656	4469	5116
Hydrocephalus	6604	9296	14 972
Diseases of the brain	22 692	40 065	49 840
Diseases of the heart and dropsy	1304	1507	2038
Diseases of the lungs	27 884	41 476	79 893
Diseases of the stomach and liver	4431	4778	4874
Violent deaths	4232	5175	17 107
Other causes	50 401	61 131	103 765

Out of 100 children born in Norway, 83 attain the age of five years, in Sweden 80, in Denmark 80, including Schleswig and Holstein down to the Elbe, the country of the Angles of old, in England 74, in Belgium 73, in France 71, in Prussia 68, in Holland 67, in Austria 64, in Spain 64, in Russia 62, in Italy 61.

Thus the chance is always in favour of the life; but here it is eight to two, there only three to two.

What is the proportion of deaths under the age of five out of 100 children that see the light? In Norway 17, Denmark 20, Sweden 20, England 26, Belgium 27, France 29, Prussia 32, Holland 33, Austria 36, Spain 36, Russia 38, Italy 39. Thus Death, drawing lots for the lives of children, has in one part of Europe two, in another four out of ten in his favour.

Out of 100 children born in addition to the number 17 dying in Norway, three die in Denmark, three in Sweden, nine in England, 10 in Belgium, 12 in France, 15 in Prussia, 16 in Holland, 19 in Austria, 19 in Spain, 21 in Russia, 22 in Italy. Thus in the sunny climate of the south, Death carries off two children from Italians for every one he takes in high latitudes from Norwegians.

In all England 26 children under five years of age die out of 100 born; but in her healthy districts she loses only 18, nearly the same number as Norway; while in her 30 large town districts, 36 perish. There is the same contrast between the country and the city as there is between Norway and Italy. In France I find contrasts of the same sort in the departments.

If we turn to particular classes the mortality presents still larger contrasts: according to the peerage records, out of 100 children born alive, 90 survive; 10 die in the first five years of age. The deaths among the children of the clergy are nearly in the same proportion. The proportions have been reversed in some foundling hospitals.

For reasons which I have explained, the rate of mortality is only exactly determined by comparing the average numbers living with the deaths in a given time. That we can do for 11 of the States of Europe.

We are able in some States to marshal our little troops in three regiments, the first of babes under one, the second children of one to three, the third of children of three to five.

By the English Life Table, of 100 children born, 15 die in the first year, five in the second, three in the third year, two in the fourth and one in the fifth; making 26 in the five years of age. Of the 15 who die in the first year, five die in the first month of life, two in the second and one in the third.

The annual rate of mortality in the first week of life in France is 154 per cent; and the greater the mortality in any country generally, the greater is its excess in the first days of life.

Acknowledgement

Farr, W. (1885) Infant and child mortality. From *Vital Statistics: a Memorial Volume of Selections from the Reports and Writings of William Farr, MD, DCL, CB, FRS.* London: Offices of the Sanitary Institute, 188–209.

ENDEMIC CRETINISM OF RECENT ONSET IN NEW GUINEA

Introduction

The definition of endemic cretinism has been the source of some controversy, but the prevailing view is that it is a syndrome of organic neurological damage arising congenitally and occurring in association with endemic goitre.[1-3] The salient features of the disorder are mental retardation, deaf mutism and cerebral diplegia. These abnormalities may all exist in the same patient, although deafness, mutism and mental retardation may be observed in the absence of conspicuous abnormal clinical neurological signs. In a region where endemic goitre occurs, the presence of deaf mutism alone can be taken as an index of the prevalence of endemic cretinism.[4] A decline in the prevalence of endemic cretinism in many countries has been noted,[5-7] and this has been correlated with the introduction of iodine prophylaxis for endemic goitre.[8] In some cases evidence has been produced that socioeconomic changes with improved living conditions resulted in a diminished prevalence of endemic cretinism, even without prophylactic iodine supplementation.[9,10] McCarrison[3] had been of the opinion that endemic cretinism appeared only in families who had experienced a high prevalence of goitre over several generations, but occasionally outbreaks of endemic cretinism had been noted in previously unaffected populations. In Yugoslavia[11] a severe focus of endemic cretinism was observed in a migrant community that settled in an iodine-deficient region, and Norris[12] had described an outbreak in an English village as long ago as 1847.

A high prevalence of endemic cretinism associated with goitre has been described in the Jimi Valley of New Guinea.[13] The visible-goitre rate in the area was 12 per cent, and investigations disclosed a mean serum-protein-bound-iodine of 2.0 μg per 100 ml with a thyroidal ^{131}I uptake greater than 60 per cent, accompanied by very low urinary iodine excretion values.[14] The prevention of endemic cretinism by intramuscular injections of iodine in oil in the Jimi Valley has already been reported.[15,16] The epidemiological characteristics of endemic cretinism in the valley in the period prior to iodine prophylaxis are now described.

Materials and methods

Village censuses have been conducted by the Government in the Jimi Valley biennially since 1956. The names and approximate ages of the inhabitants of every village were recorded, as well as such vital events as births, migration and deaths. Although inaccuracies in estimation of age in association with such censuses are notorious, it is unlikely that the error in ageing of children born since the first census in 1956 is greater than two years. In 1966 a thorough village census and medical patrol was conducted in the whole valley. The previous records were reviewed and reconciled with the 1966 population, in which the assessment and the prevalence of both goitre and endemic cretinism were determined prior to the trial of iodine in the prevention of endemic cretinism.[15] In subsequent years medical patrols have been frequently undertaken in the region and have provided opportunities for critical evaluation of the previous demographic records. The information obtained in response to specific inquiries concerning disorders of hearing and speech has permitted the amplification of the observations made during the censuses.

Specimens of water for chemical analysis were collected in plastic containers previously washed in deionised water, and one container refilled with deionised water was used as a control. Sodium was estimated by direct aspiration into a flame photometer; chloride was estimated by titration against a standard silver nitrate solution using potassium chromate as an indicator; total salt content was derived by compounding sodium and chloride values; iodine determinations, by a modification of the Zak wet ash method, were effected in the Boston Medical Laboratories by courtesy of Professor J. B. Stanbury.

Results

The population of the middle Jimi Valley was 8000 at the time of the medical census in 1966. Examination at the time of census and subsequent inquiries suggest that there were 148 people with hearing and speech abnormalities. Of these, 120 (81 per cent) have been clinically examined and the nature of the abnormalities has already been

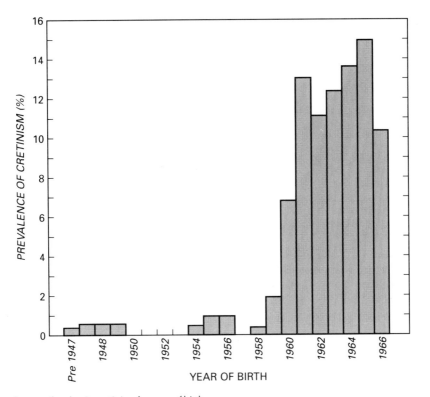

Fig. 1 Numbers of cases of endemic cretinism by year of birth.

described.[17] The majority (80 per cent) had signs of cerebral diplegia, and the remainder gross abnormalities of hearing and speech, most being deaf mutes. The remaining 28 (19 per cent) who were not seen were regarded as cases of endemic cretinism on the basis of the clear descriptions provided by the village leaders and local health workers.

If the population is grouped in age cohorts, the prevalence of endemic cretinism in the years prior to 1966 can be determined. These results are shown in Figure 1. Among those who were born prior to 1953 there were only rare cases of hearing/speech abnormality with a prevalence of approximately 0.1 per cent. A sharp rise in prevalence can be discerned in the late 1950s, and by 1965 over 15 per cent of the children born in that year were affected. Since 1966 endemic cretinism has not been observed in the offspring of people treated with iodine in oil.[15]

Anecdotal evidence of endemic cretinism was collected from village leaders and councillors in the regions studied. All informants agreed that the inhabitants of the valley were not familiar with individuals suffering from the stigmata of endemic cretinism prior to European contact.

One councillor from a village which has experienced a high incidence of the disease – Kwima – remarked that the disease had occurred only since the White man came to the valley and it was present only in the children of the present generation, not having been observed in his own contemporaries or those of the previous generation.

Table 1 summarises changes in the ecology of the Jimi Valley in the years since 1950. The increasing prevalence of endemic cretinism parallels profound changes in the socioeconomic and cultural life of the valley which have accompanied increasing contact with Western culture.

Discussion

The epidemiological evidence suggests that an epidemic of endemic cretinism has occurred in the Jimi Valley with an increasing prevalence of cases up until 1966, when the introduction of iodine prevented further occurrence of the disorder. Although many changes in the way of life of the inhabitants have coincided with the increasing prevalence of endemic cretinism, the general pattern of shifting agriculture based on a slash-and-burn horticultural cycle

177

Table 1 Ecological changes in the Jimi Valley

Year	Event
Pre-1950	Stone Age shifting agriculturists, tribal warfare, and absence of medical facilities
1953	Initial European exploration of the area
1956	Establishment of first Administration patrol post at Tabibuga in the Jimi Valley
1958	Closure of salt ovens
1959	Opening of first airstrip at Tabibuga
1960	Anglican and Nazarene mission stations opened
1965	Mission trade stores opened. Regular maternal and infant welfare services commenced
1970	Opening of road giving vehicular access to the valley

has not been materially altered. The diet is still based on root crops, although some new plants – tomatoes, peas and improved strains of taro – have complemented the previous staples of yams, sweet potato and native taro. Cooking methods have changed slightly. Food is usually roasted over the ashes of an open fire, but is occasionally steamed over heated stones in a primitive earth oven. Metal saucepans now permit food to be cooked by boiling, but this practice is infrequently adopted. Some tinned food – meat and fish, as well as refined sugar – have become available in the valley recently, but their presence was not significant before 1964 or 1965.

A change in the variety of salt consumed followed the first European contact in 1953. At that time Europeans frequently purchased goods and services on a barter basis, and patrols through the area carried rock salt for this purpose. The later establishment of Government and mission stations increased consumption of this commodity, which quickly supplanted salt manufactured by traditional methods. Rock salt of the type used is known to be grossly deficient in iodine. Inquiries as to the type and nature of the traditional salt used in the valley produced some interesting and relevant information. The Jimi people valued salt highly, and they obtained it by trade from the Simbai Valley on the farther side of the Bismarck mountain range, either travelling directly to manufacture the salt or obtaining it secondhand in exchange for stone axes and pigs. This native salt was manufactured by the distillation of water obtained from three salt springs at the villages of Tumbi, Sangen and Gai. The manufacturing process involved the construction of a crude still which consisted of a pyramid of stones topped by a large disc-like stone. This supported a container formed from banana leaves and clay in which water was evaporated. A fire and a continued replenishment of

water over a period of weeks enabled the production of appreciable quantities of salt. The process was discontinued as soon as imported rock salt became readily available in the Jimi Valley. Two of the salt springs still exist – one of them has recently been obliterated by a landslide. Water from the salt springs at Tumbi contained 15 800 salt parts per million with an iodine content of 4.4 parts per million, giving an iodine/salt ratio of 1/3600, while the Sangen spring contained 19 500 parts of salt per million with 6 parts of iodine per million and an iodine/salt ratio of 1/3250 (Table 2).

There seems no doubt, therefore, that salt rich in iodine was available and used by the Jimi people prior to European influence. The degree of salt iodisation introduced in various countries ranges from 1 part per 10 000 to 1 part per 200 000,[18] so that the salt available to the inhabitants of the Jimi Valley was appreciably richer in iodine than that usually commercially available. It is impossible to estimate the amount of traditional salt which would have been consumed daily by the inhabitants of the valley. Presumably, because of the scarcity of the commodity, it would be less than optimal.[19] However, 100 mg of the traditional salt certainly provided 15–20 µg of iodine per day – a minimum requirement which has been regarded as critical to the appearance of endemic cretinism in a goitre region.[20]

A similar phenomenon relating to endemic goitre was observed in the canton of Vaud in Switzerland, where salt from a mine at Bex, which was naturally iodised at 1 part per 100 000, was consumed.[21]

It could be argued that the increasing prevalence of endemic cretinism in the Jimi Valley was the result of the cessation of tribal fighting. Warfare was likely to create a state of social instability which would militate against the survival of severely neurologically disabled individuals. Furthermore, the influence of mission teaching, Government laws concerning homicide and the availability of such effective medical agents as penicillin and antimalarials would also increase the survival of the disabled. It is, however, a fact that in West New Guinea, in the

Table 2 Salt and iodine content of spring and control waters

Source	Total salt (p.p.m.)	Iodine (p.p.m.)	Iodine/ salt ratio
Spring-water:			
Tumbi	15 800	4.4	1/3600
Sangen	19 500	6.0	1/3250
Control (deionised water)	99	ND	

ND, not detected.

Mulia Valley, endemic cretinism was observed to be common in the context of a traditional New Guinea culture unaffected by external contact.[22] Missionaries noted cretinism in adults in a society where warfare was still a prominent component. The chronological events also suggest that the prevalence of endemic cretinism had changed before medical services were improved.

An alternative possibility concerned the infanticide of affected infants, but so far as can be determined this practice, which was common in the Jimi Valley and elsewhere in traditional Papua New Guinean communities, involved only the offspring of multiple births. Besides, the Jimi people are unable to accurately diagnose cretinous children in the immediate post-partum months. They deny that affected children were ever deliberately killed, and their present behaviour involves much solicitude and attention to the infants' welfare, suggesting that such children have never been regarded as a disgrace or embarrassment.

Although the epidemic occurrence of neurological damage in the Jimi Valley coincided with a variety of ecological changes, the overall evidence suggests that an alteration in the type of salt used by the people has been of paramount importance in disrupting a delicate ecological balance, with disastrous consequences.

References

1 Querido, A. in *Endemic Goiter*. PAHO scientific publication no. 193, 1968, 85.
2 Stanbury, J.B. in *Human Development and the Thyroid Gland* (edited by J.B. Stanbury and R.L. Kroc). New York, 1972.
3 McCarrison, R. *Lancet,* 1908, ii, 1275.
4 Stanbury, J.B., Ermans, A.M., Hetzel, B.S., Pretell, E.A. and Querido, A. *Wld Hlth Org. Chron.* 1974, 28, 220.
5 Greenwald, I. *Tex. Rep. Biol. Med.* 1957, 15, 874.
6 Stott, H., Bhatia, B., Lal, R.S. and Rai, K.C. *Indian J. med. Res.* 1930, 18, 1059.
7 Stanbury, J.B., Brownell, G.L., Riggs, D.S., Perinetti, H., Itoiz, J. and del Castillo, E.G. Harvard University monograph in medicine and public health no. 12, 1954, 86.
8 Wespi, H.J. *Schweiz med. Wschr.* 1945, 75, 625.
9 Costa, A., Cottino, F., Mortara, M. and Vogliazzo, U. *Panminerva med.* 1964, 6, 250.
10 Koenig, M.P. and Veraguth, P. in *Advances in Thyroid Research*, 1961, 294.
11 Kicic, M., Milutinovic, P., Djordjevic, S. and Ramzin, S. *ibid,* p. 301.
12 Norris, H. *Med. Times, Lond.*, 1847, 17, 257.
13 Pharoah, P.O.D. in *Endemic Cretinism*. Institute of Human Biology, Papua New Guinea monograph series no. 2, 1971, 109.
14 Buttfield, I.H. *ibid.*, p. 94.
15 Pharoah, P.O.D., Buttfield, I.H. and Hetzel B.S. *Lancet,* 1971, i, 308.
16 Pharoah, P.O.D., Buttfield, I.H. and Hetzel B.S. in *Human Development and the Thyroid Gland* (edited by J.B. Stanbury and R.L. Kroc). New York, 1972.
17 Pharoah, P.O.D. MD thesis, University of London, 1972.
18 Matovinovic, J. and Ramalingaswami, V. *Wld Hlth Org. Monogr. Ser.* 1960, 44, 385.
19 Clarke, W.C. *Place and People: an Ecology of a New Guinean Community*. Canberra, 1971.
20 Querido, A. in *Endemic Cretinism*. Institute of Human Biology, Papua New Guinea monograph series no. 2, 1971, 30.
21 Eggenberger, H. and Messerli, F.M. Transactions of the Third International Goiter Conference, 1938, 64.
22 Choufer, J.C., van Rhijn, M., Querido, A. *J. Clin. Endocrin. Metab.* 1965, 25, 385.

Acknowledgement

Pharoah, P.O.D. and Hornabrook, R.W. (1974) Endemic cretinism of recent onset in New Guinea. *Lancet,* ii, 1038–40.

11   *Professor Richard Schilling*

Tiller, J.R., Schilling, R.S.F. and Morris, J.N. (1968) Occupational toxic factor in mortality from coronary heart disease. *British Medical Journal*, iv, 407–11.

Nurminen, M. and Hernberg, S. (1985) Effect of intervention on the cardiovascular mortality of workers exposed to carbon disulphide: a 15 year follow up. *British Journal of Industrial Medicine*, 42, 32–5.

INTRODUCTION

Our own paper is an example of a combined study by a plant physician collecting data and academics, not only providing epidemiological expertise for its analysis, but also ensuring that resistance to its publication was overcome. Such cooperative research can add importantly to knowledge and give a bit of glamour and purpose to a factory doctor's job.

Clinical studies and animal experiments, describing 'atherosclerotic changes' following exposure to CS_2, encouraged us to study mortality from cardiovascular disease in a group of male workers exposed to CS_2 in three British viscose rayon factories. At the outset, death rates could not be calculated because the number at risk was not available. Instead, as a preliminary reconnaissance, the proportion of deaths from cardiovascular disease among process workers (most exposed to CS_2), non-process workers (least exposed to CS_2) and local men were compared. It revealed a highly significant excess of deaths from coronary heart disease (CHD) in the process workers. Proportional mortality has shortcomings as a measure of risk. Eventually we found that the most modern of the three factories in the preliminary investigation had detailed employment records which made a cohort study possible. This demonstrated that viscose spinners most exposed to CS_2 had significantly high death rates from CHD but not from other cardiovascular disease.[1] As management resisted further study, we were not able to proceed to the next step, which should have been a prospective clinical and environmental survey of the workforce and their exposure levels to CS_2.

Such a study was undertaken in Finland. Coronary mortality, morbidity and coronary risk factors were studied among a group of viscose rayon workers who were individually matched with controls from a paper mill. Confounding factors such as age, smoking habits, physical activity and obesity were taken into account. During the first five year follow-up there was an excess of coronary deaths, non-fatal infarctions, a history of angina and abnormal ECGs in the exposed subjects. This provided strong evidence of the causal role of CS_2 in developing CHD (Tolonen *et al.*, *British Journal of Industrial Medicine*, 1975, 32, 1–10).

The most interesting feature of the Finnish study is the intervention programme described in the elected other paper. It included a reduction in CS_2 exposure levels and removal of all workers with coronary risk factors from further exposure. The mortality excess from CHD among the CS_2 exposed workers was eliminated. Preventive action, based on environmental and clinical surveillance, saved an estimated 40 lives.

These studies exemplify the use of epidemiology in identifying work-related factors in the aetiology of a disease of common occurrence and in setting a hygiene standard. Following the Finnish study the occupational exposure limit for carbon disulphide was reduced from 20 to 10 p.p.m.

Note

1 The same cohort, studied by Sweetman *et al.* for an extended period, revealed similar patterns of mortality (*British Journal of Industrial Medicine*, 1987, 44, 20).

OCCUPATIONAL TOXIC FACTOR IN MORTALITY FROM CORONARY HEART DISEASE

Causes of death in three factories

In the manufacture of viscose rayon some workers are exposed to carbon disulphide (CS_2) and hydrogen sulphide (H_2S). The hazards of exposure to CS_2 were first recognized during the nineteenth century, when it was used as a softening agent in the cold curing of rubber. Many cases of psychosis, encephalopathy and polyneuritis were reported (Bruce, 1884; Ross, 1886; Oliver, 1902; Legge, 1934). High concentrations of H_2S cause death by respiratory paralysis, but the effects of long-term exposure to low concentrations have not been investigated.

Viscose rayon was first manufactured commercially in 1906. Cellulose is produced from wood pulp and is then mixed with CS_2 in churns to make cellulose xanthate; this is dissolved in caustic soda to form viscose and the men involved may be exposed to CS_2. The viscose solution is then spun into rayon yarn by extruding it through the fine holes of a jet into a bath of sulphuric acid and the yarn is washed and dried. Men who work in the spinning process may be exposed to both CS_2 and H_2S.

From the outset attention was given to the ventilation of workrooms and the enclosure of the processes; later a system of routine monitoring of factory atmospheres for CS_2 and H_2S was developed. In this country poisoning by CS_2 on the scale previously observed in the rubber industry has not occurred in the manufacture of rayon. Since CS_2 poisoning became notifiable in 1924, 30 cases have been reported – 13 in the rayon industry (Ministry of Labour, 1926–66).

During the past 15 years there have been several reports from other countries of viscose rayon workers developing 'atherosclerotic disease' at a relatively early age (Browning, 1965). Vigliani (1954) described cerebrovascular damage with 'focal lesions of atherosclerosis' in 43 rayon workers. Thirty-nine of these came from two factories where many cases of polyneuritis due to CS_2 had previously occurred. Others have reported 'generalized atherosclerosis', sometimes associated with renal lesions in severely poisoned workers (Attinger, 1948; Nanziante Cesaro, 1953). Alpers and Lewy (1940) observed atherosclerosis in cerebral vessels, as well as polyneuritis in animals exposed to CS_2. Rabbits exposed to CS_2 200 parts per million for 10 to 20 minutes a day for up to eight months showed changes in the coronary vessels, such as thickening of the endothelium, extramural haemorrhages with hyalinization and sclerosis of the intima (Guarino and Arciello, 1954).

We have not found any report of an occupational risk of coronary heart disease in viscose rayon workers (Ministry of Labour, 1926–66; Vigliani, 1954, Registrar General, 1958; Goldwater, 1960; Warshaw, 1960; Brieger, 1961; Browning, 1965; Brieger and Teisinger, 1967). In view of the clinical observations and animal experiments summarized above we were asked to make a study of mortality from cardiovascular disease in a group of British viscose rayon workers. Since the number at risk was not then available, *death rates* could not be calculated. Instead, the *proportion of deaths* among various rayon workers from cardiovascular disease to be expected on national experience was calculated and compared with the number actually observed among these workers. Thus each group being studied was separately compared with an independent standard.

Methods

The death registers of a municipal borough and the surrounding county in which there were three rayon factories provided the initial data. One factory started manufacturing viscose rayon about 1918 and the other two in 1928 and 1935, respectively.

We extracted for the 30 years 1933 to 1962 the names of all men aged 35 to 64 years at death whose occupation was recorded as rayon worker; exact occupations were obtained from the records of these factories. Of 397 men identified, 223 had been *process workers* employed in the viscose making or spinning processes. The remaining 174 were *non-process workers* – tradesmen, clerks and general labourers – who in general must have had much less exposure to either CS_2 or H_2S. In terms of physical activity of occupation the process workers on average were probably the more active.

For 'controls' we used the 561 deaths of other local men aged 35 to 64 in social classes III, IV and V (excluding agricultural workers) in the registers of the municipal borough. The male deaths for cardiovascular diseases in the area of England and Wales in which the factories are situated are somewhat higher than the national rates, perhaps because the drinking-water is very soft (Crawford *et al.*, 1968). We then classified the certified deaths of rayon process workers, other rayon workers and other local men under three headings: coronary heart disease, other cardiovascular, including cerebrovascular disease, and other causes.

Deaths were next allocated to three age groups – 35–44, 45–54, and 55–64 years – in each of the six quinquennial periods between 1933 and 1962. The deaths to be expected from coronary heart disease and from other diseases were calculated from corresponding national mortality data of the Registrar General for each five-year period. For example, in England and Wales there were 116 381 deaths of men aged 45–54 in 1948–52; of these, 18 473 were certified as from coronary heart disease. Over the same period there were 18 deaths in this age range of rayon process workers from all causes in the town and surrounding county that we were studying. The 'expected' number of deaths from coronary heart disease at ages 45–54 is $(18\,473 \div 116\,381)$ x 18; that is, 2.9. The number actually 'observed' was nine.

Results

Over the 30-year period 42 per cent of all the deaths of these rayon process workers were certified to *coronary heart disease*; the proportion was 24 per cent for other rayon workers ($P < 0.001$) and 17 per cent for the other local men. Nationally, this fraction was 14 per cent. The proportion among the process workers is higher from 1943, but by 1958–62 is only slightly in excess of that for other local men (see Figure 1).

Coronary heart disease

Table 1 gives the observed and expected deaths from coronary heart disease for each quinquennial period; an excess of deaths was found in all three occupational groups. The excess is greatest in the rayon process workers and statistically significant in each age group ($P < 0.001$). In the other rayon workers the excess is small and significant only for all ages combined. Coronary deaths among the other local men show similar trends to the rayon non-process workers, but the excess observed is statistically significant at 45–54 years and for all ages together.

Other cardiovascular disease

Rayon process workers aged 35–44 had eight deaths against 3.3 expected ($P < 0.02$); this was the only statistically excess observed in any of these groups. The rayon process workers had 19 deaths from *cerebrovascular disease* against 15.6 expected, but this excess might well have occurred by chance.

Older rayon workers

Deaths of rayon workers at ages 65–74 were also extracted; there was no excess of certified deaths from coronary or cerebrovascular disease in either the process or the non-process workers.

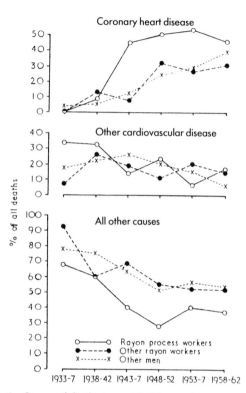

Fig. 1 Causes of death at ages 35–64 years in rayon workers and other men in social classes III, IV and V between 1933 and 1962. Deaths have been extracted from the local registers in an area in which three viscose rayon factories are situated. They have been classified under three main causes, using the International Classification of Diseases codes, as follows: coronary heart disease, 420; other cardiovascular diseases, 330–334, 400–416, 421–468.

Further test

In a small viscose rayon factory in another county the records of the personnel department showed that 38 employees had died between 1951 and 1960, and all but two of the death certificates were traced. Fourteen had been process workers, and nine of them aged 31 to 58 died of coronary heart disease. Four of the 22 deaths in non-process workers were certified as coronary heart disease, at ages 56 to 77. The difference between these proportions is significant ($P < 0.01$).

Comment

This preliminary reconnaissance of cardiovascular mortality is defective in several respects. 'Process' workers had to be treated as a homogeneous group and the relative risk in the viscose making and spinning processes

182

Table 1 Observed and expected deaths from coronary heart disease in rayon workers and other local men

Period	35–44 years		45–54 years		55–64 years		35–64 years	
	O	E	O	E	O	E	O	E
Rayon process workers								
1933–7	0	0.1	0	–	0	0.2	0	0.3
1938–42	0	0.2	2	0.6	0	0.4	2	1.2
1943–7	1	0.2	7	0.9	1	0.6	9	1.7
1948–52	3	0.5	9	2.9	8	2.8	20	6.2
1953–7	2	0.3	10	3.3	16	8.0	28	11.6
1958–62	0	0.2	8	4.9	27	15.4	35	20.5
1933–62	6	1.5	36	12.6	52	27.42	94	41.5
	$P < 0.001$		$P < 0.001$		$P < 0.001$		$P < 0.001$	
Other rayon workers								
1933–7	0	–	0	0.1	0	0.5	0	0.6
1938–42	0	–	0	0.2	2	0.7	2	0.9
1943–7	1	0.1	1	0.6	0	1.7	2	2.4
1948–52	2	0.2	4	1.1	5	4.4	1i	5.7
1953–7	0	0.4	4	2.4	8	6.7	12	9.5
1958–62	0	0.4	3	3.8	11	7.6	14	11.8
1933–62	3	1.1	12	8.2	26	21.6	41	30.9
							$P < 0.05$	
Other local men in social classes III, IV and V								
1933–7	0	0.4	1	1.5	3	2.7	4	4.6
1938–42	1	0.2	4	2.4	1	4.6	6	7.3
1943–7	1	0.5	3	2.1	7	6.1	11	8.7
1948–52	0	0.4	9	4.4	13	9.5	22	14.4
1953–7	0	0.7	11	5.9	13	11.6	24	18.2
1958–62	2	1.6	9	5.2	19	13.5	30	20.2
1933–62	4	3.9	37	21.5	56	48.0	97	73.4
			$P < 0.001$				$P < 0.01$	

'Expected' deaths derived from the proportion (coronary heart disease deaths/all deaths) in England and Wales (for details see text). Each excess of deaths was tested for statistical significance by χ^2, using the difference between the observed and expected deaths from other causes as well as coronary heart disease. The expected deaths from coronary heart disease may be calculated by another method (Doll, 1958). Deaths from other causes are multiplied by the ratio of deaths from coronary heart disease to deaths from other causes in England and Wales. This gives a lower 'expected' figure. In this and subsequent tables P values are given only when less than 0.05.

was not assessed. Moreover, we did not examine risk in relation to length of exposure.

'Other males' from the same area were not altogether suitable as controls, since they included men who had previously been process workers in the rayon factories. The exact number of these is not known, because it was impracticable to link all death register entries with factory employment records. However, superficial examination of records back to 1948 showed that at least nine men of the 'control' group who died of coronary heart disease at ages 45 to 64 were employed at one time as rayon

process workers. Some of the excess of deaths in the controls when they were compared with the national figures conceivably could be accounted for by ex-rayon process workers.

There could be another explanation of the excess mortality from coronary heart disease among the rayon process workers – namely, that they are protected from *other* diseases and therefore have a higher proportional mortality from coronary heart disease (Morris, 1967) (see Figure 1). This seems unlikely, but the occupational risk of coronary heart disease, if there is one, can be proved only by direct measurements of actual death rates in a defined population of rayon workers. Eventually we found that such a study could be made in the most modern of the three factories reported on above. This is described next.

Death rates in one factory

The factory which started manufacturing rayon in 1935 kept detailed employment records that made it possible to identify and trace some 2000 men and calculate appropriate death rates of those employed in the viscose making and spinning processes.

Methods

Choice of population
The population chosen comprised the men employed in the factory for one year or more at any time from 1 January 1945 to 31 December 1949. The analysis of mortality was confined to those aged 45 to 64 from 1 January 1950 to 31 December 1964. The number of men who were within these ages at any time during this 15-year period was 2129. Almost a third were still employed in the factory in 1964 and from information already obtained in the first part of this investigation many of the rest were known to have died. Others were sought through the Central Register of the National Health Service. In all, 1980 (93 per cent) were traced; 1731 were alive and 249 dead by the end of 1964. Over 97 per cent of those with more than ten years' service in the industry were traced, and we are reporting only on them.

Occupational classification
For each of the men we obtained date of birth, dates of employment and occupations in the industry, and, where applicable, the date and certified cause of death. We next divided the men into three occupational groups: (1) process workers who had worked in the department making *viscose* but not in the spinning department; (2) process workers who had worked in the *spinning* department; and (3) *non-process* workers, including men who had spent less than one month in a process department. Men of foreman grade or higher were classified as 'staff' and the remainder as operatives; the staff employed on process work cannot be subdivided into viscose and spinning groups, since most had worked in both as part of their training. Finally, we calculated for each of these occupational groups the number of man-years[1] lived at ages 45–49, 50–54, 55–59 and 60–64 during each of three quinquennial periods, 1950–4, 1955–9 and 1960–4.

Calculation of death rates
We obtained all causes of death from death certificates and classified them as coronary heart disease, other cardiovascular disease or other causes. Knowing the man-years at risk in each group in each quinquennial period it was possible to calculate the corresponding death rates per 1000 man-years for these various rayon workers. The corresponding rates for the home population of England and Wales were calculated from the Registrar General's Tables. Thus the experience of the various occupations is first compared with the national experience. Later we compare the death rates in occupations within the factory.

Comparison with national figures

Process operatives
The death rate from coronary heart disease of operatives in the viscose making department was 2.2 against an expected rate of 3.2 per 1000 man-years; they had 22 deaths from all causes against 28.5 expected (Table 2). There is no evidence of an occupational mortality hazard in this department. The operatives in the spinning department with more than ten years' employment had higher death rates than expected from coronary heart disease, other cardiovascular disease and other causes. The death rate from coronary heart disease was 6.1 against 3.2 expected (Table 2); this excess is highly significant ($P < 0.001$); and all age groups over 50 contribute to it, particularly men aged 50–54 years. There are three sections in the spinning department – spinning itself, washing and drying – and it is possible to get an indication of their relative risk by examining the mortality of men who spent at least 90 per cent of their employed time in a particular section. Twice as many of the actual spinners died of coronary heart disease as expected (10 against 4.5, $P < 0.01$). The excess among men in the washing section (5 observed against 2.2 expected) was similar but not significant; there was no excess in the drying section. These numbers are very small, but they do point to an occupational risk in the spinning section and possibly also in washing.

Non-process operatives
Two hundred and eighty-one non-process operatives with more than 10 years' employment in rayon factories showed no significant deviations from the expected mortality rates (Table 2). Forty-one fitters have been excluded from this group because they had probably spent much of their time in the spinning department maintaining machinery. Six of them died of coronary heart disease against an expected number of 1.8.

Table 2 Observed and expected deaths and death rates among operatives and staff, aged 45–64, with more than 10 years' employment in rayon factories

Occupation	Man-years at risk	Coronary heart disease				Other cardiovascular disease		Other causes	
		Deaths		Rates per 1000 man-years		Deaths		Deaths	
		O	E	O	E	O	E	O	E
Operatives									
Viscose making	2221	5	7.2	2.2	3.2	2	5.0	15	16.3
Viscose spinning	4585	28	14.6[b]	6.1	3.2	15	9.9	40	33.1
Non-process[a]	1997	6	8.0	3.0	4.0	10	6.1	14	18.6
Staff									
Spinning	1502	9	4.3[c]	6.0	2.9	1	2.8	11	9.7
Non-process	752	3	2.3	4.0	3.0	2	1.6	3	5.2

Expected figures are based on the national rates for England and Wales. [a] Excludes 41 fitters. [b] $\chi^2 = 12.2$; $P < 0.001$. [c] $\chi^2 = 5.2$; $P < 0.05$.

Staff

All but one of the 254 members of staff who were employed for more than 10 years were traced. Nine of the 163 who had service in the spinning department died of coronary heart disease, against 4.3 expected ($P < 0.05$) (Table 2).

Length of service and mortality rate

The proportion of men traced was high enough in the spinning plus wash sections to assess also the mortality risk of those who had less than 10 years' employment. With seven observed against 2.4 deaths expected from coronary heart disease ($P < 0.01$) the occupational risk does not seem to be confined to men with long service.

Mortality in spinning and other departments

We have found, therefore, that compared with the national experience both operatives and staff in the spinning department with more than 10 years' employment had a significantly higher death rate than expected from coronary heart disease. By contrast, the men who had not worked in the spinning department had death rates from coronary heart disease lower than expected. Next, therefore, we compared directly the mortality of all men in the spinning and all men in other departments, by means of the death rates per 1000 man-years, standardized for age and for year of death to allow for the secular changes in mortality.

These death rates from coronary heart disease are respectively 6.6 and 2.7 per 1000 man-years for all men in the spinning room and all men in other departments

($P < 0.01$) (Table 3). It is mostly accounted for by a significantly higher death rate from coronary heart disease in spinning room operatives compared with other operatives. Men employed in the spinning room also showed higher death rates for other cardiovascular diseases and from other causes, but the differences are not significant.

CS₂ and H₂S exposures

Routine monitoring for CS_2 and H_2S has been undertaken in this factory for at least 20 years and the results of a fair sample of the tests made between 1946 and 1963 were available. Concentrations of CS_2 were lower in viscose making than in spinning. In the viscose making department 17 per cent of tests in the churn rooms showed more than 20 p.p.m., the threshold limit value for CS_2 (Ministry of Labour, 1965). Exposure occurs almost entirely in the churn rooms, in which about a quarter of the viscose workers are employed at any one time; since many rotate their jobs, men spend most of their time in workrooms where there is no CS_2. Thus overall exposure was considerably lower than indicated by these figures. There is no exposure to H_2S in the viscose making department.

In the spinning department nearly half of the sample tests showed more than the threshold limit value for CS_2. Exposures to H_2S were relatively low; few of the tests were above the threshold limit value of 10 p.p.m.

There are at least three possible explanations of an occupational risk of coronary heart disease occurring in the *spinning department* but not in the department making viscose; it could be caused by the higher exposures to CS_2 in the spinning department, or by

185

Table 3 Standardized death rates per 1000 man-years for staff and operatives aged 45–64 years with more than 10 years' employment in rayon factories

Occupation	Standardized death rates per 1000 man-years[a]		
	Coronary heart disease	Other cardiovascular disease	Other causes
Employed in spinning			
Staff	7.1	0.9	9.0
Process operatives	6.4[b]	3.8	9.6
Total	6.6[c]	3.2	9.5
Not employed in spinning			
Staff	4.4	3.2	4.6
Viscose operatives	2.3[b]	1.0	7.3
Non-process operatives[d]	2.5[b]	4.1	6.0
Total	2.7[c]	2.8	6.3

[a] Standardized death rate = observed deaths ÷ expected deaths × crude death rate for males aged 45–64 in England and Wales for 1950–64.
[b] Normal deviate: 2.98, $P < 0.01$. [c] Normal deviate: 2.82, $P < 0.01$. [d] Excludes fitters, many of whom are likely to have worked from time to time in the spinning department; their standardized death rate from coronary heart disease was 11.5 per 1000 man-years.

exposures to H_2S which do not occur in viscose making, or by the combination of the two.

To investigate whether or not CS_2 itself is producing the risk in the spinning rooms, we recalculated the proportional mortality from coronary heart disease of men who worked *only* in the viscose making departments of the three factories studied in the first part of this paper. The factory built in 1935 was equipped with modern churns, and their viscose makers probably had much lower exposures to CS_2 than those in the other two factories. The men in the most modern factory had 6 observed and 5.0 expected deaths from coronary heart disease, whereas the men in the two older factories had 13 deaths against 4.6 expected. This supports the suggestion that exposure to CS_2 is a likely cause of the excess mortality in the spinning room of the most modern factory, and that exposure of viscose makers in its churn room have been low enough not to constitute a mortality risk from coronary heart disease.

Discussion

We have identified an occupational risk in men exposed to CS_2 in three viscose rayon factories; there is evidence of a similar risk in a fourth factory in another county. Apart from the risk of angina pectoris and sudden death in workers exposed to nitroglycol and nitroglycerin reported by several workers and recently again by Lund *et al.* (1968), this seems to be the only 'hard' evidence of an occupational toxic factor in the aetiology of ischaemic heart disease and related conditions.

Occupational hazards are often recognized without much difficulty. Thus industrial lead-poisoning or pneumoconiosis occur in limited groups of workers, present characteristic signs and symptoms, and the diagnosis may be confirmed by a biological test or specific X-ray changes. To identify a specific occupational risk of coronary heart disease is altogether another matter, because the disease is widespread among middle-aged men, and meanwhile nothing specific is known on the clinical presentation of the disease in this occupation. On present evidence there are multiple causes of coronary heart disease, and occupational exposure in viscose rayon manufacture appears to be another.

If CS_2 is in fact the responsible agent, discovery of its mode of action might help to clarify the aetiology of atherosclerosis and coronary heart disease, and such a search should be related to the present interest in the role of trace elements in this disease (Crawford *et al.*, 1968). Several studies in other countries have already suggested a link between CS_2 exposure, lipid metabolism and atherogenesis. High blood cholesterol levels have been reported in viscose rayon workers, with an increase usually in the β-lipoprotein fraction, but these have not been consistent findings (Brieger and Teisinger, 1967). Szendzikowski and Patelski (1962) found in rats that CS_2 reduced the lipolytic activity of the aorta *in vitro* and also the concentration of the non-esterified fatty acids in the plasma *in vivo*.

The first part of the present investigation showed that the excess of coronary deaths in the process workers did not occur before 1943, was highest in 1943–7, then fell gradually and was slight in 1958–62. The risk may therefore have arisen from wartime conditions and subsequently diminished with improving ventilation and the installation of modern churns. Furthermore, with reduced exposures to CS_2 in the churn rooms, following improvements in methods of work, the risk seems to have been confined to the spinning rooms. While the most likely agent is CS_2, the relatively low exposures to H_2S that occur in spinning rooms cannot be dismissed.

Workers who may be exposed to CS_2 in the viscose rayon industry are periodically examined by the factory medical service. Prospective surveys now are also needed, and could take into account several of the postulated causes and precursors of modern epidemic coronary heart disease, such as cigarette smoking, physical inactivity and obesity. Serial blood lipid, blood pressure and electrocardiographic observations should be made in such groups and in appropriate 'controls'. We would also like to see a detailed retrospective search of the clinical and necropsy reports of viscose rayon workers who have died of coronary heart disease for evidence of any special features of its natural history.

We cannot say whether men entering the viscose rayon industry today have an above-average risk of coronary heart disease. However, by examining the quantitative relationship between coronary heart disease mortality and the concentrations of CS_2 since 1945 it should be possible to decide whether there is any remaining mortality hazard and also to indicate the maximum concentration free of risk. The present threshold limit value for CS_2 of 20 p.p.m. relates only to its short-term toxic action and its acute systemic effects (American Conference of Governmental Industrial Hygienists, 1966), and is clearly an insufficient guide.

Note

1 These calculations were based on whole years. So man-years have been slightly underestimated, but the error is small and can be ignored.

References

Alpers, B.J. and Lewy, F.H. (1949) *Arch. Neurol. Psychiat.* (Chic.), 44, 725.

American Conference of Governmental Industrial Hygienists (1966) *Documentation of Threshold Limit Values.* Cincinnati.

Attinger, E. (1948) *Schweiz. Med. Wschr.,* 78, 667.

Brieger, H. (1961) *J. Occup. Med.,* 3, 302.

Brieger, H. and Teisinger, J. (editors) (1967) *Toxicology of Carbon Disulphide,* Excerpta Medica Foundation, Monograph No. 2. Amsterdam.

Browning E. (1965) *Toxicity and Metabolism of Industrial Solvents.* Amsterdam.

Bruce, A. (1884) *Edinb. Med. J.,* 29, 1009.

Crawford, M.D., Gardner, M.J. and Morris, J.N. (1968) *Lancet,* 1, 827.

Doll, R. (1958) *Brit. J. Industr. Med.,* 15, 217.

Goldwater, L.J. (1960) *Arch. Industr. Hyg.,* 21, 509.

Guarino, A. and Arciello, G. (1954) *Atti XI Congresso Internazionale di Medicine del Lavoro,* 2, 385. Naples.

Legge, T.M. (1934) *Industrial Maladies,* edited by S.A. Henry. London.

Lund, R.P., Haggendal, J. and Johnsson, G. (1968) *Brit. J. Industr. Med.,* 25, 136.

Ministry of Labour (1926–66) *Annual Reports of Chief Inspector of Factories,* 1925–65. HMSO, London.

Ministry of Labour (1965) *Dust and Fumes in Factory Atmospheres,* Safety Health and Welfare Booklet, New Series, No. 8. HMSO, London.

Morris, J.N. (1967) *Uses of Epidemiology,* 2nd edn. Edinburgh.

Nunziante Cesaro, A. (1953) *G. Clin. Med.,* 34, 731.

Oliver, T. (1902) *Dangerous Trades.* London.

Registrar General (1958) *Decennial Supplement England and Wales,* 1951, *Occupational Mortality,* Part II. HMSO, London.

Registrar General, *Statistical Review, England and Wales, Tables, Part I Medical,* 1933 *et seq.* HMSO, London.

Ross, J. (1886) *Med. Chron.,* 5, 257.

Szendzikowski, S. and Patelski, J. (1962) *Proceedings of Fourth International Congress of Angiology,* 202.

Vigliani, E.C. (1954) *Brit. J. Industr. Med.,* 11, 235.

Warshaw, L.J. (1960) *The Heart in Industry.* New York.

Acknowledgement

Tiller, J.R., Schilling, R.S.F. and Morris, J.N. (1968) Occupational toxic factor in mortality from coronary heart disease. *British Medical Journal,* iv, 407–11.

EFFECTS OF INTERVENTION ON THE CARDIOVASCULAR MORTALITY OF WORKERS EXPOSED TO CARBON DISULPHIDE: A 15 YEAR FOLLOW UP

The pathological effects of exposure to carbon disulphide (CS_2) on the heart have been investigated epidemiologically in our department since 1967.[1] After finding an excess of coronary heart disease over a five year period among workers exposed to CS_2 in a viscose rayon plant,[2] we began a vigorous intervention programme. The programme comprised, *inter alia,* such preventive measures as the transfer of workers with symptoms and signs of coronary heart disease to exposure-free work areas. Thereafter, we decided to monitor mortality among the established cohort to investigate the trend in the risk of death from cardiovascular diseases. A reanalysis of the first five year data yielded a significant exposure–response relation (as measured by the Mantel extension test, one sided $P = 0.003$[8]). With the non-exposed referent group as the standard (and no exposure level being scored as zero), the age standardised mortality rate ratio estimates in the low exposure (average level score 1.2), medium exposure (score 2.9) and high exposure (score 5.3) categories were 4.5, 6.8 and 7.4, respectively. If the non-exposed category were excluded from the analysis of a trend, however, the pattern of the exposure–response relation was flat. The follow up mortality studies[3–5] indicated that the higher risk of the rayon plant workers was levelling off when compared with the risk among a reference cohort of unexposed paper mill workers. This paper presents a fifteen year update of the impact of cardiovascular disease on the risk of death, with an allowance for deaths due to other causes.

Design of study

As a review of the project has been published elsewhere,[6] only an outline of the essential features will be given.

Study populations

The index cohort comprised 343 men with five or more years exposure to CS_2 at any time (median duration of exposure 11 years) at the onset of the prospective follow up in 1967. In all, 62 per cent of the cohort continued to be exposed at work, the remainder having changed to jobs in which they were no longer exposed to CS_2. A reference cohort of equal size was selected from a nearby paper mill. The referents had had no or insignificant (less than six months) exposure to CS_2 or other industrial intoxicants. The two cohorts were matched with respect to the most influential confounders – namely, age, district of birth and type of job. Their smoking habits, physical fitness and use of medicines proved to be almost the same.

Exposure

The concentrations of CS_2 have varied greatly over time. In most departments the exposure concentrations have been decreasing since 1945. (The company was founded in 1942.) A notable decline in the average concentrations

took place after 1972–3 (Figure 1). Furthermore, in 1972 only half (53 per cent) and in 1977 only one-fifth (19 per cent) of the members of the original index cohort continued to be exposed at work, as those with indications of incipient coronary disease (electrocardiographic changes, angina, hypertension or hyperlipidaemia) had been systematically removed from exposure.

Methods of mortality analysis

At the end of the 15 year period in 1982 there were no losses to follow up. Copies of the death certificates were obtained for all the dead subjects and coded uniformly according to the 1965 revision of the International Classification of Disease, Injuries, and Causes of Death.[7] Ischaemic heart disease (category numbers 410–414 or A83), other heart diseases (420–429 or A84) and cerebrovascular diseases (430–438 or A85) were tabulated as separate disease entities and grouped hierarchically.

The statistical problem of competing causes of death was handled by the actuarial or density method, which collects the man-years of follow up contributed by each subject during a set calendar time and age subinterval. Estimation of the mortality rate ratio was based on a large sample test statistic with an assumption of a binomial model (see reference 8 for details). A log–linear model (log (rate ratio) $= a + b$ (years)) was fitted to the annual data (grouped into five strata) to describe the relationship. The maximum likelihood estimates of the model parameters were then used, firstly, to evaluate the hypothesis

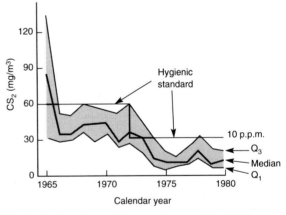

Fig. 1 Median value and interquartile range (Q_3–Q_1) of average concentrations of carbon disulphide (mg/m³) in air of rayon stable fibre factory from 1965 to 1980; Q_1, Q_2, Q_3 = first, second (median), third quartile. Finnish hygienic standards (60 mg/m³ (22 p.p.m.) before 1972 and 30 mg/m³ (10 p.p.m.) after 1972) are also shown.

Table 1 Number of deaths between 1967 and 1982 according to selected causes of death (ICD)

Cause of death	Cohort	
	Rayon plant workers (n = 343)	Paper mill workers (n = 343)
Ischaemic heart disease (A83)	32	24
Other forms of heart disease (A84)	6	1
Cerebrovascular disease (A85)	4	2
Neoplasms (A45–61)	14	19
All other causes	12	10
All causes	67	56

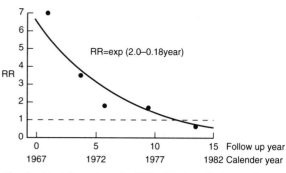

Fig. 2 Mortality rate ratio (RR) of ischaemic heart disease among workers exposed to carbon disulphide relative to unexposed workers during 5 year follow up period.

that no functional trend existed – that is, that $b = 0$ or the rate ratio was constant over the study period – and, secondly, to test the tenability of the model. Finally, the relative mortality rates of the cohorts were expressed with the corresponding Finnish national death rates for 1975 (the median year of death) as the standard.[9] As the sampling errors associated with the standard population are negligible, the statistical testing was based on a Poisson distribution.[8]

Results

As the compared cohorts were equal in size when the follow up began, the absolute numbers of deaths for the entire 15 year period are informative in themselves; see Table 1. Vascular diseases caused more deaths in the exposed cohort (63 per cent) than in the unexposed cohort (48 per cent), but this was counterbalanced by a higher number of deaths due to cancer among the paper mill workers (34 per cent) than the rayon plant workers (21 per cent). The preponderance of cardiovascular and cerebrovascular deaths was 1.6 times greater in the exposed cohort than in the unexposed cohort, and the rate ratio was almost significant (Table 2). The more than twofold excess of deaths due to lung cancer among the paper mill workers failed to reach statistical significance, however.

The estimated overall mortality rate ratio for ischaemic heart diseases in the rayon plant workers was affected by changes in exposure. Figure 2 shows how the raised mortality of the exposed cohort in the period preceding the intervention (carried out in 1973 to 1974) descended to the level of the referents. The test for the trend was significant ($\chi^{2(1)} = 7.0$, $P < 0.01$) and the exponential model did not deviate appreciably from the period specific estimates of the rate ratio ($\chi^{2(3)} = 3.2$).

Table 2 Mortality rates[a] (per 1500 man-years) and rate ratios for vascular diseases and neoplasms in the 15 year prospective follow up

Cause of death	Cohort		Rate ratio	Confidence limits (95%)	P value (two sided)
	Rayon plant workers (4685 man-years)	Paper mill workers (4830 man-years)			
Cardiovascular and cerebrovascular disease (A83–A85)	13.4	8.4	1.6	1.0–2.6	0.05
Cardiovascular disease (A83–A84)	12.2	7.8	1.6	0.9–2.6	0.08
Ischaemic heart disease (A83)	10.2	7.5	1.4	0.8–2.3	0.24
Neoplasms (A51–A61)	4.5	5.8	0.76	0.4–1.5	0.44
All causes	21.5	17.4	1.2	0.9–1.8	0.24

[a] Incidence densities

189

When national rates were used as the standard (equal to 100), the exposed cohort still had an unfavourable mortality rate for ischaemic heart diseases (relative mortality rate 130), whereas the unexposed cohort was relatively better off (rate 79).

Discussion

We have provided epidemiological evidence that indicates that the levelling off of the cardiovascular risk among a group of workers exposed to CS_2 was brought about by the measures taken to exclude the toxic substance from the environment. The striking parallelism between the course of the average level of exposure (Figure 1) and the estimated mortality rate (Figure 2) supports the contention that the cardiotoxic effect of CS_2 is reversible. Perhaps the strongest decisive factor, however, was the gradual withdrawal of cohort members from work where exposure occurred.

If we contrast, somewhat arbitrarily, the incidence figures for cardiovascular deaths during the first seven years of follow up with the figures for the latter eight year period we find that the relative death rates were 3.2 and 1.0, respectively. To evaluate the impact of the intervention measures, we can compute the (hypothetical) number of deaths from ischaemic heart disease that would have occurred among the index cohort had the same rate of mortality that prevailed before 1975 continued after 1975.

On the basis of the rates for the referents, this number was estimated to be 59 instead of 19, the number observed. Thus the fraction of prevented or postponed cardiovascular deaths among the formerly exposed workers becomes $(59 - 19)/59 = 68$ per cent.

The rate ratio function approached unity, a result perhaps slightly affected by the ageing of the cohorts, as the national incidence of cardiac arrest increases with age. It is also possible that exposure to CS_2 hastens death in people prone to coronary heart disease. If so the survivors at the fifteenth year of follow up are those with a lower risk of coronary death than either the reference cohort or the general population of the same age structure.

In conclusion, our results suggest that the cardiotoxic effects of CS_2 are reversible in the sense that the cessation of, or a radical decrease in, exposure reduces the risk of cardiovascular mortality to background levels. Because the exposure of most cohort members had ceased our results cannot be used to specify a safe level of exposure; this would require follow up studies of workers with steady, low level exposure.

References

1 Hernberg, S., Partanen, T., Nordman, C.H., Sumari, P. Coronary heart disease among workers exposed to carbon disulphide. *Br. J. Ind. Med.* 1970; 27, 313–25.

2 Tolonen, M., Hernberg, S., Nurminen, M., Tiitola, K. A follow-up study of coronary heart disease in viscose rayon workers exposed to carbon disulphide. *Br. J. Ind. Med.* 1975; 32, 110.

3 Hernberg, S., Tolonen, M., Nurminen, M. Eight-year follow-up of viscose rayon workers exposed to carbon disulphide. *Scan. J. Work Environ.* 1976; 2, 27–30.

4 Tolonen, M., Nurminen, M., Hernberg, S. Ten-year mortality of workers exposed to carbon disulphide. *Scand. J. Work Environ. Health* 1979; 5, 109–14.

5 Hernberg, S., Tolonen, M. Epidemiology of coronary heart disease among viscose rayon workers. *G. Ital. Med. Lav.* 1981; 3, 49–52.

6 Nurminen, M. Occurrence of ischaemic heart disease among male industrial workers exposed to carbon disulphide: a recollection of an epidemiologic study in occupational health. In Karvonen M.J. and Mikheeu, M.I. (eds) *Manual on epidemiology of occupational health.* Geneva: World Health Organisation. November 1986.

7 World Health Organisation. *International classification of diseases, injuries, and causes of death,* 8th rev. Geneva: World Health Organisation, 1965.

8 Rothman, K.J., Boice, J.D. Jr. *Epidemiological analysis with a programmable calculator.* Washington: US Department of Health, Education and Welfare, National Institute of Health, 1979.

9 Central Statistical Office of Finland. *Causes of death in Finland 1975. Official statistics of Finland, VI B: 131.* Helsinki CSO, 1979.

Acknowledgement

Nurminen, M. and Hernberg, S. (1985) Effect of intervention on the cardiovascular mortality of workers exposed to carbon disulphide: a 15 year follow up. *British Journal of Industrial Medicine,* 42, 32–5.

12 *Professor Mervyn Susser*

Stein, Z., Susser, M., Saenger, G. and Marolla, F. (1973) **Nutrition and mental performance.** *Science*, 178, 708–13.

Smith, C.A. (1947) **The effect of wartime starvation in Holland upon pregnancy and its products.** *American Journal of Obstetrics and Gynecology*, 53, 599–606.

INTRODUCTION

The subject of the paper I have chosen was the first result of a study conceived by Zena Stein and myself. We aimed to test the hypothesis, newly fashionable in the mid–1960s and largely accepted as fact, that nutritional deprivation early in development depressed mental ability. We thought an idea of such huge importance, especially to the less developed world, needed definitive tests (something we were bolder and more sanguine about than we would be now).

Poor nutrition in free-ranging human beings is nearly always thoroughly confounded by poverty, social class and their surrogates. Experimental data in rats localized an irreversible effect on brain development of acute and severe deprivation[1] during a 'critical period' equivalent in humans to the second half of pregnancy and perhaps the first months of life. Our hypothesis followed: namely, that foetal growth retardation owing to poor nutrition would irreversibly retard mental development.

We mounted two studies with designs we believed might be strong enough to meet the challenge of confounding, as none had been up to then. One was a randomized trial of prenatal food supplements among the poor black women of Harlem in New York.[2] Neither we nor any funding agencies were prepared to wait for the ultimate outcome of the development of their offspring until they had reached adulthood. For the second study, therefore, we searched for situations in which we might capture older individuals who had experienced early and severe food deprivation.

Twenty years before we began this line of work, the American paediatrician Clement Smith had published the paper that is here the companion to ours. His observations, cleverly analysed with the help of statistician Jane Worcester, stemmed from his tour as a member of the team of nutritionists who were charged with the welfare of the people of liberated Holland at the tail end of the Second World War. The Allied forces had just relieved Western Holland from a devastating famine punitively created by the Nazis. The famine was well demarcated in time and place by the transport embargo that caused it, and sharp both in onset and termination. These unnatural circumstances, however, were conducive to a natural experiment. While Smith's data from a Rotterdam maternity clinic were not the first to be reported,[3] they were crucial for us. They localized a distinct effect of famine exposure on foetal growth, manifested in birth weight, to the third trimester.

We could be reasonably secure, therefore, that exposure to prenatal nutritional deprivation in Dutch cities had been severe enough to retard foetal growth. I went to Holland to find if the other crucial elements for a cogent natural experiment could be met. We would solve our design problem if we could find a national check point through which all young people must pass, and where date and place of birth were recorded. Those basic requirements could define the intra-uterine famine exposure of the successive cohorts of a historical cohort design.

We salvaged riches beyond anything we had a right to expect. The Dutch had been dedicated record keepers on a national scale ever since Napoleon established his Batavian Republic in 1795, with population registers in every locality to keep track of the growth and movement of the population. The core data reported in this paper were records of military induction to which all 19-year-old men were then subject. In the result, we were also able to assemble relevant data, for the birth cohorts of interest, on the exposure in terms of quantitative food rations as well as time and place, and on the outcomes in terms of fertility, maternity and birth outcome, subsequent mortality and, at age 19, morbidity and physique together with mental state and performance. We had come upon a national famine unique in the history of the world for both its clear boundaries and the detail of its documentation. The study was also rendered unique by its capacity to follow several aspects of the development of a historical cohort from birth through two decades.

This first result, reprinted here, refuted the hypothesis at issue. No single result is sufficient, however, to eliminate a hypothesis. In this instance, the ecological design imposed by confidentiality and the form of some of the data sets could raise initial doubts, even though the design met many criteria for a rigorous ecological study.[4] But to eliminate alternative hypotheses is always a requirement of sound inference. We therefore brought all our data sources to bear for this purpose; the results, assembled in a book,[5] supported the refutation. Enough time has passed, too, for subsequent studies to help validate a number of the results in a variety of ways.[6–12] Perhaps the main moral of this study is that epidemiologists do well to seek and seize opportunity on the Willie Sutton principle. When this now legendary New York robber was asked why he always and only robbed banks, he replied: 'That's where the money is.'

References

1 Winick, M. and Noble, A. (1966) Cellular response in rats during malnutrition at various ages. *Journal of Nutrition*, 89, 300–6.

2 Rush, D., Stein, Z. and Susser, M. (1980) Diet in pregnancy: a randomized controlled trial of nutritional supplements. *March of Dimes Birth Defects: Original Article Series*. Vol. 16:3. New York: Alan R. Liss. **See also** Rush, D., Stein, Z. and Susser, M. (1980) A randomized controlled trial of prenatal nutritional supplementation. *Pediatrics*, 65, 683–97.

3 Sindram, I. S. (1945) De invloed van ondervoeding op de groei van de vrucht. *Ned. T. Verlosk.*, 45, 30–48.

4 Susser, M. (1993) The logic in ecologic. *American Journal of Public Health*, in press.

5 Stein, Z., Susser, M., Saenger, G. and Marolla, F. (1975) *Famine and Human Development: The Dutch Hunger Winter of 1944/45*. Oxford: Oxford University Press.

6 Milunsky, A., Jick, H., Jick, S., Abruell, C.L., MacLaughlin, D.J., Rothman, K.J. and Willet, W. (1989) Multivitamin/folic acid supplementation in early pregnancy reduces the prevalence of neutral tube defects. *JAMA*, 262, 2847–52.

7 MRC Vitamin Study Research Group (1991) Prevention of neutral tube defects: results of the Medical Research Council vitamin study. *Lancet*, 338, 131–7.

8 Susser, M. (1989) The challenge of causality: human nutrition, brain development and mental performance. *Bulletin of the New York Academy of Medicine*, 65, 1032–49.

9 Susser, M. (1991) Maternal weight gain, infant birth weight, and diet: causal sequences. *American Journal of Clinical Nutrition*, 53, 1384–96.

10 Jones, A.P. and Friedman, M.I. (1982) Undernourished during pregnancy. *Science*, 215, 1518–19.

11 Aaby, P., Seim, E., Knudsen, K., Bukh, J., Lisse, I.M. and da Filda M. C. (1990) Increased post-perinatal mortality among children of mothers exposed to measles during pregnancy. *American Journal of Epidemiology*, 132, 531–9.

12 Aaby, P., Bukh, J., Lisse, I.M., Seim, E. and da Filda M.C. (1988) Increased perinatal mortality among children of mothers exposed to measles during pregnancy. *Lancet*, i, 516–19.

NUTRITION AND MENTAL PERFORMANCE:
Prenatal exposure to the Dutch famine of 1944–1945 seems not related to mental performance at age 19

Nutrition is one among the complex of factors embraced by social class that may account for the influence of social class on intelligence. Despite the attention given to the influence of malnutrition on mental performance through its effect on the developing brain (1), the evidence to establish this causal sequence in humans is lacking. Published studies have suffered from flaws in design or execution; many have not had adequate control groups; and both specifying and assessing nutritional intake in human populations is very difficult (2). The circumstances of the *hongerwinter* in the Netherlands in 1944–5 have enabled us to isolate the experience of famine from other elements of the social environment. Here we relate material starvation during pregnancy to the mental status of the offspring in adult life.

The Dutch famine was remarkable in three respects: (i) famine has seldom if ever struck where extensive, reliable and valid data allow the effects to be analysed within specified conditions of the social environment; (ii) the famine was sharply circumscribed in both time and place; (iii) the type and the degree of nutritional deprivation

Table 1 Rations of calories, protein, fats and carbohydrates in 3-month averages for the period June 1944 to August 1946 inclusive

Area	June–Aug. 1944	Sept.–Nov. 1944	Dec.–Feb. 1944–45	Mar.–May 1945	June–Aug. 1945	Sept.–Nov. 1945
Calories						
West	1512	1414	740	670	1757	2083
North	1512	1450	1345	1392	1755	2083
South	1512	1403	1375	1692	1864	2083
Protein (grams)						
West	42	40	21	14	55	61
North	42	42	38	43	53	61
South	42	42	44	50	58	61
Fats (grams)						
West	32	25	15	12	54	50
North	32	26	23	26	39	50
South	32	25	21	28	38	50
Carbohydrates (grams)						
West	275	253	127	119	268	333
North	275	259	237	237	283	333
South	275	251	245	300	317	333

during the famine were known with a precision unequalled in any large human population before or since.

On 17 September 1944 British paratroops landed at Arnhem in an effort to force a bridgehead across the Rhine. At the same time, in response to a call from the Dutch government-in-exile in London, Dutch rail workers went on strike. The effort to take the bridgehead failed, and the Nazis in reprisal imposed a transport embargo on western Holland. A severe winter froze the barges in the canals, and soon no food was reaching the large cities (3).

Several indices attest to the severity of the famine in the cities of western Holland:

1 At their lowest point the official food rations reached 450 calories per day, a quarter of the minimum standard. In cities outside the famine area, rations almost never fell below 1300 calories per day (Table 1). The supply of food gradually declined during the first six weeks of the embargo, until in November 1944 the deficiency became severe. The famine continued into the first week in May 1945 when the Allied armies crossed the Rhine and liberated Holland. Fats, carbohydrates and protein were concurrently and almost equally affected.

2 The death rate in the affected cities rose sharply, and many deaths were certified as due to starvation.

3 Clinical reports made during the famine noted a high frequency of hunger oedema and osteomalacia, and frequent loss of as much as 25 per cent of total body weight.

4 Sample surveys made immediately after the famine by specialist nutrition teams brought in by the liberating armies confirmed the severity of the effects reported during the famine.

Sources of data and study design

The famine affected the large cities of western Holland. The people of rural areas and small towns were better off than those in cities because they could reach food-producing areas. In the Netherlands south of the Rhine the Allied armies were in occupation; the east and the north had better access to food. This geographic demarcation was used in our study design; we compared seven famine-stricken cities of the west (Amsterdam, Leiden, Haarlem, Utrecht, s'Gravenhage, Rotterdam, Delft) with eleven control cities in the south, east and north (Maastricht, Heerlen, Breda, Tilburg, Eindhoven, Enschede, Helmond, Hengelo, Zwolle, Leeuwarden, Groningen). The study and control cities comprised all those in the affected and unaffected parts of the country with a population greater than 40,000 (except Arnhem and Nijmegen, which, at the time of famine, were disrupted by warfare). Three of the affected cities, but none of those unaffected, had populations greater than 500 000.

We chose to carry out a retrospective cohort study. This we did by reconstructing birth cohorts exposed to famine and comparing them with cohorts not so exposed. To execute this design we sought out epidemiological checkpoints in the life arc of the affected individuals. The criteria for these checkpoints were three:

1 All the members of the cohort at risk who passed through the checkpoint could be identified in terms of an outcome variable of interest to the study.
2 Date of birth was recorded for each individual.
3 The place of birth was recorded for each individual.

Given date and place of birth, we could assign individuals to exposed and unexposed groups. By far the best checkpoint proved to be military induction procedures of males at age 18. Routinely, all those capable of appearing are medically examined and psychologically tested. Some 98 per cent of males surviving and resident in the Netherlands are included in our study.

The study population comprises 125 000 males born in the selected famine and control cities in the three year period 1 January 1944 to 31 December 1946, who were inducted by the military at about 19 years of age. Twenty thousand of these, we inferred from their date of birth and place of birth, were exposed to the famine through maternal starvation.

Dependent variables

Three dependent variables, all concerned with intellectual performance, are reported below.

1 Severe mental retardation. This variable is defined by the clinical diagnosis assigned at examinations, and coded according to the International Classification of Diseases Codes (1948) as 3250 (idiot), 3251 (imbecile) and 3254 (mongoloid).
2 Mild mental retardation. This variable is also defined by the clinical diagnosis assigned at examination and the International Classification of Diseases Code 3252 (debilitas mentis).
3 Intelligence quotient. This variable represents the score on the Raven Progressive Matrices (Dutch version). This test is the most sensitive measure of mental performance available for this study, and virtually every individual has a score. The data we used were scores grouped in six levels. Across the country the average proportions in each group, from highest to lowest scores, were 1, 17.7 per cent; 2, 28.4 per cent

3, 20.2 per cent; 4, 13.6 per cent; 5, 9.9 per cent; 6, 4.8 per cent; not known, 5.3 per cent.

The clinical levels of severe and mild retardation are consistent with the usual standards; that is, a division around IQ 50 separates the two levels of severity. The data are derived from the military induction examinations. These examinations, carried out at seven centres in Holland, are standardized procedures which include clinical examination and physical, psychological and educational tests. Ninety-five per cent of those inducted had intelligence test scores coded from their records. Residents of institutions are not directly examined, but reports on them are obtained and included in the files. Rejections for any condition, including mental retardation, are the responsibility of the medical officer in charge of the induction centre. He reviews every record, and where necessary obtains the clinical records of handicapped persons in institutions.

Independent variables

The independent study variable, or hypothesized cause, was exposure to famine.

A postulated moderator variable was the stage of growth and development of the fetus on exposure to famine: namely, the fetal age of the cohort at the time of exposure. This variable has importance in terms of the hypothesis of critical periods. The hypothesis states that developing organ systems are most vulnerable at the period of maximum growth; interruption of development at a critical period (specifically, when cell number is increasing) is likely to be irreversible or, at the least, subsequent development is likely to be retarded (4). On this hypothesis, stage of growth is a moderator variable that specifies conditions in which interaction with the causal variable will be found. We therefore designated birth cohorts by their stage of gestation at the time of exposure to famine.

Figure 1 shows the basic elements in the design of the study. In Figure 1, each horizontal bar represents a cohort of births in a one month period: the beginning of the bar represents the month of conception; the end of the bar, the month of birth. The dates of conception are inferred from dates of birth. The average error in these estimates is bound to be small because, on the average, the reduction in the duration of gestation during the famine was not more than four days (5).

The cohorts, grouped by the stage of gestation and exposure, are defined below. Cohorts A1 (births between January and July 1944) and A2 (births between August

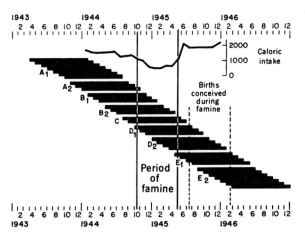

Fig. 1 Design of study. Cohorts by month of conception and month of birth, in the Netherlands, 1943–1946, related to calories in the rations of famine cities. Solid vertical lines bracket the period of famine and broken vertical lines bracket the period of births conceived during famine.

and October 1944) were conceived and born before the famine. Cohorts B1 (births between November 1944 and January 1945) and B2 (births between February and April 1945) were conceived before the famine and born during the famine; B1 was exposed for the third trimester of gestation, and B2 was exposed for the second trimester as well as the third. Cohort C (births in May or June 1945), conceived before and born after the famine, was exposed during the middle six months of gestation. Cohort D1 (birth between July and September 1945) and D2 (births between October 1945 and January 1946) were conceived during the famine; D1 was exposed during the first and second trimesters of gestation, D2 was exposed for only the first. Finally, cohorts E1 (births between February and May 1946) and E2 (births between June and December 1946) were never exposed to famine.

Early postnatal exposure to famine can be examined as well as prenatal exposure by comparisons among the birth cohorts for which the postwar period and unaffected areas are used as controls.

Birth weight is a second potential moderator variable of importance to this study. The period crucial for birth weight, the third trimester, is also a time of high velocity of brain growth in the human infant (6). Although our own studies, among others, show that the role of birth weight in perinatal mortality is a strong one (7), its role in child development is still obscure (8). The Dutch famine afforded an opportunity to try to elucidate this role. The mean birth weight curve in Figure 2 is drawn from data on

851 singleton births taken from hospitals in Heerlen (control city), and 862 singleton births from hospitals in Rotterdam (famine city). The famine curve is much the same in the data reported by Smith, by Sindram and by Stroink (5). Because most births took place at home, birth weights could not be obtained for the individual members of the military induction cohorts. These data therefore serve as collateral indicators of their experience. The social attributes of home and hospital births are not known, but the hospital births include all social classes and the results are consistent between hospitals in both affected and unaffected areas.

Two confounding variables, fertility and social class, have been controlled in analysis. A marked decline in fertility occurred in the famine cities but was absent in control cities. We found that the decline affected all social classes at more or less the same time, but the loss of fertility in each social class was different in degree. Manual workers were affected more than non-manual workers. The consequence was to produce proportions of social classes among the birth cohorts that differed according to their time of exposure to famine. This difference was not found for the control cities.

The distribution by social class of births conceived in the postwar period reverses the distribution found for births conceived during the famine. This is the mirror image of the famine period; it is evidently a rebound phenomenon which, in epidemiological terms, represents the effect of a greater risk for conception; that is, it is the consequence of susceptibility to pregnancy in the postwar period that differed among the social classes because of their different rates of fertility during the famine.

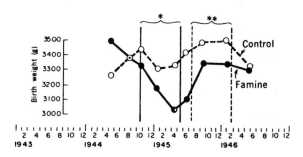

Fig. 2 Mean birth weight in maternity hospitals selected from famine and control cities (Rotterdam and Heerlen, respectively) by cohort of birth. Solid vertical lines bracket the period of famine, and broken vertical lines show the period of births conceived during famine.

Table 2 Results of a survey of mental performance in male birth cohorts from famine and control cities, at age 19. The categories manual and non-manual refer to occupational status of the fathers. These comprise 92.6 per cent of the birth cohorts at military induction. The total includes also those others with fathers in agricultural occupations (1.6 per cent), fathers dead more than 6 years (2.6 per cent) and those with no known occupations of fathers (3.2 per cent). The cohorts are defined in the text

Category	Group	Birth cohorts								
		A1	A2	B1	B2	C	D1	D2	E1	E2
Mental retardation by grade of severity (rates per thousand)										
Severe										
Total	Famine	3.11	2.40	2.55	3.83	4.02	5.29	3.76	3.33	4.37
	Control	3.49	2.00	3.18	4.79	4.66	3.75	3.41	4.85	2.94
Mild										
Manual	Famine	42.2	37.9	39.2	51.2	45.1	48.3	42.4	49.9	54.7
	Control	71.1	61.1	69.5	60.4	46.9	53.8	64.6	62.7	67.6
Non-manual	Famine	10.4	11.8	10.0	11.5	9.9	5.1	8.0	10.3	12.0
	Control	7.1	8.8	16.6	7.2	6.8	12.0	10.3	9.9	10.3
Total	Famine	34.90	32.68	31.44	37.75	36.19	35.70	31.40	36.89	40.16
	Control	55.20	45.58	59.04	47.94	39.58	40.90	52.93	47.65	52.14
Mean scores of the cohorts on Raven progressive matrices test										
Manual	Famine	2.74	2.67	2.67	2.67	2.61	2.63	2.58	2.65	2.74
	Control	2.86	2.73	2.87	2.79	2.84	2.77	2.81	2.76	2.79
Non-manual	Famine	2.17	2.15	2.10	2.11	2.13	2.10	2.06	2.13	2.19
	Control	2.19	2.15	2.14	2.13	2.11	2.10	2.14	2.11	2.12
Total	Famine	2.54	2.48	2.47	2.45	2.43	2.45	2.38	2.45	2.52
	Control	2.67	2.56	2.65	2.60	2.60	2.56	2.62	2.54	2.57
Numbers at risk										
Manual	Famine	6856	2980	2856	2772	1750	2050	1889	6371	10 272
	Control	1683	800	663	839	588	837	1071	1612	2322
Non-manual	Famine	4437	1956	1805	2001	1212	1377	1493	4566	7778
	Control	3486	1474	1353	1605	959	1579	2075	2663	4054
Total	Famine	12 522	5416	5089	5219	3233	3781	3726	12 008	19 920
	Control	5725	2501	2202	2712	1718	2665	3514	4743	7134

Results

Table 2 sets out the rates of severe and mild mental retardation, the mean score on the matrices, the numbers at risk in two classes of father's occupation and the total numbers at risk for each birth cohort, in famine and control cities (Figures 3 to 5).

The frequency of severe mental retardation among survivors of the birth cohorts is related neither to conception nor to birth during the famine (Figure 3).

A slight rise in frequency of severe mental retardation in the famine cities parallels the decline in birth weight, but must be discounted as an effect of the famine in the west, because a concurrent rise in frequency occurred in the control cities. The rise in the D1 cohort, we found, was almost entirely due to Down's syndrome. The famine was mild at the time of D1 conceptions, when the chromosomes might have been vulnerable to insult, and the

distribution of the syndrome across the whole period does not suggest that the cluster in the D1 cohort was due to the famine.

The frequency of mild mental retardation too is related neither to conception nor to birth during the famine (Table 2). Control city rates are always higher than famine city rates. Although the rise in the total frequency of mild mental retardation in famine cities during the famine is parallel to the decline in birth weights of cohorts B2 and C, the rise is far exceeded among births conceived after the famine and born in 1946.

The D2 cohort, conceived at the height of the famine, actually shows a decline in the rate of mild mental retardation. This decline in frequency can be explained by the confounding due to the differential fertility among the social classes referred to above. Frequencies by father's occupation show, as expected, that sons of fathers in manual work have a far higher rate of mild

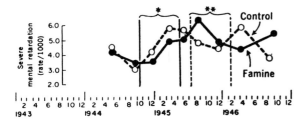

Fig. 3 Rates of severe mental retardation in Dutch men examined at age 19, by cohort of birth in famine and control cities. Solid vertical lines bracket the period of famine, and broken vertical lines show the period of births conceived during famine.

mental retardation than sons of fathers in non-manual work (Figure 4). No systematic relation with prenatal famine experience is seen in the two occupational classes, and the decline in the D2 cohort seen in the total rate almost disappears.

The later postwar rise in the frequency of mild mental retardation in cohorts E1 and E2 can be accounted for partly by the rebound fertility of the lower classes after the famine.

For the Raven matrices data, a numerically higher score signifies a poorer performance, according to the Dutch method of scoring. Once more we failed to find an association with the period of famine (Table 2).

By far the most striking variation is between mean grouped scores of the non-manual and manual classes (Figure 5). The influence of the social class variable is further underlined by the sensitivity of the measure to differential fertility among the social classes referred to above. Again, for the D2 cohort, conceived at the height

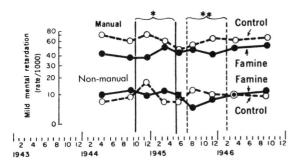

Fig. 4 Rates of mild mental retardation in Dutch men examined at age 19, for manual and non-manual classes according to father's occupation, by cohort of birth in famine and control cities. Solid vertical lines bracket the period of famine, and broken vertical lines show the period of births conceived during famine.

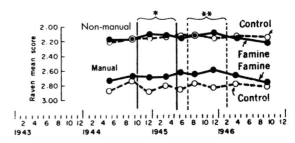

Fig. 5 Mean grouped scores on Raven progressive matrices test of Dutch men examined at age 19, for manual and non-manual classes according to father's occupation, by cohort of birth in famine and control cities. Solid vertical lines bracket the period of famine, and broken vertical lines show the period of births conceived during famine.

of the famine, there is a slight rise in intelligence (that is, a lower numerical score). An analysis within nine occupational classes, however, removed almost all of the rise in IQ. This supports the explanation that this rise reflects an under-representation of the manual classes among the births of the D2 cohort.

Interpretation

A number of reservations must be considered before inferences are drawn from the above results.

1 Completeness of the birth cohorts examined in the military sample at induction. For the purpose of validation, we made a follow-up through the records of the local population registers of a randomly selected 2000 births, all from two separate cities. Ninety-six per cent were located in records of death, migration or military induction.

2 Ecological fallacies. The exposure to famine can be determined from rations for groups defined by time and place of birth, and the analysis must rely on group performance related to group exposures. Where variations in performance within groups are considered, uniformity or variation in exposure to famine can only be assumed.

3 The comparability of the famine and control cities. There are differences other than exposure to the famine between the famine and control cities, particularly in size, religion and occupational composition. It is conceivable, but we believe most unlikely, that some factors related to the differences acted only during the period of the famine to suppress or distort the results among survivors.

4 Adequacy of measures of mental ability. The extensive

197

literature on IQs need not be reviewed here. In our view, IQs are more reliable than most epidemiological measures, despite their limitations. The matrices scores and the clinical criteria are consistent for the particular range of abilities they reflect.

5 Adequacy of the military induction examinations. We personally observed examinations at one of the seven centres. They were carried out in a standard fashion, and with the large number of subjects involved they seem adequate for our purposes.

6 The use of males alone as subjects. By most developmental criteria, females are less sensitive to insult than males. It is unlikely, although possible, that they would show effects where males did not.

7 Nature of the nutritional insult. In our study we examine the effects of acute starvation involving all components of the diet in a population of pregnant mothers previously reasonably well nourished. The results should not be generalized to the effects of chronic malnutrition with a different set of dietary deficiencies such as often occurs in developing countries, nor to nutritional insult in postnatal life.

Taking all these reservations into account, we believe that the results point to three conclusions about the measures of adult mental performance described. (i) Starvation during pregnancy had no detectable effects on the adult mental performance of surviving male offspring. (ii) Mental performance in surviving adult males from a total population had no clear association with changing levels of mean birth weight in a selected hospital sample of that population. (iii) The association of social class with mental performance was strong.

Alternative hypotheses to explain the absence of detectable effects of famine on mental performance must be considered.

Selective survival. Survivors of the famine-affected cohorts might have been selected from fetuses unimpaired by maternal starvation, whereas the deaths in the affected cohorts were selected from those who were impaired.

This hypothesis implies an all-or-none effect: the exposed fetus either survived unimpaired or died from the insult. In support of the hypothesis one might cite the high death rates of mentally retarded populations early in life, and the sensitivity of these rates to environment. An analysis of deaths undertaken to examine this interpretation is yet to be completed.

Compensatory experience. Postnatal learning in the period from birth to military induction might have compensated for neurological impairment of the fetus induced *in utero* by the famine. This hypothesis, if proved

correct, would controvert the critical period hypothesis. Since postnatal learning seems closely related to social environment, on this hypothesis we might expect to find interaction between the effects of social environment and famine. None was evident in the data relating mental performance to social class and exposure to famine.

The results are positive in two respects. First, they point either to a high order of protection afforded the fetus *in utero*, or to great resilience of the fetus in the face of nutritional insult, or to both. Second, the results affirm the association of social environment and mental performance. Among these birth cohorts there are considerable variations, not reported here, on the matrices and in the frequency of mild mental retardation between large cities and small, between town and country, between religious groups and between birth orders. These variations in mental performance point to effects of postnatal experience that are likely to be crucial and demand continued testing.

References and Notes

1 J. Cravioto., M.S. De Licardie., H.G. Birch, *Paediatrics* 1966; 38 (suppl.): 319. D.B. Coursin, *Fed. Proc.* 1967; 26: 134. M. Winick, *J. Pediat.* 1969; 74: 667. H.F. Eichenwald and P.C. Fry, *Science* 1969; 163: 644.

2 Z. Stein and H. Kassab, in *Mental Retardation*, J. Wortis, ed. (Grune & Stratton, New York, 1970), p. 92.

3 W. Warmbrunn, *The Dutch under German Occupation, 1940–1945* (Stanford University Press, Stanford, 1963). L. De Jong, *De Bezetting* (Querido, Amsterdam, 1965), five volumes. For a contemporary account of the declining food situation and the rationing see: N. W. Posthumus, ed., *Ann. Amer. Acad. Pol. Soc. Sci.* 1946; 245. C. Banning, *ibid.,* p. 93; J. Breunis, *ibid.,* P.J. Maliepaard, *ibid.,* p. 48. M.J.L. Dols and D.J.A.M van Arcken, *Milbank Mem. Fund Quart.* 1946; 245: 319. For a description of the nutritional state of the population during and immediately after the famine see: G.C.E. Burger, J.C. Drummond, H.R. Sandstead, eds., *Malnutrition and Starvation in Western Netherlands September 1944, July 1945* (Hague General State Printing Office, The Hague, 1948), parts 1 and 2.

4 M. Winwick and A. Noble, *J. Nutr.* 1966; 89: 300. J. Dobbing, in *Applied Neurochemistry*, A.N. Davison and J. Dobbing, eds. (Blackwell, Oxford, 1968).

5 C.A. Smith, *Amer. J. Obstet. Gynecol.* 1947; 53: 599. J.A. Stroink, *Ned. Tijdschr. Verlosk.* 1947; 47: 101. I.S. Sindram, *ibid.* 1953; 53: 30.

6 M. Winick and P. Rosso, *Pediat. Res.* 1969; 3: 181. J. Dobbing, *Amer. J. Dis. Child.* 1970; 120: 411.

7 J. Ashford, J. Fryer, F. Brimblecombe, *Brit. J. Prev. Soc. Med.* 1969; 23: 164. L. Bergner and M. Susser, *Paediatrics* 1970; 46: 946.

8 H. Knobloch and B. Pasamanick, *Amer. J. Public Health* 1959; 49: 1164. A. McDonald, *Brit. J. Prev. Soc. Med.* 1964; 18: 59. H.G. Birch, S.A. Richardson, D. Baird, G. Horobin, R. Illsley, *Mental Subnormality in the Community* (Williams & Wilkins, Baltimore, 1970).

Acknowledgement

Stein, Z., Susser, M., Saenger, G. and Marolla, F. (1973) Nutrition and mental performance. *Science*, 178, 708–13. Copyright 1973 by the AAAS.

THE EFFECT OF WARTIME STARVATION IN HOLLAND UPON PREGNANCY AND ITS PRODUCTS

The association of maternal malnutrition with improper growth or development of the fetus, prematurity, stillbirth and neonatal death, and with toxaemia during pregnancy, has been strongly indicated by numerous researches.[1-13] Nevertheless, proof is needed that this relationship is actually one of cause and effect. Unsatisfactory pregnancies may, of course, occur in ill-nourished women merely because women of suboptimal health and hygiene tend to eat improper diets.[12] Test circumstances in which maternal diet is the only variable are obviously needed. The mass malnutrition in western Holland during the 'hunger winter' of 1944–5 seemed likely to offer useful data of this type. Results of a study made in Rotterdam and The Hague are presented elsewhere insofar as their effects upon the newborn infant are concerned.[14] The present paper amplifies certain of those data and describes the effects upon the mother during pregnancy as well.

The causes and other details of the Dutch starvation period need not be discussed here, so that space will be given only to a brief account of the type and duration of nutritional inadequacy. The food situation began to deteriorate in October 1944, and in December reached a low level rather steadily maintained until liberation of the country in May 1945. Therefore, the critical period lasted at least five months, but not more than eight. Thus, pregnancies ending just before relief of hunger had begun in relatively good nutritional circumstances; on the other hand, those beginning during hunger were ended after relief. The data of Table 1 show probably the most reliable estimate of food available to pregnant women in representative months of the hunger period.[15] It is noteworthy that what occurred was a relatively brief period of severe, generalized undernutrition, not outstandingly poor for any single dietary element. The main sources of data used for analysis of the results upon pregnancy were the records of the National School for Midwives at Rotterdam, and the Obstetrical Service of the Zuidwal Hospital at The Hague. Since the major findings from both institutions showed parallel trends, they will be grouped together in most of this presentation. Numerous less formal investigations and interviews were made to check specific points.

Upon pregnancy in general an outstanding effect of hunger was a fall to one-third of the expected number of births representing conceptions during the undernutrition period. This period was marked by amenorrhoea in about 50 per cent of women, with normal menstruation reported only in about 30 per cent.[16-18] The nutritional basis of 'war amenorrhea' has been investigated by others,[19-21] and in Sydenham's recent study[21] seems suggestively connected with insufficient protein intake. Menstruation in the Dutch women, as in those of other studies mentioned, was regularly resumed with the return of food. The gross interference with this function, with its striking result upon later birth rate, testifies to the stringency of nutritional conditions during the hunger winter. All of the pregnancies whose records were used in this study were analysed to determine whether maternal age or parity were altered from the normal. No significant change occurred in these underlying factors. Therefore, though fewer women conceived during the months of undernutrition, those who did so, or who gave birth, at that time were not essentially different from the patients of pre-hunger or post-hunger times who served as controls.

As a paediatrician, the author can only record his findings and those of Dutch obstetricians in general upon toxaemia of pregnancy with a minimum of speculation. Although a number of German authors reported a decrease in toxaemia during starvation in the former war,[22] the nutritional significance of their conclusions has been criticized.[23] More recently, the general consensus has been that a definite reciprocal relation exists between nutrition – especially protein nutrition – and frequency of toxaemia states.[4,10,24,25] It was therefore distinctly surprising to learn that all Dutch obstetricians had seen less than the expected amount of toxaemia during the hunger period. Review of records from the Midwifery School substantiated this impression. Results are given briefly in Table 2, in the preparation of which three diagnostic criteria were used. The first (A) includes every diagnosis of toxaemia of whatever degree. To restrict the diagnosis to a more definite one, cases were excluded unless they showed a blood pressure rise to 140 mm or more, albuminuria or oedema of at least grade 2 plus, or

Table 1 Nutrition available for pregnant women (The Hague and Leiden)[a] from evaluation by H. M. Sinclair, Oxford Nutrition Survey, for SHAEF[15]

Item	Recommended daily allowance[b]	September 1944	February 1945	April 1945
Calories	(2500)	1925	731	912
Protein (g) (vegetable)		38	24	28
(animal)	(85)	23	9	11
Fat (g)		50	11	14
Calcium (mg)	(1500)	1075	649	517
Iron (mg)	(15)	16.3	9.6	10.7
Vitamin A (i.u.)	(6000)	1260	445	766
Thiamin (mg)	(1.8)	1.1	1	0.6
Niacin (mg)	(18)	9.2	3.0	4.1
Riboflavin (mg)	(2.5)	1.2	0.5	0.5
Ascorbic acid (mg)	(100)	59	34	53

[a] Reasonably similar in Rotterdam.
[b] Food and Nutrition Board, 1945.

Table 2 Undernutrition and toxaemia (Midwifery School, Rotterdam)

Period	Pre-war (1938–9)	Immediately pre-hunger (1944)	Hunger (1944–5)	Immediately post-hunger (1945)
Number of patients at risk (5–9 months pregnant)	3360	975	2254	875
A Per cent diagnosed toxaemia (unqualified)	3.2	3.4	1.9	3.8
B Per cent diagnosed toxaemia, with BP at least 140, or albumin at least ++, or oedema at least ++, or convulsions	2.2	2.4	1.1	2.2
C Per cent diagnosed toxaemia, with albumin at least ++, or oedema at least ++, or convulsions	0.8	0.75	0.6	1.7

convulsions. This resulted in the second line of figures (B) in Table 2. Finally, the criterion of blood pressure was removed altogether because of the prevailing hypotension due to undernutrition,[26] and either marked albuminuria or oedema, or convulsions, were required for the case to be included in the figures of line C. It will be noted that by none of these manipulations could the data be made to show any increase of toxaemia during the under-nutrition period. For two of the categories used in Table 2 (A and B) a statistically significant decline in this condition appears to have occurred.

Though decline in toxaemia was not assignable to any change in maternal age or parity, a factor difficult to evaluate was the definite scarcity in table salt available during the hunger period. The concurrent reduction of toxaemia suggests that future studies of nutrition and toxaemia must be carefully evaluated with regard to salt intake as well as to specific type and duration of maternal food habits. To say that a 'good' diet will reduce the incidence of toxaemia and a 'poor' one increase it is futile until one can specify the exact elements constituting goodness and poorness in this regard.

Effects of maternal nutrition upon the birth weight of infants born in Rotterdam and at The Hague are shown in Figure 1. Representation by percentiles (explained in the legend) shows that at the beginning of the critical period birth weights were distributed over about the same range as in the previous winter. The decline in birth weight which followed was steeper among the constitutionally larger infants (upper percentiles) than among the smaller ones, a fact equally notable in the rise after liberation and return of food. From the 50 percentile or median line, which is of most significance statistically, it appears that babies born just before return of food weighed scarcely less than those born two to three months earlier. Since the undernutrition of mothers giving birth just before the

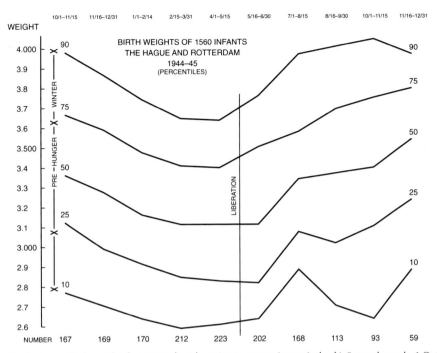

Fig. 1 Change in distribution of birth weights for 1560 infants born in ten successive periods of 1.5 months each, 1 October 1944 to 31 December 1945, The Hague and Rotterdam. Lines connect the same percentile, crosses on the left indicate the same percentiles for infants born during the previous winter.

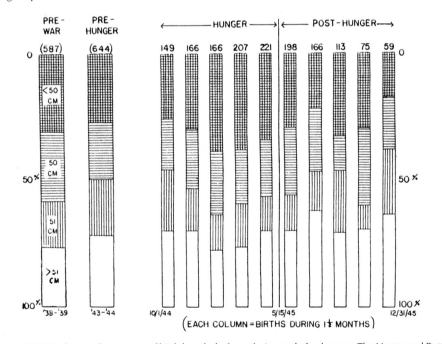

Fig. 2 Percentages of 1533 infants in four ranges of birth length, before, during and after hunger, The Hague and Rotterdam. The ten narrower columns represent the same ten successive periods used in Figure 1. The number of infants measured is given at the top of each column.

liberation must have begun much earlier in pregnancy, it is apparent that birth weight reflects the nutrition of late pregnancy rather than that earlier in gestation. Finally, it must be stressed that individual pregnancies showed exceptions to these findings. Only in the analysis of fairly large groups does the fundamental relation between maternal nutrition and fetal weight gain clearly appear.

Although accurate figures as to birth length are not so easy to obtain, those from the two clinics (Figure 2) showed a relatively greater number of short babies during the months of hunger than before or thereafter. As hunger progressed the changes did not follow the same smooth curve from period to period as did those for weight. Nevertheless, the total group of infants born under hunger circumstances were shorter by a statistically significant degree than the total group born previously, or born after the return of food. Since length is only one dimension while weight is the product of three, changes in the former cannot be expected to be as sharp as those in the latter.

Statistics upon various undesirable outcomes of pregnancy are presented in Table 3 under four groupings according to maternal circumstances. The 674 pre-war pregnancies of 1938–9 (from the Rotterdam source only) represent a normal control period uninfluenced by war or malnutrition. The 830 pre-hunger deliveries from both clinics portray the fourth winter of Nazi occupation but a year before the hunger winter, whose figures are given by the third column. Finally, the last column was added to include infants born several months after the return of food, but conceived at the worst phase of starvation. The small number of births in this last group testifies to reduced fertility during the hunger period.

Figures for abortion and miscarriage are included to satisfy the reader's curiosity, but there is no reason to assume that they are accurate or that conclusions can be drawn from them. Only the data from the Rotterdam clinic have been listed, as those from The Hague were even less serviceable. Prematurity, which was much more reliably recorded, was based in this analysis upon a weight criterion only, all infants of less than 2250 g (5 lb) being so diagnosed. The slight increase in prematurity in the Rotterdam clinic during hunger was practically nullified by the actual decrease shown in data from The Hague. For both clinics, the largest incidences occur in the post-hunger months, whose total case material is dangerously small for statistical purposes. Certainly during circumstances of marked nutritional inadequacy, no significant increase in premature births was recorded.

It was possible to confirm data for stillbirth by consulting municipal records from the cities of Rotterdam and The Hague as a whole. These were in agreement with

Table 3 in showing no increase in incidence of stillbirth during the hunger winter. The tendency to increase in post-hunger months is probably related to the concurrent rise in percentage of premature births. Neonatal death occurred actually less commonly in the hunger period than before or after. Although the municipal statistics on this point were in disagreement with the hospital data, the former were largely based upon infants born at home and thus subject to all sorts of unusual privations. The hospital figures are more useful for our purposes.

Data as to congenital malformations do show a slight increase in the last column, but unfortunately the small number of properly timed pregnancies renders the difference of no statistical significance. Further investigations[14] also resulted unsatisfactorily in failing to define a relationship between maternal nutrition and malformations, largely because of low fertility at the critical period of nutritional stringency.

Lactation, judged solely by the percentage of mothers nursing their babies during the hunger period, was singularly unaffected.[14] There was no means of knowing the cost in maternal tissue involved, but the evidence indicated that a woman not receiving adequate food could still secrete milk enough to sustain a desperately hungry baby.

General comment and summary

The severe undernutrition of the winter of 1944–5 in Northwestern Holland was marked by the following effects upon pregnancy and the fetus: (1) amenorrhoea and infertility were so common as to reduce strikingly the expected number of births; (2) infants conceived before the hunger months but born during them were significantly below the expected weight and height (evidence suggests the correlation of this effect with maternal nutrition during the last half or last trimester of pregnancy); (3) toxaemia was not increased and by certain criteria was actually reduced in comparison with expected frequency; (4) prematurity and congenital malformations were slightly but not significantly increased in occurrence; (5) no effect was noted upon the incidence of stillbirth, neonatal death or lactation, when the last is limited solely to the secretion of sufficient milk to support an infant.

These findings are surprising in view of the numerous recent studies suggesting a significant and clear-cut relation between maternal nutrition and almost all aspects of the course and product of pregnancy.[1–3] Of the various interpretations which suggest themselves, the first is that reports from Dutch cities were false, and that there was no

Table 3 Results of pregnancy (Rotterdam and The Hague)

Period →		Pre-war	Pre-hunger	Hunger	Conceived in hunger
Born during →		1938–9	1/10/1943 to 1/5/1944[a]	1/12/1944 to 15/5/1945	1/10 to 31/12/ 1945
Births	Rotterdam	674	659	412	135
	The Hague	–	171	342	47
	Total	674	830	754	182
Per cent abortion and miscarriage	Rotterdam	1.67	5.6	2.2	8.33
Per cent prematurity, less than	Rotterdam	5.27	4.98	6.3	8.4
2250 g	The Hague	–	8.2	6.4	11.0
	Total	5.27	5.7	6.3	9.1
Per cent stillbirth	Rotterdam	3.5	3.2	1.8	4.03
	The Hague	–	2.9	0.3	4.25
	Total	3.5	3.16	1.0	4.1
Per cent neonatal death	Rotterdam	1.55	3.0	2.36	5.05
	The Hague	–	6.1	1.77	4.65
	Total	1.55	3.66	2.05	4.94
Per cent malformed	Rotterdam	1.36	1.6	0.5	2.42
	The Hague	–	0	1.82	4.44
	Total	1.36	1.26	0.97	2.95

[a] 1/11/1943 to 1/4/1944 for The Hague

lack of adequate food for pregnant women. This is certainly not true. The manifest decrease in birth weight during the hunger period should dispose of any doubts on that point.

A second interpretation is that these data from Holland are of real significance, whereas investigations working elsewhere[4–10,24,25] have mistaken association for aetiology. This is considered to be unlikely, particularly in view of reports in which improvement in the course and product of pregnancy appears to have coincided with directed improvement of nutrition in a controlled group of patients.[7–10] The difficulty of proving that untoward results of pregnancy in ill-nourished women are the direct consequences of their nutritional status is, however, a real and challenging one.

A third interpretation, believed to be nearer the truth, is that the nutritional circumstances of the Dutch situation were not comparable to those of other studies in American, Canadian and British obstetric clinics.[4–10,24,25] The Dutch women had been reasonably well fed until subjected to a brief period of acute general undernutrition. By contrast, the other studies usually involve women who have nourished themselves, more or less indefinitely as a rule, upon diets adequate in calories but insufficient in certain individual food elements. Quite possibly acute undernutrition may result in one way while chronic malnutrition may result in another. The need for careful analysis of the time factor in nutritional studies of

pregnancy is strongly suggested. It is also obvious that fetal growth may be related to maternal caloric intake of late pregnancy, whereas fetal development and viability may rest, nutritionally speaking, as much upon the maternal circumstances before conception as upon those of pregnancy itself.

References

1 Burke, B.S., *J. Am. Diet. A.* 1944; 20: 735.
2 Williams, P.F., *JAMA* 1945; 127: 1052.
3 Lund, C.J., *JAMA* 1945; 128: 344.
4 Burke, B.S., Beal, V., Kirkwood, S.B. and Stuart H.C. *Am. J. Obst. & Gynaec.* 1943; 46: 38.
5 Burke, B.S., Harding, V.V. and Stuart H.C., *J. Pediat.* 1943; 23: 506.
6 Burke, B.S., *Am. J. Pub. Health* 1945; 35: 334.
7 Ebbs, J.H., Tisdall, F.F. and Scott W.A., *J. Nutrition* 1941; 22: 515.
8 Ebbs, J.H., Brown, A., Tisdall, F.F., Moyle, W.J. and Bell, M. *Canad. M.A.J.* 1942; 46: 1.
9 Interim Report of the People's Health League, *Lancet* 1942; 2: 10.
10 Balfour, M.L., *Lancet* 1944; 1: 208.
11 Warkany, J., *J. Pediatr.* 1944; 25: 476.
12 Warkany, J., *Manifestations of Prenatal Nutritional Deficiency, Vitamins and Hormones* (edited by R.S. Harris and K.V. Thimann), Vol. 3, New York, 1945, Academic Press.

203

13 Baird, D., *J. Obst. & Gynaec. Brit. Emp.* 1945; 52:217 and 340.
14 Smith, C.A., *J. Pediatr.* 1947; 30:229.
15 Sinclair, H.M. (Director), Oxford Nutritional Survey – Preliminary Report on Nutritional Surveys in the Netherlands, May and June, 1945, Oxford.
16 v. Boudijk Bastiaanse, M.A., personal communication.
17 Holmer, A., personal communication.
18 de Snoo, K., personal communication.
19 Kurtz, C. *Monatschr. f. Geburtsh. u. Gynäk.* 1920; 52:367.
20 Whiteacre, F.E. and Barrera, B., *JAMA* 1944; 124:399.
21 Sydenham, A., *Brit. Med. J.* 1946; 2:159.
22 Editorial Note. *JAMA* 1917; 68:732.
23 Ehrenfest, H., *Am. J. Obst. & Gynec.* 1920; 1:214.
24 Tompkins, W.T., *J. Internat. Coll. Surgeons* 1941; 4:147.
25 Holmes, O.M., *West. J. Surg.* 1941; 49:56.
26 Lups, S. and Francke, C., *Nederl. tijdschr. v. geneesk.* 1946; 90:764 (abstract *JAMA* 1946; 132:958).

Acknowledgement

Smith, C.A. (1947) The effect of wartime starvation in Holland upon pregnancy and its products. *American Journal of Obstetrics and Gynecology*, 53, 599–606. Permission by Copyright Licensing Agency Ltd.

Index